Study Guide

Clinical Procedures
for Medical Assistants

Eleventh Edition

Kathy Bonewit-West, BS, MEd
Professor Emeritus
Medical Assistant Program
Hocking College
Nelsonville, Ohio

Former Member, Curriculum Review Board of the
American Association of Medical Assistants

ELSEVIER

3251 Riverport Lane
St. Louis, Missouri 63043

STUDY GUIDE FOR CLINICAL PROCEDURES FOR MEDICAL
ASSISTANTS, ELEVENTH EDITION

ISBN: 978-0-323-75882-6

Notice

Content Director: Kristin Wilhelm
Content Strategist: Laura Klein
Content Development Manager: Luke Held
Senior Content Development Specialist: Rae L. Robertson
Publishing Services Manager: Deepthi Unni
Project Manager: Thoufiq Mohammed
Design Direction: Gopalakrishnan Venkatraman

Printed in United States of America

Last digit is the print number: 9 8 7 6 5 4 3 2 1

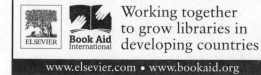

Preface

Outcome-based education prepares individuals to perform the prespecified tasks of an occupation under real-world conditions at a level of accuracy and speed required of the entry-level practitioner of that profession. Outcome-based education plays an important role in medical assisting programs in preparing qualified individuals for careers in medical offices, clinics, and related health care facilities. The *Study Guide for Clinical Procedures for Medical Assistants* has been developed using a thorough outcome-based approach. It meets the criteria stipulated by the Commission on Accreditation of Allied Health Education (CAAHEP) Standards and Guidelines for the Medical Assisting Educational Programs and the Accrediting Bureau of Health Education Schools (ABHES) Programmatic Evaluation Standards for Medical Assisting. Instructors should find this Study Guide a valuable teaching aid for training students who are able to think critically and to perform competently in the clinical setting.

Each study guide chapter is organized into the following sections:

1. *ASSIGNMENT SHEETS*: The Study Guide Assignment Sheets indicate the assignments required for each chapter, along with a space provided for the student to document the following: the date each assignment is due, completion of the assignment, and points earned for each assignment. The Laboratory Assignment Sheet indicates the procedures required for each chapter, along with the textbook and Study Guide reference pages, the number of practices required to attain competency, and a space for documenting the score earned on the Performance Evaluation Checklist.

2. *PRETEST AND POSTTEST*: These tests have been included for each chapter using true/false questions that allow the student to test his or her acquisition of knowledge for each chapter before and after completing the chapter. These tests can be used as a study guide to prepare for chapter tests.

3. *KEY TERM ASSESSMENT*: This section provides the student with an assessment of his or her knowledge of the medical terms covered in each chapter. This section also includes an assessment of the word parts of the medical terms (prefixes, suffixes, and combining forms) to evaluate the student's knowledge of the meaning of the medical term through its word parts.

4. *EVALUATION OF LEARNING*: These questions help the student evaluate his or her progress throughout each chapter. After the student has completed these questions and checked them for accuracy, they provide an ongoing review of the textbook material. Individuals preparing for a certification examination will find the completed Evaluation of Learning sections useful study aids for the clinical aspect of the examination.

5. *CRITICAL THINKING ACTIVITIES*: In this section, the student performs activities that enhance his or her ability to think critically. Some situations require the student to become involved in a game or play a role; others require the student to use independent research to answer questions posed by a patient. Independent research helps the student become familiar with resources available to acquire additional knowledge and skills outside the classroom.

6. *PRACTICE FOR COMPETENCY*: This section consists of worksheets that provide the student with a guide for the practice of each clinical skill presented in the textbook.

7. *EVALUATION OF COMPETENCY*: This section includes two components. The first component is the Performance Objective, which provides an exact description of what the learner must be able to demonstrate to attain competency for each procedure presented in the textbook. A performance objective consists of the (1) outcome, (2) conditions, and (3) standards. The second component is the Performance Evaluation Checklist, which evaluates the student's performance against an established set of performance standards.

8. *SUPPLEMENTAL EDUCATION*: Several medical assisting content areas are more complex and require a more detailed study. Because of this, two supplemental education sections have been incorporated into this manual. The section "Taking Patients' Symptoms" provides supplemental education for Chapter 1 (The Medical Record and Health History) in the textbook; the section "Drug Dosage Calculation" provides supplemental education for Chapter 11

(Administration of Medication). In these two sections, a step-by-step, self-directed approach has been used, beginning with basic concepts and advancing to more difficult ones. The student should find that this type of approach facilitates the process of becoming proficient in these areas.

9. *EVOLVE SITE*: The Evolve site (http://evolve.elsevier.com/Bonewit) offers many opportunities for students to apply the theory and skills learned throughout the textbook. Organized by chapter, the Evolve site includes several games (e.g., Quiz Show, Road to Recovery) to provide entertainment while the student is learning important concepts related to selected chapters, matching exercises, labeling exercises, identification exercises, and other helpful activities. Of particular importance on the Evolve site are the following:

   a. *Apply Your Knowledge*: These multiple-choice questions allow the student to test his or her acquisition of practical knowledge for each chapter. These test questions can be used as a study guide to prepare for chapter tests and for a national certification examination.

   b. *Practicum Activity worksheets*: Practicum Activity worksheets are completed by the student at his or her practicum site. These worksheets assist the student in relating classroom knowledge to the real-world setting of the medical office.

   c. *Procedural Videos*: These step-by-step procedural videos directly correlate to procedures found in the textbook. They give students a visual representation of the reading material and reinforce how to perform correct clinical procedures.

   d. *Video Evaluation:* The video evaluation quizzes assess the student's knowledge of key points in the clinical skills presented in the procedural videos presented on the Evolve site (http://evolve.elsevier.com/Bonewit).

I want to thank the staff at Elsevier for their assistance and support in preparing this Study Guide. I would also like to express my appreciation to the following individuals who provided encouragement and friendship throughout this endeavor: Daniel Baldwin, Marlene Donovan, Dawn Shingler, Deborah Murray, Rob Bonewit, Hollie Bonewit-Cron, and Tristen West.

Kathy Bonewit-West, BS, MEd

Message to the Student

This Study Guide has been designed to facilitate the attainment of competency in the clinical theory and procedures in your textbook. Each chapter of the manual has been organized into the ten components outlined below. By completing each component, it is hoped that your ability to assimilate the theory and perform the clinical skills will be greatly enhanced.

1. **TEXTBOOK AND STUDY GUIDE ASSIGNMENT SHEETS**
   A. Each time your instructor makes an assignment from the textbook, Study Guide, or Evolve site, document the date due in the appropriate space on the Textbook or Study Guide Assignment Sheet.
   B. Complete each assignment by the due date. Place a checkmark in the appropriate space on the Textbook or Study Guide Assignment Sheet after completing each assignment.
   C. Grade the assignment according to the directions stipulated by your instructor.
   D. Record your points earned in the appropriate space on the Textbook or Study Guide Assignment Sheet.

2. **LABORATORY ASSIGNMENT SHEET**
   A. Your instructor will assign the procedures to be completed for each laboratory practice session. Check the assigned procedures in the appropriate space on the Laboratory Assignment Sheet.
   B. Refer to the page numbers on the Laboratory Assignment Sheet for the Practice for Competency and Evaluation of Competency worksheets required for each procedure your instructor assigned.
   C. Remove the worksheets from the Study Guide required for each procedure to be performed, and bring them to your laboratory practice session.
   D. Record the score you earned on the Evaluation of Competency Performance Evaluation Checklist in the appropriate space on the Laboratory Assignment Sheet. This will provide you with a record of your progress on clinical procedures.

3. **PRETEST AND POSTTEST**
   A. Complete the Pretest before beginning a study of each chapter. Complete the Posttest after completing your study of the chapter. Place a checkmark in the appropriate space on the Study Guide Assignment Sheet after completing each test.
   B. Check your work for accuracy against the textbook, and correct any errors.
   C. Grade the tests according to the directions stipulated by your instructor.
   D. Record the points you earned in the appropriate space on the Study Guide Assignment Sheet.
   E. Review the Pretest and Posttest before taking your chapter test.

4. **KEY TERM ASSESSMENT**
   A. Study the Terminology Review section located at the end of each chapter in the textbook.
   B. Match the medical terms with the definitions and complete the word parts table. Place a checkmark in the appropriate space on the Study Guide Assignment Sheet after completing the exercise.
   C. Check your work for accuracy against the textbook, and correct any errors.
   D. Grade the exercise according to the directions stipulated by your instructor.
   E. Record the points you earned in the appropriate space on the Study Guide Assignment Sheet.
   F. Review the Key Term Assessment before taking your chapter test.

5. **EVALUATION OF LEARNING QUESTIONS**
   A. Read the textbook chapter.
   B. Complete the Evaluation of Learning questions. Place a checkmark in the appropriate space on the Study Guide Assignment Sheet after completing the questions.
   C. Check your work for accuracy against the textbook, and correct any errors.
   D. Grade the questions according to the directions stipulated by your instructor.
   E. Record the points you earned in the appropriate space on the Textbook Assignment Sheet.
   F. Review the Evaluation of Learning questions before taking your chapter test.

6. **CRITICAL THINKING ACTIVITIES**
   A. Review the information required to complete the Critical Thinking Activities.
   B. Obtain any additional materials or resources required.
   C. Complete each Critical Thinking Activity. Place a checkmark in the appropriate space on the Study Guide Assignment Sheet after completing each assigned activity.
   D. Grade each Critical Thinking Activity according to the directions stipulated by your instructor.
   E. Record the points you earned in the appropriate space on the Textbook Assignment Sheet.

7. EVOLVE SITE ACTIVITIES
A. Complete each Evolve site activity listed on the Study Guide Assignment Sheet. Place a checkmark in the appropriate space on the Assignment Sheet after completing each assigned activity.
B. Record the points you earned in the appropriate space on the Assignment Sheet.

8. VIDEO EVALUATION
A. View the procedural videos assigned by your instructor (available on the Evolve site).
B. Complete the Video Evaluation questions on the Evolve site, and place a checkmark in the appropriate space on the Study Guide Assignment Sheet.
C. Check your work for accuracy, and correct any errors.
D. Grade the questions according to the directions stipulated by your instructor.
E. Record the points you earned in the appropriate space on the Study Guide Assignment Sheet.
F. Review the Video Evaluation questions before being evaluated on each clinical skill by your instructor.

9. PRACTICE FOR COMPETENCY
A. Your instructor will assign procedures to be completed for each laboratory practice session. For each procedure assigned, place a checkmark in the appropriate space on the Laboratory Assignment Sheet.
B. Refer to the page numbers on the Laboratory Assignment Sheet for the Practice for Competency and Evaluation of Competency sheets required for each procedure your instructor assigned. Locate and tear out the sheets required for each procedure to be performed, and bring them to your laboratory practice session.
C. Practice each assigned procedure the required number of times indicated on the Laboratory Assignment Sheet or as designated by your instructor. Use the following guidelines when practicing the procedure to attain competency over each procedure:
1. Information indicated on the Practice for Competency sheet
   a. Record your practices in the chart provided.
2. Procedure as presented in your textbook
3. Video of the procedure (on the Evolve site)
   a. View each procedure several times to make sure you understand the correct technique and theory.
4. Evaluation of Competency Performance Checklist
   a. Ensure that you can perform each procedure according to the criteria stipulated under conditions and standards.
5. Peer evaluation
   a. If directed by your instructor, obtain a peer evaluation using the Evaluation of Competency Performance Evaluation Checklist.
D. Bring the completed Practice for Competency sheet to your laboratory testing session, and present it to your instructor for his or her review before testing on the procedure.

10. EVALUATION OF COMPETENCY PERFORMANCE CHECKLIST
A. Write your name and date in the space indicated on the Evaluation of Competency Performance Evaluation Checklist.
1. Do not chart the procedure (in advance) on the Evaluation of Competency sheet. You do this after you have been tested on the procedure.
B. For each procedure being evaluated, bring the following to your laboratory testing session, and present them to your instructor:
1. Completed Practice for Competency sheet
2. Evaluation of Competency Performance Checklist
3. Outcome Assessment Record
C. Demonstrate the proper procedure for performing the clinical skill for your instructor.
D. Document results (if required) in the chart provided on the Evaluation of Competency Checklist.
E. Obtain your instructor's initials on your Outcome Assessment Record, indicating you have performed the procedure with competency.
F. Record the score you earned in the appropriate space on your Laboratory Assignment Sheet.

After you have completed each chapter in this Study Guide, place the perforated sheet into a three-ring notebook. This will provide an ongoing record of your academic progress. The notebook provides a classroom reference and a certification examination review resource.

I hope that this Study Guide will assist in your attainment of competency in clinical medical assisting procedures and will facilitate your transition from the classroom to the workplace.

Kathy Bonewit-West, BS, MEd

Outcome Assessment Record

This list of outcomes is used to maintain an ongoing record of classroom and practicum outcome assessment. Your instructor should initial each outcome when you have performed it with competency in the classroom. When you have performed the outcome with competency at your externship facility, it should be initialed by your practicum supervisor. Space is provided for three externship experiences in the event that you extern at more than one practicum site.

Name_____	Classroom Performance	Practicum	Practicum	Practicum
THE MEDICAL RECORD AND HEALTH HISTORY				
Complete or assist the patient in completing a health history form.				
Obtain and document a patient's symptoms.				
MEDICAL ASEPSIS AND THE OSHA STANDARD				
Perform handwashing.				
Apply an alcohol-based hand sanitizer.				
Apply and remove disposable exam gloves.				
Demonstrate the proper use of a sharps container.				
Prepare regulated waste for pickup by an infectious waste service.				
STERILIZATION AND DISINFECTION				
Sanitize instruments.				
Wrap an instrument for autoclaving.				
Sterilize items in an autoclave.				
VITAL SIGNS				
Measure oral body temperature.				
Measure axillary body temperature.				
Measure rectal body temperature.				
Measure aural body temperature.				
Measure temporal artery body temperature.				
Measure radial pulse and respirations.				
Measure apical pulse.				
Perform pulse oximetry.				
Measure blood pressure.				

Name_____	Classroom Performance	Practicum	Practicum	Practicum
THE PHYSICAL EXAMINATION				
Measure weight and height.				
Demonstrate proper body mechanics.				
Position and drape a patient.				
Transfer a patient from and to a wheelchair.				
Prepare an examining room.				
Prepare a patient for a physical examination.				
Assist the provider with a physical examination.				
EYE AND EAR ASSESSMENT AND PROCEDURES				
Assess distance visual acuity.				
Assess color vision.				
Perform an eye irrigation.				
Perform an eye instillation.				
Perform an ear irrigation.				
Perform an ear instillation.				
PHYSICAL AGENTS TO PROMOTE TISSUE HEALING				
Apply a heating pad.				
Apply a hot soak.				
Apply a hot compress.				
Apply an ice bag.				
Apply a cold compress.				
Apply a chemical cold and hot pack.				
Apply a hot and cold gel pack.				
Assist with the application and removal of a cast.				
Instruct a patient in proper cast care.				
Apply a splint.				
Apply a brace.				
Measure a patient for axillary crutches.				
Instruct a patient in mastering crutch gaits.				
Instruct a patient in the use of a cane.				
Instruct a patient in the use of a walker.				

Name_____	Classroom Performance	Practicum	Practicum	Practicum
THE GYNECOLOGIC EXAMINATION AND PRENATAL CARE				
Provide patient instructions for a breast self-examination.				
Provide instructions for a patient-collected vaginal specimen.				
Assist with a gynecologic examination.				
Assist with a prenatal examination.				
THE PEDIATRIC EXAMINATION				
Carry an infant in the following positions: cradle and upright.				
Measure the weight and length of an infant.				
Measure the head circumference of an infant.				
Measure the chest circumference of an infant.				
Measure the blood pressure of a child.				
Plot and calculate pediatric growth measurements.				
Administer an intramuscular injection to an infant.				
Administer a subcutaneous injection to an infant.				
Collect a urine specimen using a pediatric urine collector.				
Collect a specimen for a newborn screening test.				
MINOR OFFICE SURGERY				
Apply and remove sterile gloves.				
Open a sterile package.				
Add an item to a sterile field from a peel-apart package.				
Pour a sterile solution into a container on a sterile field.				
Change a sterile dressing.				
Remove sutures.				
Remove surgical staples.				
Assist the provider with the application of a topical tissue adhesive.				
Apply and remove skin closure tape.				

Name_____	Classroom Performance	Practicum	Practicum	Practicum
Set up a tray for minor office surgery.				
Assist the provider with minor office surgery.				
Apply the following bandage turns: circular, spiral, spiral-reverse, figure-eight, and recurrent.				
ADMINISTRATION OF MEDICATION				
Prepare and administer oral medication.				
Prepare an injection from a vial.				
Prepare an injection from an ampule.				
Reconstitute a powdered drug.				
Administer a subcutaneous injection.				
Locate the following intramuscular injection sites: deltoid, vastus lateralis, ventrogluteal, and dorsogluteal.				
Administer an intramuscular injection.				
Administer an injection using the Z-track method.				
Administer an intradermal injection.				
Administer a tuberculin skin test and read the test results.				
CARDIOPULMONARY PROCEDURES				
Run an electrocardiogram.				
Instruct a patient in the guidelines for wearing a Holter monitor.				
Apply a Holter monitor.				
Perform a spirometry test.				
Measure a patient's peak flow rate.				
COLORECTAL AND MALE REPRODUCTIVE TESTS AND PROCEDURES				
Instruct a patient for a fecal occult blood test.				
Develop a fecal occult blood test.				
Instruct a patient in the preparation for a sigmoidoscopy.				
Assist the provider with a sigmoidoscopy.				
Instruct a patient in the preparation for a colonoscopy.				

Name_____	Classroom Performance	Practicum	Practicum	Practicum
Provide instructions for a testicular self-examination.				
RADIOLOGY AND DIAGNOSTIC IMAGING				
Instruct a patient in the proper preparation required for each of the following x-ray examinations: mammogram, bone density scan, upper GI study, lower GI study, and intravenous pyelogram.				
Instruct a patient in the proper preparation required for each of the following: ultrasonography, computed tomography, magnetic resonance imaging, and nuclear medicine study.				
INTRODUCTION TO THE CLINICAL LABORATORY				
Operate an emergency eyewash station.				
Complete a laboratory request form.				
Collect a specimen for transport to an outside laboratory.				
Review a laboratory report.				
URINALYSIS				
Instruct a patient in clean-catch midstream urine specimen collection.				
Instruct a patient in 24-hour urine specimen collection.				
Assess the color and appearance of a urine specimen.				
Perform a CLIA-waived chemical assessment of a urine specimen.				
Prepare a urine specimen for microscopic analysis by a provider.				
Perform a CLIA-waived urine pregnancy test.				
PHLEBOTOMY				
Perform a venipuncture using the vacuum tube method.				
Perform a venipuncture using the butterfly method.				
Separate serum from a blood specimen.				
Collect a capillary blood specimen.				

Name_____	Classroom Performance	Practicum	Practicum	Practicum
HEMATOLOGY				
Perform a CLIA-waived hemoglobin determination.				
Perform a CLIA-waived hematocrit determination.				
Prepare a blood smear for transport to an outside laboratory.				
Perform a CLIA-waived PT/INR test.				
BLOOD CHEMISTRY AND IMMUNOLOGY				
Perform a CLIA-waived blood glucose test.				
Perform a CLIA-waived blood chemistry test.				
Perform a CLIA-waived rapid mononucleosis test.				
MEDICAL MICROBIOLOGY				
Use a microscope.				
Collect a throat specimen.				
Collect a nasopharyngeal specimen.				
Collect a specimen using a collection and transport system.				
Perform a CLIA-waived rapid strep test.				
Perform a CLIA-waived rapid influenza test.				
NUTRITION				
Instruct a patient according to a patient's special dietary needs.				
EMERGENCY PREPAREDNESS AND PROTECTIVE PRACTICES				
Demonstrate proper use of a fire extinguisher.				
Participate in a mock exposure event.				
ADDITIONAL OUTCOMES (List)				

Name_____	Classroom Performance	Practicum	Practicum	Practicum

Contents

The Medical Record and Health History

CHAPTER ASSIGNMENTS

√ After Completing	Date Due	Study Guide Pages	STUDY GUIDE ASSIGNMENTS (CTA = Critical Thinking Activity)	Possible Points	Points You Earned
		5	Pretest	10	
		6	Term Key Term Assessment	11	
		6-12	Evaluation of Learning questions	58	
		13	CTA A: Medical Abbreviations	20	
		13	CTA B: Chief Complaint	6	
		14	CTA C: Crossword Puzzle	23	
			Evolve: Road to Recovery: Medical Abbreviations (Record points earned)		
		22-28	Taking Patient Symptoms: Supplemental Education for Chapter 1 (10 points for each problem)	60	
			Evolve: Apply Your Knowledge questions	10	
			Evolve: Video Evaluation	6	
		5	Posttest	10	
			ADDITIONAL ASSIGNMENTS		
			Total points		

√ When Assigned by Your Instructor	Study Guide Pages	Practices Required	LABORATORY ASSIGNMENTS (Procedure Number and Name)	Score*
	15-17	1	**Practice for Competency**: Health History Form	
	22-28	5	**Practice for Competency** 1-1: Obtaining and Documenting Patient Symptoms	
	19-21		**Evaluation of Competency** 1-1: Obtaining and Recording Patient Symptoms	*
			ADDITIONAL ASSIGNMENTS	

Notes

Name: _____   Date: _____

True or False

_____ 1. The medical record serves as a legal document.

_____ 2. PHI includes health information in any form that contains patient-identifiable information.

_____ 3. A therapeutic service report documents the assessment and treatment designed to restore a patient's ability to function.

_____ 4. An example of a hospital document is a discharge summary report.

_____ 5. Diabetes mellitus is an example of a familial disease.

_____ 6. The medical assistant should make sure to document a procedure before performing it.

_____ 7. A symptom is any change in the body or its functioning that indicates the presence of disease.

_____ 8. A feeling of dizziness or light-headedness is known as vertigo.

_____ 9. Excessive perspiration is known as flatulence.

_____ 10. Pain is an example of an objective symptom.

? POSTTEST

True or False

_____ 1. The purpose of HIPAA is to provide patients with more control over the use and disclosure of their health information.

_____ 2. An example of a diagnostic procedure report is a urinalysis report.

_____ 3. A laboratory report is a report of the analysis or examination of body specimens.

_____ 4. The health history provides subjective data about a patient to assist the provider in arriving at a diagnosis.

_____ 5. The family history is a review of the health status of the patient's blood relatives.

_____ 6. The chief complaint is the symptom causing the patient the most trouble.

_____ 7. The social history includes information on the patient's lifestyle, such as health habits and living environment.

_____ 8. The patient's name must be included at the beginning of each entry documented in the patient's medical record.

_____ 9. A decrease in the amount of water in the body is known as edema.

_____ 10. Cyanosis is an example of an objective symptom.

Directions: Match each medical term (numbers) with its definition (letters).

_____ 1. Diagnosis

_____ 2. Diagnostic procedure

_____ 3. Documenting

_____ 4. Electronic health record

_____ 5. Familial disease

_____ 6. Health history report

_____ 7. Medical record

_____ 8. Objective symptom

_____ 9. Paper-based patient record

_____ 10. Subjective symptom

_____ 11. Symptom

A. A collection of subjective data about a patient

B. A symptom felt by the patient but not observed by an examiner

C. The process of recording information about a patient in the medical record

D. Any change in the body or its functioning that indicates the presence of disease

E. A medical record that is stored on a computer

F. A written record of the important information regarding a patient

G. A symptom that can be observed by an examiner

H. The scientific method of determining and identifying a patient's condition

I. A condition that occurs in or affects blood relatives more frequently than would be expected by chance

J. A procedure performed to assist in the diagnosis, management, or treatment of a patient's condition

K. A medical record in paper form

EVALUATION OF LEARNING

Directions: Fill in each blank with the correct answer.

1. List three functions of the medical record.

_____

_____

_____

2. What is the meaning of the acronym HIPAA?

_____

3. What is the purpose of the HIPAA Privacy Rule?

_____

_____

4. Who must comply with HIPAA?

_____

5. What is a Notice of Privacy Practices?

_____

_____

6. What is protected health information?

_____

_____

7. List examples of when HIPAA does not require written consent for the use or disclosure of protected health information in the following categories:

    a. Treatment: _____

    b. Payment: _____

    c. Health care operations: _____

8. What must be done before the medical office can disclose protected health information (PHI) to a business associate?

    _____

    _____

9. What are some examples of business associates to whom the medical office may disclose PHI?

    _____

    _____

10. How must medical office employees be informed of the privacy and security measures that must be followed with respect to PHI?

    _____

    _____

11. List three examples of medical office administrative documents.

    _____

    _____

12. List five examples of medical office clinical documents.

    _____

    _____

13. What is a laboratory report, and what is its purpose?

    _____

    _____

14. What is a diagnostic procedure?

    _____

    _____

15. What information is included in a diagnostic procedure report?

    _____

    _____

16. List five examples of diagnostic procedure reports.

    _____

    _____

17. What information is documented in a therapeutic service report?

_____

_____

18. List three examples of therapeutic service reports.

_____

_____

19. What is the purpose of hospital documents?

_____

_____

20. Who is responsible for preparing hospital documents?

_____

21. List five examples of hospital documents.

_____

_____

22. What are consent forms?

_____

23. List two examples of consent documents.

_____

24. What types of forms are typically included in a paper-based patient record (PPR)?

_____

_____

25. What is an EHR?

_____

_____

26. What are the general functions performed by an EHR software program?

_____

_____

27. List and describe the advantages of the electronic medical record.

_____

_____

_____

_____

28. What is a health history report?

_____

_____

29. List four functions of a health history report.

_____

_____

_____

30. What are three ways in which a health history can be entered into the EHR?

_____

_____

_____

31. State the purpose of the following sections of the health history:

   a. Identification data: _____

   b. Chief complaint: _____

   _____

   c. Present illness: _____

   _____

   d. Past history: _____

   _____

   e. Family history: _____

   _____

   f. Social history: _____

   _____

   g. Review of systems: _____

   _____

32. What is a chief complaint?

_____

33. What guidelines must be followed in documenting the chief complaint?

_____

_____

_____

34. What is the present illness, and how is this information usually obtained?

_____

_____

35. What is the past history, and how is it usually obtained?

_____

_____

36. List five examples of information included in the past medical history.

_____

_____

_____

37. List three examples of familial diseases.

_____

_____

38. Explain the importance of the social history.

_____

_____

39. What specific areas are included in the social history?

_____

_____

40. What is the review of systems (ROS)?

_____

_____

41. Explain the importance of good documentation.

_____

_____

42. What may result if the medical assistant documents information in the wrong patient's medical record?

_____

_____

43. Why is it important for the medical assistant to use the commonly accepted abbreviations, medical terms, and symbols when documenting in the medical record?

_____

_____

44. Why is it important to document immediately after performing a procedure?

_____

45. Why is it important to adhere to the following guidelines when documenting in the PPR?

    a. Use black ink: _____

    _____

    b. Write in legible handwriting: _____

    _____

    c. Draw a single line through unneeded space: _____

    _____

    d. Never erase or obliterate an entry: _____

    _____

46. What should be done if an error is made when documenting in a PPR?

    _____

    _____

47. What are progress notes?

    _____

    _____

48. What is the purpose of progress notes?

    _____

49. What is a symptom?

    _____

50. What is the difference between a subjective symptom and an objective symptom?

    _____

    _____

51. List three examples of subjective symptoms.

    _____

    _____

52. List three examples of objective symptoms.

    _____

    _____

53. In general, what information should be documented regarding a procedure performed on a patient?

    _____

    _____

54. What information should be documented regarding medication administered to a patient?

_____

_____

55. What information should be documented regarding a specimen collected from a patient?

_____

_____

56. Why is it important to document diagnostic procedures and laboratory tests ordered for a patient?

_____

_____

57. What is the importance of having a patient sign a patient instruction form?

_____

_____

58. Why is it important for the medical assistant to witness the patient's signature on an instruction sheet provided to the patient?

_____

_____

CRITICAL THINKING ACTIVITIES

A. Medical Abbreviations

Write a paragraph describing a visit to your doctor's office in the space provided using at least 20 abbreviations and symbols outlined in Table 1-1 of your textbook.

_____

_____

_____

_____

_____

_____

_____

_____

_____

_____

_____

B. Chief Complaint

Indicate whether each of the following statements is an incorrect (I) or correct (C) example of documenting a chief complaint (CC). If the example is incorrect, explain which documentation guideline is not being followed.

_____ 1. CC: Low back pain _____

_____ 2. CC: Sore throat and fever for the past 2 days _____

_____ 3. CC: Dyspnea, paleness, and fatigue, similar to that associated with anemia, that have lasted for 2 weeks_____

_____ 4. CC: Poor health for the past several months _____

_____ 5. CC: Weakness and fatigue related to poor eating habits and lack of exercise

_____

_____ 6. CC: Heart palpitations occurring after drinking coffee in the morning before work

_____

_____

13

C. Crossword Puzzle: Symptoms

Directions: Complete the crossword puzzle using the terms provided.

Across
2 Stool is hard and dry
4 Blue skin from lack of O_2
5 Nosebleed
10 Skin eruption
11 Dizziness
14 No appetite
15 Yellow skin
18 Severe itching
19 Involuntary contractions of muscles
20 Gas
21 Head pain

Down
1 Fast pulse rate
2 Shivering
3 May be productive or nonproductive
5 Fluid retention
6 Ejection of stomach contents
7 Decreased H_2O levels in the body
8 Red face
9 Elevated temp
12 Bad all over
13 Loose, watery stools
16 Sensation of stomach discomfort
17 Feeling of distress or suffering

PRACTICE FOR COMPETENCY

Health History Form

Complete the health history form (pages 15 to 17) using yourself as the patient.

Procedure 1-1: Obtaining and Documenting Patient Symptoms

Practice obtaining patient symptoms, by completing Taking Patient Symptoms: Supplemental Education for Chapter 1 (pages 22-28 in this study guide).

PATIENT HEALTH HISTORY

A | **IDENTIFICATION DATA**   Please print the following information.

Today's date _____

Name _____

_____ Male _____ Female

Address _____

_____ Married ____ Separated ____ Divorced ____ Widowed ____ Single

_____

Date of Birth _____

Telephone _____
     Home number   Work number

B | **PAST HISTORY**

Have you ever had the following: (Circle "no" or "yes"; leave blank if uncertain)

Measles ___ no yes	Heart Disease ___ no yes	Diabetes ___ no yes	Hemorrhoids ___ no yes
Mumps ___ no yes	Arthritis ___ no yes	Cancer ___ no yes	Asthma ___ no yes
Chickenpox ___ no yes	Sexually Transmitted no yes Disease	Polio ___ no yes	Allergies ___ no yes
Whooping Cough ___ no yes	Anemia ___ no yes	Glaucoma ___ no yes	Eczema ___ no yes
Scarlet Fever ___ no yes	Bladder Infections ___ no yes	Hernia ___ no yes	AIDS or HIV+ ___ no yes
Diphtheria ___ no yes	Epilepsy ___ no yes	Blood or Plasma ___ no yes Transfusions	Infectious Mono ___ no yes
Pneumonia ___ no yes	Migraine Headaches ___ no yes	Back Trouble ___ no yes	Bronchitis ___ no yes
Rheumatic Fever ___ no yes	Tuberculosis ___ no yes	High Blood ___ no yes Pressure	Mitral Valve Prolapse no yes
Stroke ___ no yes	Ulcer ___ no yes	Thyroid Disease ___ no yes	Any other disease ___ no yes
Hepatitis ___ no yes	Kidney Disease ___ no yes	Bleeding Tendency _ no yes	Please list: _____

MAJOR HOSPITALIZATIONS: If you have ever been hospitalized for any major medical illness or operation, write in your most recent hospitalizations below.

Hospitalizations	Year	Operation or illness	Name of hospital	City and state
1st Hospitalization				
2nd Hospitalization				
3rd Hospitalization				
4th Hospitalization				

TESTS AND IMMUNIZATIONS: Mark an X next to those that you have had.

Tests:
- [ ] TB Test
- [ ] Rectal/Hemoccult
- [ ] Sigmoidoscopy
- [ ] Colonoscopy

- [ ] Electrocardiogram
- [ ] Chest X-ray
- [ ] Mammogram
- [ ] Pap Test

Immunizations:
- [ ] Influenza
- [ ] Hepatitis B
- [ ] Tetanus
- [ ] MMR
- [ ] Polio

ALLERGIES: List all allergies (foods, drugs, environment). [ ] None

_____
_____
_____
_____

CURRENT MEDICATIONS: List the following that you are currently taking: Prescription medications, over-the-counter (OTC) medications, vitamin supplements, and herbal supplements. [ ] None

Medication	Frequency

ACCIDENTS/INJURIES: Describe all serious accidents, severe injuries, head injury, or fractures. Include the date each occurred. [ ] None

Accident/Injury: Date:

_____
_____
_____
_____

(Continued)

C FAMILY HISTORY

For each member of your family, follow the purple or blue line across the page and check boxes for:
1. Their present state of health
2. Any illnesses they have had

	Good Health	Poor Health	Deceased	If deceased, write in age and cause of death.	Allergies or Asthma	Diabetes	Heart Disease	Stroke	Cancer	High Blood Pressure	Glaucoma	Arthritis	Ulcer	Kidney Disease	Mental Health Problems	Alcohol/Drug Abuse	Obesity	High Cholesterol	Thyroid Disease
Father:																			
Mother:																			
Brothers/Sisters:																			

D SOCIAL HISTORY

EDUCATION _____ High school _____ College _____ Postgraduate

Occupation _____ Years _____

Previous occupations _____ Years _____

_____ Years _____

Have you ever been exposed to any of the following in your environment?

☐ Excess dust (coal, lime, rock)   ☐ Cleaning fluids/solvents   ☐ Radiation   ☐ Other toxic materials

☐ Sand   ☐ Hair spray   ☐ Insecticides

☐ Chemicals   ☐ Smoke or auto exhaust fumes   ☐ Paints

Please answer the follwing questions by placing an X in the box in front of the word Yes or No, except where you are asked for specific information. This information is obviously highly confidential and will be released to other health professionals or insurance carriers ONLY with your consent.

DIET:

Do you eat a good breakfast?	☐ Yes	☐ No
Do you snack between meals (soft drinks, chips, candy bars)?	☐ Yes	☐ No
Do you eat fresh fruits and vegetables each day?	☐ Yes	☐ No
Do you eat whole grain breads and cereals?	☐ Yes	☐ No
Is your diet high in fat content?	☐ Yes	☐ No
Is your diet high in cholesterol content?	☐ Yes	☐ No
Is your diet high in salt content?	☐ Yes	☐ No
Are you allergic to any foods?	☐ Yes	☐ No

How many glasses of water do you drink each day? _____

How would you describe your overall eating habits?   ☐ Excellent   ☐ Good   ☐ Fair   ☐ Poor

PERSONAL HISTORY:

Do you find it hard to make decisions?	☐ Yes	☐ No
Do you find it hard to concentrate or remember?	☐ Yes	☐ No
Do you feel depressed?	☐ Yes	☐ No
Do you have difficulty relaxing?	☐ Yes	☐ No
Do you have a tendency to worry a lot?	☐ Yes	☐ No
Have you gained or lost much weight recently?	☐ Yes	☐ No
Do you lose your temper often?	☐ Yes	☐ No
Are you disturbed by any work or family problems?	☐ Yes	☐ No
Are you having sexual difficulties?	☐ Yes	☐ No
Have you ever considered committing suicide?	☐ Yes	☐ No
Have you ever desired or sought psychiatric help?	☐ Yes	☐ No

EXERCISE:

Do you exercise on a regular basis?	☐ Yes	☐ No
Does your job require strenuous, sustained physical work?	☐ Yes	☐ No

SLEEP PATTERNS:

Do you seem to feel exhausted or fatigued most of the time?	☐ Yes	☐ No
Do you have difficulty either falling asleep or staying asleep?	☐ Yes	☐ No

USE OF TOBACCO/ALCOHOL/CAFFEINE/DRUGS: Amt:

How much do you smoke per day?   ☐ Cigarettes ____

☐ Don't smoke   ☐ Cigars/pipes ____

Do you take two or more alcoholic drinks per day?	☐ Yes	☐ No
Do you drink six or more cups of coffee or tea per day?	☐ Yes	☐ No
Are you a regular user of sleeping pills, marijuana, tranquilizers, painkillers, etc.?	☐ Yes	☐ No
Have you ever used heroin, cocaine, LSD, PCP, etc.?	☐ Yes	☐ No

List any country outside the United States you have visited in the past six months. _____

When did you have your last physical examination? _____

Patient's Name _____

E **REVIEW OF SYSTEMS**

HEAD AND NECK
_____ Frequent headaches
_____ Neck pain
_____ Neck lumps or swelling

EYES
_____ Wears glasses
_____ Blurry vision
_____ Eyesight worsening
_____ Sees double
_____ Sees halo
_____ Eye pain or itching
_____ Watering eyes
_____ Eye trouble

EARS
_____ Hearing difficulties
_____ Earaches
_____ Running ears
_____ Buzzing in ears
_____ Motion sickness

MOUTH
_____ Dental problems
_____ Swellings on gums or jaws
_____ Sore tongue
_____ Taste changes

NOSE AND THROAT
_____ Congested nose
_____ Running nose
_____ Sneezing spells
_____ Head colds
_____ Nosebleeds
_____ Sore throat
_____ Enlarged tonsils
_____ Hoarse voice

RESPIRATORY
_____ Wheezes or gasps
_____ Coughing spells
_____ Coughs up phlegm
_____ Coughed up blood
_____ Chest colds
_____ Excessive sweating, night sweats

CARDIOVASCULAR
_____ High blood pressure
_____ Racing heart
_____ Chest pains
_____ Dizzy spells
_____ Shortness of breath
_____ Shortness of breath at night
_____ More pillows to breathe
_____ Swollen feet or ankles
_____ Leg cramps
_____ Heart murmur

DIGESTIVE
_____ Heartburn
_____ Bloated stomach
_____ Belching
_____ Stomach pains
_____ Nausea
_____ Vomited blood
_____ Difficulty swallowing
_____ Constipation
_____ Loose bowels
_____ Black stools
_____ Gray stools
_____ Pain in rectum
_____ Rectal bleeding

URINARY
_____ Night frequency
_____ Day frequency
_____ Wets pants or bed
_____ Burning on urination
_____ Brown, black, or bloody urine
_____ Difficulty starting urine
_____ Urgency

MALE GENITAL
_____ Weak urine stream
_____ Prostate trouble
_____ Burning or discharge
_____ Lumps on testicles
_____ Painful testicles

FEMALE GENITAL
__/__/__ Last menstrual period
__/__/__ Last Pap test
_____ Postmenopausal or hysterectomy
_____ Noticed vaginal bleeding
_____ Abnormal LMP
_____ Heavy bleeding during periods
_____ Bleeding between periods
_____ Bleeding after intercourse
_____ Recent vaginal itching/discharge
_____ No monthly breast exam
_____ Lump or pain in breasts
_____ Complications with birth control

OBSTETRIC HISTORY
_____ Gravida
_____ Para
_____ Preterm
_____ Miscarriages
_____ Stillbirths
_____ Has had an abortion

MUSCULOSKELETAL
_____ Aching muscles
_____ Swollen joints
_____ Back or shoulder pains
_____ Painful feet
_____ Disability

SKIN
_____ Skin problems
_____ Itching or burning skin
_____ Bleeds easily
_____ Bruises easily

NEUROLOGICAL
_____ Faintness
_____ Numbness
_____ Convulsions
_____ Change in handwriting
_____ Trembles

F **PROGRESS NOTES**

Date	

17

Notes

Procedure 1-1: Obtaining and Documenting Patient Symptoms

Name: _____   Date:_____

Evaluated by: _____   Score:_____

Performance Objective

Outcome:	Obtain and document patient symptoms.
Conditions:	Given the following: medical record of the patient to be interviewed and a pen with black ink.
Standards:	Time: 10 minutes. Student completed procedure in _____ minutes.
	Accuracy: Satisfactory score on the Performance Evaluation Checklist.

Performance Evaluation Checklist

Trial 1	Trial 2	Point Value	Performance Standards
		•	Assembled equipment.
		•	Made sure to obtain or access the correct patient record.
		•	Went to the waiting room and asked the patient to come back.
		•	Escorted the patient to a quiet room.
		•	In a calm and friendly manner, greeted the patient and introduced yourself.
		•	Identified the patient by full name and date of birth.
		•	Asked the patient to be seated.
		•	Seated yourself facing the patient at a distance of 3 to 4 feet.
		▷	Explained the purpose of this seating arrangement.
			Used good communication skills:
		•	Used the patient's name of choice.
		•	Demonstrated genuine interest and concern for the patient.
		•	Maintained appropriate eye contact.
		•	Used terminology the patient could understand.
		•	Listened carefully and attentively to the patient.
		•	Paid attention to the patient's nonverbal messages.
		•	Avoided judgmental comments.
		•	Avoided rushing the patient.
		•	Located the progress note sheet in the PPR or progress note template in the EHR.

Trial 1	Trial 2	Point Value	Performance Standards
		•	Documented the date, time, and CC abbreviation.
		•	Used an open-ended question to obtain the chief complaint.
		▷	Explained why an open-ended question should be used.
			Documented the chief complaint in the PPR:
		•	Limited the CC to one or two symptoms.
		•	Referred to a specific rather than a vague symptom.
		•	Documented concisely and briefly.
		•	Used the patient's own words as much as possible.
		•	Included the duration of the symptom.
		•	Avoided using names of diseases.
			Documented the chief complaint in the EHR by completing each field of the chief complaint template:
		•	Obtained additional information regarding the chief complaint.
		•	Thanked the patient and proceeded to the next step in the patient workup.
		•	Informed the patient approximately how long he or she will need to wait for the provider.
		•	If using a PPR, placed the medical record in the appropriate location for review by the provider.
		■	Demonstrated critical thinking skills.
		■	Demonstrated active listening.
		★	Completed the procedure within 10 minutes.
			Totals

CHART

Date	

Evaluation of Student Performance

EVALUATION CRITERIA			COMMENTS
Symbol	**Category**	**Point Value**	
★	Critical Step	16 points	
•	Essential Step	6 points	
■	Affective Competency	6 points	
▷	Theory Question	2 points	

Score calculation: 100 points

     – ____ points missed

       ___Score

Satisfactory score: 85 or above

CAAHEP Competencies Achieved

Psychomotor (Skills)
☑ V. 2. Correctly use and pronounce medical terminology in health care interactions.

Affective (Behavior)
☑ A.1. Demonstrate critical thinking skills.
☑ A.4. Demonstrate active listening.

ABHES Competencies Achieved

☑ 3. d. Define and use medical abbreviations when appropriate and acceptable.
☑ 4. a. Follow documentation guidelines.
☑ 7. a. Collect and process documents.
☑ 7. g. Display professionalism through written and verbal communications.
☑ 8. b. Obtain and document chief complaint, patient history, and vital signs.

Taking a patient's symptoms is a frequent and important responsibility of the medical assistant, who must have a thorough knowledge of symptoms and related terminology. A **symptom** is defined as any change in the body or its functioning that indicates the presence of disease. The medical assistant can observe **objective symptoms** presented by the patient, such as coughing, rash, and swelling. The medical assistant must rely on information relayed by the patient to obtain data on **subjective symptoms**. Examples of subjective symptoms include pain, pruritus, and vertigo.

This section is designed as supplemental education for Chapter 1 (The Medical Record) in your textbook. Completion of the exercises in this section can assist you in documenting a patient's symptoms effectively and thoroughly, which is essential to an accurate diagnosis by the provider.

Learning Objectives

After completing this chapter, you should be able to do the following:
1. Explain the purpose of analyzing a symptom.
2. State the seven basic types of information that must be obtained to analyze a symptom.
3. Analyze a symptom by using direct questions.

Analysis of a Symptom

Before a symptom can be analyzed, the **chief complaint** (CC) must first be identified. The chief complaint is the patient's reason for seeking care or the symptom causing the patient the most trouble. An open-ended question should be used to elicit the chief complaint from the patient, and it should be documented following the documentation guidelines presented in your textbook. The next step is to analyze the chief complaint in detail from the time of its onset. The purpose of this is to provide a complete description of the current status of the chief complaint.

Analyzing the chief complaint requires a combination of good listening and writing skills. The medical assistant must know what information should be documented for each symptom and the questions to ask the patient to obtain this information. A list of symptoms, explanation of the information required for each symptom, and examples of questions to ask the patient are provided.

Type of Information Required

The following information is needed for each symptom to provide a full description of the current status of the chief complaint:

1. Location of the symptom. This refers to the specific area of the body where the symptom is located. Locating the symptom is the first step in determining the cause of the patient's disease. The patient may refer to the location in general terms, such as the head, arm, stomach, or back. The medical assistant must be more specific than this and determine the exact location using descriptions, such as "occurs in the lower back" or "occurs under the sternum." Several questions can assist in accomplishing this.
   - Where exactly does it hurt?
   - Can you show me where it hurts?
   - Do you feel it anywhere else?

2. Quality of the symptom. The quality of the symptom includes a complete and concise description of the symptom. The medical assistant should use informative terms to describe the character of each symptom. For example, if the patient complains of pain, the character of the pain must be included. Several terms can be used to describe pain.
   - Burning
   - Aching
   - Sharp
   - Dull
   - Throbbing
   - Cramplike
   - Squeezing

   If the patient has vomited, the medical assistant should indicate the color, odor, and consistency of the vomitus. If the patient has a cough, the medical assistant should indicate whether it is productive or nonproductive and whether blood is present. Refer to the list of terms on pages 27 and 28 of this manual, which can assist in describing symptoms. Specific examples of questions that are helpful in determining the quality of the symptom are as follows:
   - Describe it (the symptom) to me as fully as possible.
   - What is it (the symptom) like?

3. Severity of the symptom. Severity refers to the quantitative aspect of the symptom. It includes the following:
   - Intensity of the symptom (e.g., mild, moderate, severe)
   - Number (e.g., of convulsions, of nosebleeds)
   - Volume (e.g., of vomitus, of blood, of mucus)
   - Size or extent (e.g., of the rash, edema, lumps, or masses)

   This information assists the provider in determining the extensiveness or seriousness of the illness. Questions to determine severity are often specific to that symptom. For example, if the patient has a productive cough, the medical assistant should determine how much phlegm is being coughed up (e.g., teaspoon, half of a cup). At first, this area may appear difficult, but as you practice taking symptoms, you will learn what questions to ask the patient, and it eventually will become automatic. The examples at the end of this section and the student practice problems provide guidance in developing skill in this area. Some examples of general questions that can be used to determine the severity of a symptom are as follows:
   - How bad is it (the symptom)?
   - Does it (the symptom) limit your normal activities?

4. Chronology and timing of the symptom. Chronology and timing include a sequential account of the symptom up to the time the patient came to the medical office for treatment. This information is important in determining the duration of the symptom and change in it since it first occurred. Chronology and timing include the following four areas:
   a. Date of onset: The date of onset of the symptom should be indicated, if possible, as a calendar date and clock time. The patient may need some time to recall this information. Examples of questions that help obtain this information are as follows:
      - When did you experience this (the symptom) for the first time?
      - Exactly when did this begin?
   b. Duration: The duration of the symptom refers to how long the symptom lasts after it occurs, for example: 10 minutes, 2 hours, continuously. Examples of questions to obtain this information are as follows:
      - How long does it last after occurring?
      - For what length of time do you experience this symptom?
   c. Frequency: The frequency of the symptom refers to how often the symptom occurs, such as twice daily or a single attack every 2 weeks. Examples of questions to obtain this information are as follows:
      - How often does it occur?
      - How often has the symptom recurred?
   d. Change over time: This area refers to any change in the symptom since it first occurred. A change in a symptom reflects the nature of the underlying disease, which assists the provider in making a diagnosis. Examples of questions to obtain this information are as follows:
      - Has the symptom changed since it first occurred?
      - Is it (the symptom) getting better, worse, or staying the same?

5. Manner of onset. The manner of onset refers to what the patient was doing when the symptom first occurred and exactly what was experienced by the patient when the symptom began. These data help provide information on the pathologic process responsible for the symptom. For example, the patient may have been lifting a heavy object before experiencing low back pain. This information helps the provider in making an accurate diagnosis. Examples of questions that are helpful in determining the manner of onset are as follows:
   - What exactly did you experience when it (the symptom) first occurred?
   - What was the first thing you noticed?
   - Did it (the symptom) come on suddenly or gradually?
   - What were you doing when it (the symptom) began?
   - Where were you when this happened?
   - How were you feeling before it (the symptom) began?

6. Modifying factors. Symptoms are often influenced by activities or physiological processes such as physical exercise, change in weather, bodily functions (e.g., bowel movements, eating, coughing), pregnancy, emotional states, and fatigue. Some activities may aggravate the symptom, while others may alleviate it. These influences may help to determine what is causing the problem. For example, pain that becomes worse after the patient eats, but is relieved after taking an antacid assists the provider in focusing on gastrointestinal disorders. Questions to assist in determining modifying factors are as follows:
   - Does anything make it (the symptom) better?
   - Does anything make it worse?
   - What have you done to make it better?
   - What did you do to help it?
   - Are you taking any medication for it? Did it help?

23

7. Associated symptoms. There is usually more than one symptom associated with a disease process. Determining these additional symptoms gives the provider a complete picture of the illness. Examples of questions that help to identify the presence of additional symptoms are as follows:
  ■ Are you having any other symptoms?
  ■ What other problems have you noticed since you became ill?

Examples

The following examples illustrate how to analyze a symptom. The chief complaint is listed first, followed by questions to ask the patient from the seven basic categories of information.

Example: Chief complaint: Headaches that began 2 months ago.

1. Using your finger, point to the location of the headache.
2. Describe the pain. Is it sharp, dull, throbbing?
3. Are you able to carry on normal activities when you have a headache?
4. Is it sometimes more severe than usual?
5. When exactly did your headaches begin?
6. How long does your headache last when it occurs?
7. How often do you get a headache?
8. Since your headaches began, have they gotten better or worse, or have they stayed the same?
9. What were you doing the first time you experienced a headache?
10. What was your health status before your headaches began?
11. Do you get a headache before, during, or after a particular activity, such as reading or watching TV?
12. Does anything make your headache better?
13. Are you taking any medication for your headache? Does it help?
14. Have you had any other problems since your headaches began, such as nausea, vomiting, dizziness, or problems with vision?

Example: Chief complaint: The patient has been coughing for the past 3 days.

1. Does it hurt when you cough? Where? Show me with one of your fingers.
2. What is the cough like?
3. Can you cough for me?
4. Do you bring up any phlegm when you cough? What color is it? Is blood present?
5. Describe the pain. Is it sharp, dull, squeezing?
6. Do you become exhausted when you cough?
7. How much phlegm do you bring up? A teaspoon? Half a cup?
8. How much blood is present in the phlegm?
9. When did your cough first begin?
10. Does it seem like an attack? How long does the attack last?
11. How often do you get a coughing attack?
12. Does your cough seem to be getting better or worse?
13. What was the first thing you noticed when you became ill?
14. How were you feeling before your symptoms began?
15. Is there anything that makes your cough better?
16. Is there anything that makes your cough worse?
17. Do you cough more at night or during the day?
18. Are you taking any medication for it? Does it help?
19. Are you having any other problems?

Practice Problems

In the space provided, indicate examples of direct questions to ask the patient to obtain the necessary information for the symptoms presented in the chief complaint.

Problem 1

Chief complaint: Earache and fever for the past 2 days.

Questions:

_____

_____

_____

_____

_____

_____

_____

_____

Problem 2

Chief complaint: Rash with itching that began 3 days ago.

Questions:

_____

_____

_____

_____

_____

_____

_____

_____

_____

Problem 3

Chief complaint: Pain during urination that began yesterday.

Questions:

_____

_____

_____

_____

_____

_____

_____

_____

Problem 4

Chief complaint: Low back pain for the past 3 months.

Questions:

_____

_____

_____

_____

_____

_____

_____

_____

Problem 5

Chief complaint: Sore throat and fever for the past 24 hours.

Questions:

_____

_____

_____

_____

_____

_____

_____

_____

Chapter **1 The Medical Record and Health History**

Problem 6

> *Chief complaint: Chest pain that occurred this morning.*

Questions:

_____

_____

_____

_____

_____

_____

_____

_____

_____

Terms for Describing Symptoms

Pain

    Burning, aching, sharp, dull, throbbing, cramping, squeezing

    Radiating, transient, constant

    Localized, superficial, deep

Respirations

    Rapid, irregular, shallow, deep, labored, gasping, noisy, wheezing

    Apnea, dyspnea, orthopnea

    Discomfort, pain, cyanosis, cough

Cough

    Nonproductive, productive

    Persistent, dry, hacking, barking, spasmodic

    Phlegm: color, consistency, presence or absence of blood

    Exhausting or painful

Cardiovascular system

    Pain, palpitations

    Sharp, radiating

    Dyspnea, orthopnea

    Cyanosis

Gastrointestinal system

    Abdomen: flaccid, rigid, distended

    Appetite: anorexia, intolerance to foods

    Heartburn, pain after eating, belching, nausea, vomiting, flatulence, change in bowel habits, constipation, diarrhea, black stools

Chapter **1** **The Medical Record and Health History**

Urine or Stool

    Abnormality: color, odor, consistency, frequency

    Contents: sediment, mucus, blood

    Elimination: urgency, nocturia, pain, burning

Skin

    Rash: pruritus, red, swelling, distribution

    Lesions: color, character, distribution

    Pallor: flushing, jaundice, warm, dry, cold, clammy

    Ecchymosis, petechiae, cyanosis, edema

    Pruritus, sweating, change in color, bruises easily

Ears

    Pain, loss of hearing, tinnitus, vertigo

    Discharge, infection

Eyes

    Itching, burning, blurry vision, seeing double, photophobia

    Discharge, watering, infection

2 Medical Asepsis and the OSHA Standard

CHAPTER ASSIGNMENTS

√ After Completing	Date Due	Study Guide Pages	STUDY GUIDE ASSIGNMENTS (CTA = Critical Thinking Activity)	Possible Points	Points You Earned
		33	Pretest	10	
		34-35	Term Key Term Assessment A. Definitions B. Word Parts (Add 1 point for each key term)	27 15	
		35-42	Evaluation of Learning questions	67	
		43	CTA A: Infection Process Cycle	5	
		43	CTA B: Handwashing	8	
		44	CTA C: Personal Protective Equipment: Gloves	8	
		44-45	CTA D: OSHA Standard	10	
		46	CTA E: Discarding Medical Waste	20	
			Evolve: Discard It! (Record points earned)		
		47	CTA F: Crossword Puzzle	25	
			Evolve: Quiz Show (Record points earned)		
			Evolve: Apply Your Knowledge questions (Record points earned)	10	
			Evolve: Video Evaluation	56	
		33	Posttest	10	
			ADDITIONAL ASSIGNMENTS		
			Total points		

29

√ When Assigned by Your Instructor	Study Guide Pages	Practices Required	LABORATORY ASSIGNMENTS (Procedure Number and Name)	Score*
	49	5	**Practice for Competency** 2-1: Handwashing	
	51-52		**Evaluation of Competency** 2-1: Handwashing	*
	49	4	**Practice for Competency** 2-2: Applying an Alcohol-Based Hand Sanitizer	
	53-54		**Evaluation of Competency** 2-2: Applying an Alcohol-Based Hand Sanitizer	*
	49	3	**Practice for Competency** 2-A: Determination of Exam Glove Size	
	55-56		**Evaluation of Competency** 2-A: Determination of Exam Glove Size	*
	49	5	**Practice for Competency** 2-3: Application and Removal of Disposable Exam Gloves	
	57-58		**Evaluation of Competency** 2-3: Application and Removal of Disposable Exam Gloves	*
	49	3	**Practice for Competency** 2-B: Proper Use of a Sharps Container	
	59-60		**Evaluation of Competency** 2-B: Proper Use of a Sharps Container	*
	49	3	**Practice for Competency** 2-C: Disposal of Hazardous Material	
	61-62		**Evaluation of Competency** 2-C: Disposal of Hazardous Material	*
			ADDITIONAL ASSIGNMENTS	

Chapter **2** **Medical Asepsis and the OSHA Standard**

Notes

Name: _____ Date: _____

True or False

_____ 1. A microorganism is a tiny living plant or animal that cannot be seen with the naked eye.

_____ 2. A disease-producing microorganism is known as a nonpathogen.

_____ 3. Microorganisms grow best in an acidic environment.

_____ 4. Coughing and sneezing help to force pathogens from the body.

_____ 5. An alcohol-based hand sanitizer should be used to sanitize hands that are visibly soiled.

_____ 6. OSHA stands for Occupational Safety and Health Administration.

_____ 7. A biohazard warning label must be fluorescent orange or an orange-red color.

_____ 8. Prescription eyeglasses are acceptable eye protection when handling blood.

_____ 9. Hepatitis B is an infection of the liver caused by a virus.

_____10. HIV cannot be transmitted through casual contact.

? POSTTEST

True or False

_____ 1. Bacteria and viruses are examples of microorganisms.

_____ 2. An anaerobe can exist only in the presence of oxygen.

_____ 3. The optimum growth temperature is the temperature at which a microorganism grows the best.

_____ 4. Medical asepsis refers to practices that inhibit the growth and hinder the transmission of pathogenic microorganisms.

_____ 5. Resident flora are picked up in the course of daily activities and are usually pathogenic.

_____ 6. The purpose of the OSHA Standard is to prevent exposure of employees to bloodborne pathogens.

_____ 7. OSHA requires the Exposure Control Plan to be updated annually.

_____ 8. An engineering control includes all measures and devices that isolate or remove the bloodborne pathogens hazard from the workplace.

_____ 9. A reagent strip that has been used to test urine is an example of regulated medical waste.

_____10. Patients with chronic hepatitis B face an increased risk of developing pancreatitis.

A. Definitions

Directions: Match each key term with its definition.

_____ 1. Acute infection

_____ 2. Aerobe

_____ 3. Anaerobe

_____ 4. Antiseptic

_____ 5. Chronic infection

_____ 6. Bloodborne pathogens

_____ 7. Cilia

_____ 8. Contaminated

_____ 9. Exposure incident

_____ 10. Hand hygiene

_____ 11. Infection

_____ 12. Medical asepsis

_____ 13. Microorganism

_____ 14. Nonintact skin

_____ 15. Nonpathogen

_____ 16. Occupational exposure

_____ 17. Opportunistic infection

_____ 18. Optimum growth temperature

_____ 19. Parenteral

_____ 20. Pathogen

_____ 21. pH

_____ 22. Postexposure prophylaxis

_____ 23. Regulated medical waste

_____ 24. Reservoir host

_____ 25. Resident flora

_____ 26. Sharps

_____ 27. Transient flora

A. A disease-producing microorganism

B. Microorganisms that reside on the superficial skin layers and are picked up in the course of daily activities

C. A microorganism that needs oxygen to live and grow

D. Reasonably anticipated skin, eye, mucous membrane, or parenteral contact with bloodborne pathogens or other potentially infectious materials that may result from the performance of an employee's duties

E. Practices that are employed to inhibit the growth and hinder the transmission of pathogenic microorganisms

F. Piercing of the skin barrier or mucous membranes, such as through needlesticks, human bites, cuts, and abrasions

G. Skin that has a break in the surface

H. The temperature at which an organism grows best

I. The degree to which a solution is acidic or basic

J. A specific eye, mouth, or other mucous membrane, nonintact skin, or parenteral contact with blood or other potentially infectious materials that results from an employee's duties

K. Pathogenic microorganisms in human blood that can cause disease in humans

L. The condition in which the body, or part of it, is invaded by a pathogen

M. Medical waste that may contain infectious materials posing a threat to health and safety

N. Slender, hairlike projections that constantly beat toward the outside to remove microorganisms from the body

O. A microorganism that does not normally produce disease

P. A microscopic plant or animal

Q. A microorganism that grows best in the absence of oxygen

R. The presence or reasonably anticipated presence of blood or OPIM on an item or surface

S. The organism that becomes infected by a pathogen and also serves as a source of transfer of pathogens to others

T. An infection that takes advantage of an opportunity not normally available such as the weakened immune system of an HIV-infected individual.

U. An agent that inhibits the growth of or kills microorganisms

V. The process of cleansing or sanitizing the hands

W. Treatment administered to an individual after exposure to an infectious disease to prevent the disease

X. Objects that can penetrate the skin such as needles and lancets

Y. An infection that develops suddenly and lasts for a short period of time.

Z. An infection that develops slowly and may worsen over an extended period of time.

AA. Microorganisms that reside on the skin and normally do not cause disease.

B. Word Parts

Directions: Indicate the meaning of each word part in the space provided. List as many medical terms as possible that incorporate the word part in the space provided.

Word Part	Meaning of Word Part	Medical Terms That Incorporate Word Part
1. aer/o		
2. an-		
3. anti-		
4. -septic		
5. a-		
6. micro-		
7. non-		
8. path/o		
9. -gen		
10. para-		
11. enter/o		
12. -al		
13. post-		
14. pro-		
15. -phylaxis		

EVALUATION OF LEARNING

Directions: Fill in each blank with the correct answer.

1. List four examples of types of microorganisms.

_____

_____

2. Define medical asepsis in terms of pathogens and nonpathogens.

_____

_____

3. List the six growth requirements needed by microorganisms to survive.

_____

_____

_____

4. What is the difference between an autotroph and a heterotroph?

_____

_____

5. What is the difference between an aerobe and an anaerobe?

_____

_____

_____

6. Why do most microorganisms prefer a neutral pH?

_____

_____

7. List three examples of how a microorganism can be transmitted from one person to another.

_____

_____

8. List five examples of how microorganisms can enter the body.

_____

_____

9. List four examples of factors that would make a host more susceptible to the entrance of a pathogen.

_____

_____

10. List five protective devices of the body that prevent the entrance of microorganisms.

_____

_____

_____

11. List three techniques for sanitizing the hands in the medical office?

_____

_____

12. What is the difference between resident flora and transient flora?

_____

_____

_____

13. How does handwashing sanitize the hands?

_____

_____

14. List three examples of when handwashing should be performed in the medical office.

_____

_____

15. How does antiseptic handwashing sanitize the hands?

_____

_____

16. List five examples of when an alcohol-based hand sanitizer may be used to sanitize the hands.

_____

_____

_____

17. What are the advantages and disadvantages of alcohol-based hand sanitizers?

Advantages:

_____

Disadvantages:

_____

18. When does the CDC recommend gloves be worn in the medical office?

_____

_____

19. What is a disadvantage of latex gloves?

_____

20. What are the symptoms of a mild and severe allergic reaction to latex gloves?

a. Mild allergic reaction: _____

_____

b. Severe allergic reaction: _____

_____

21. What are the advantages and disadvantages of nitrile gloves?

_____

_____

22. What are the advantages and disadvantages of vinyl gloves?

_____

_____

23. What may occur if the medical assistant's gloves are too small or too large?

a. Too small: _____

_____

b. Too large: _____

_____

24. What guidelines should be followed when working with gloves?

_____

_____

_____

25. List six medical aseptic practices the medical assistant should follow in the medical office to control infection.

_____

_____

_____

_____

26. What does the acronym OSHA stand for, and what is the purpose of OSHA?

_____

_____

27. What is the purpose of the OSHA Occupational Exposure to Bloodborne Pathogens Standard?

_____

_____

28. Who must follow the OSHA Bloodborne Pathogens Standard? List examples.

_____

_____

_____

29. What is occupational exposure?

_____

_____

30. What are sharps? List examples of sharps.

_____

_____

31. List five examples of other potentially infectious materials (OPIMs).

_____

_____

_____

32. List examples of nonintact skin.

_____

_____

33. What is an exposure incident? List examples of exposure incidents.

_____

_____

_____

34. What is the purpose of the exposure control plan (ECP)? How often must it be updated?

_____

_____

35. List three examples of items to which a biohazard warning label must be attached.

_____

_____

36. What is the purpose of a sharps injury log? What types of offices must maintain this log?

_____

_____

37. Define an engineering control, and list three examples of engineering controls.

_____

_____

_____

38. What is a safer medical device?

_____

_____

39. What is a work practice control?

_____

40. List examples of work practice controls required by the OSHA Standard.

_____

_____

_____

39

41. What should you do if you splash blood in your eyes?

_____

42. What is personal protective equipment (PPE)? List examples of PPE.

_____

_____

_____

43. List six guidelines that must be followed when using PPE.

_____

_____

_____

_____

44. List examples of housekeeping procedures required by the OSHA Standard.

_____

_____

_____

45. List four guidelines that must be followed with respect to biohazard sharps containers.

_____

_____

_____

46. Who must be offered the hepatitis B vaccination?

_____

47. When does an employer *not* have to offer the hepatitis B vaccine to medical office personnel?

_____

_____

48. What must be done if a medical office employee declines the hepatitis B vaccination?

_____

49. What is regulated medical waste? What are examples of regulated medical waste?

_____

_____

_____

50. Explain how to prepare regulated medical waste for pickup by a medical waste service.

_____

_____

_____

51. How should regulated medical waste be stored while waiting for pickup by the medical waste service? Explain why.

_____

_____

_____

52. What information is included on a regulated medical waste tracking form?

_____

_____

53. What is the difference between an acute infection and a chronic infection?

_____

_____

54. What are the symptoms of acute hepatitis B?

   a. Mild symptoms: _____

   _____

   b. Severe symptoms: _____

   _____

55. What types of liver disease can result from chronic hepatitis B?

_____

56. What is the most likely means of contracting hepatitis B in the health care setting?

_____

_____

57. What side effects may occur after the administration of a hepatitis B vaccine?

_____

_____

58. What postexposure prophylaxis (PEP) is recommended for an unvaccinated individual who has been exposed to hepatitis B?

_____

_____

41

59. What may eventually occur in a patient with chronic hepatitis C?

_____

60. How is the hepatitis C virus transmitted?

_____

61. What is the treatment for chronic hepatitis C?

_____

62. What is the difference between HIV and AIDS?

_____

_____

63. How is HIV transmitted? How is it not transmitted?

_____

_____

_____

64. What is an opportunistic infection?

_____

65. What are the characteristics of AIDS?

_____

_____

66. What are three types os tests used to screen for the presence of HIV?

_____

67. How do AIDS antiretroviral medications control HIV infection?

_____

CRITICAL THINKING ACTIVITIES

A. Infection Process Cycle

Carefully review the infection process cycle and the requirements for growth needed by microorganisms. Create an environment in a medical office that would function to interrupt the infection process cycle and discourage the growth of pathogens.

_____

_____

_____

B. Handwashing

Using the principles outlined in the handwashing procedure, explain what may happen under the following circumstances:

1. The medical assistant's uniform touches the sink during the handwashing procedure.

_____

_____

2. The hands are not held lower than the elbows during the handwashing procedure.

_____

_____

3. Friction is not used to wash the hands.

_____

_____

4. Water is splashed on the medical assistant's uniform during the handwashing procedure.

_____

_____

5. The medical assistant continually uses water that is too cold to wash hands.

_____

_____

6. The medical assistant turns off the running water with his or her bare hands.

_____

_____

7. The medical assistant does not clean his or her fingernails daily.

_____

_____

8. The medical assistant's skin becomes chapped.

_____

_____

Chapter **2** **Medical Asepsis and the OSHA Standard**

C. Personal Protective Equipment: Gloves

In which of the following situations does OSHA require the use of clean disposable gloves? Indicate your answer by placing a check mark in the space provided.

_____ 1. Performing a urinalysis on a urine specimen that contains blood.

_____ 2. Sanitizing operating scissors for sterilization.

_____ 3. Performing a finger puncture.

_____ 4. Performing a vision screening test on a school-aged child.

_____ 5. Cleaning up a blood spill on a laboratory worktable.

_____ 6. Drawing blood from an elderly patient.

_____ 7. Measuring the weight of a college student.

_____ 8. Testing a blood specimen for glucose.

D. OSHA Standard

The following situations may occur in the medical office. For each situation, indicate an appropriate action to take that complies with the OSHA Bloodborne Pathogens Standard.

1. **Situation:** You apply gloves in preparation for performing a venipuncture and notice the left glove has a small tear in it.

   Action:

   _____

   _____

2. **Situation:** You are getting ready to apply gloves and notice that you have a cut on your finger.

   Action:

   _____

   _____

3. **Situation:** You accidentally get some blood on your bare hands while removing your gloves.

   Action:

   _____

   _____

4. **Situation:** A part-time clinical medical assistant was just hired. She is not immunized against hepatitis B.

   Action:

   _____

   _____

5. **Situation:** A clinical medical assistant who has worked at the office for 5 years changes her mind and decides she wants the hepatitis B vaccine.

   Action:

   _____

   _____

6. **Situation:** You are wearing a protective laboratory coat over your scrubs. While performing a laboratory test, some blood splashes onto your lab coat, but it does not penetrate through to your scrubs.

   Action:

   _____

   _____

7. **Situation:** You go into an examining room and notice that the biohazard sharps container in that room is completely full.

   Action:

   _____

   _____

8. **Situation:** You have collected three tubes of blood from a patient using glass tubes. You accidentally drop one of the blood tubes, and it breaks.

   Action:

   _____

   _____

9. **Situation:** You are wearing a protective lab coat over your scrubs, and you are getting ready to leave for the day.

   Action:

   _____

   _____

10. **Situation:** You remove your gloves after giving an injection to a patient and accidentally discard them into the biohazard sharps container.

    Action:

    _____

    _____

45

E. Discarding Medical Waste

Indicate where each of the following (used) items should be discarded using these acronyms:

RWC: regular waste container
BSC: biohazard sharps container
BB: biohazard bag waste container

_____ 1. Urine testing strip

_____ 2. Lancet

_____ 3. Gloves with blood on them

_____ 4. Blood tube

_____ 5. Tongue depressor

_____ 6. Razor blade

_____ 7. Capillary pipet

_____ 8. Dressing saturated with blood

_____ 9. Patient drape

_____ 10. An empty urine container

_____ 11. Sutures caked with blood

_____ 12. Thermometer probe cover

_____ 13. Patient gown

_____ 14. Disposable diaper

_____ 15. Dressing saturated with a purulent discharge

_____ 16. Clean disposable gloves

_____ 17. Disposable vaginal speculum

_____ 18. An outdated vaccine

_____ 19. Syringe and needle

_____ 20. Examining table paper

F. Crossword Puzzle: Medical Asepsis and the OSHA Standard

Directions: Complete the crossword puzzle using the clues provided.

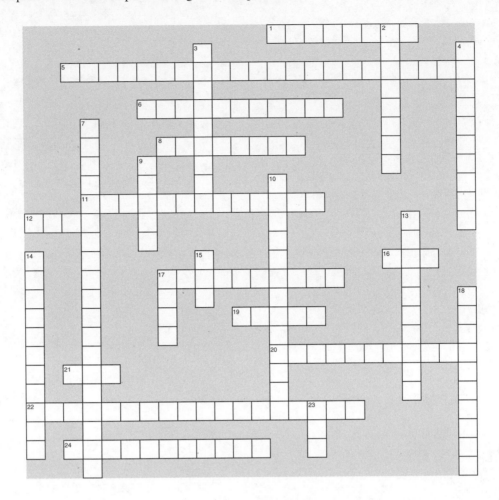

Across

1 Grows best without oxygen
5 Infection resulting from a weakened immune system
6 HBV serious complication
8 Microorganism that causes disease
11 Normally live on the skin
12 Vaginal secretions (example)
16 Protector of public health
17 Can live dry for 1 week
19 Traps microorganisms
20 Low resistance
21 After exposure: may prevent disease
22 Isolates or removes bloodborne pathogens hazard
24 Eats "live stuff"

Down

2 Example of a microorganism
3 Body invasion by a pathogen
4 Found in antimicrobial soap
7 Way to prevent needlestick injuries
9 HIV screening test
10 Broken skin
13 No. 1 chronic viral disease in the United States
14 No. 1 aseptic practice
15 Scrubs are not this
17 Hepatitis B passive immunizing agent
18 Piercing of the skin barrier
23 Discard in a biohazard container

Notes

PRACTICE FOR COMPETENCY

Procedure 2-1: Handwashing

Perform the handwashing procedure. List five medically aseptic steps that must be followed during this procedure.

1. _____

2. _____

3. _____

4. _____

5. _____

Procedure 2-2: Applying an Alcohol-Based Hand Sanitizer

Apply an alcohol-based hand sanitizer. Practice applying a gel and a foam hand sanitizer. List the brand name of each hand sanitizer, and the percentage of alcohol making up the sanitizer.

_____

_____

Procedure 2-A: Determination of Glove Size

Determine your glove size for both surgical and exam gloves and record the results in the space provided.

Surgical glove size: _____

Exam glove size: _____

Procedure 2-3: Application and Removal of Disposable Exam Gloves

Apply and remove disposable exam gloves. In the space provided, list ways in which contamination can occur from improper removal of the gloves.

_____

_____

Procedure 2-B: Proper Use of a Sharps Container

Demonstrate the proper use of a sharps container by discarding contaminated sharps into the sharps container. In the space provided, indicate the items you discarded into the sharps container.

_____

_____

Procedure 2-C: Disposal of Hazardous Material

Handle and prepare regulated medical waste for pickup by a medical waste service. In the space provided, list examples of regulated medical waste.

_____

_____

Notes

✅ EVALUATION OF COMPETENCY

Procedure 2-1: Handwashing

Name: _____   Date: _____

Evaluated by: _____   Score: _____

Performance Objective

Outcome:	Perform handwashing.
Conditions:	Using a sink.
	Given liquid soap and paper towels.
Standards:	Time: 5 minutes. Student completed procedure in _____ minutes.
	Accuracy: Satisfactory score on the Performance Evaluation Checklist.

Performance Evaluation Checklist

Trial 1	Trial 2	Point Value	Performance Standards
		•	Removed watch or pushed it up on the forearm.
		•	Removed rings.
		▷	Stated the reason for removing rings.
		•	Stood at sink with clothing away from edge of sink.
		•	Turned on faucets with paper towel.
		▷	Explained the reason for turning on faucets with paper towel.
		•	Adjusted the water to a warm temperature.
		•	Discarded paper towel into trash can.
		•	Wet hands and forearms with water.
		•	Held hands lower than elbows at all times.
		▷	Explained why the hands should be held lower than elbows.
		•	Did not touch the inside of sink with hands.
		•	Applied soap to hands.
		•	Washed palms and backs of hands with 10 circular motions and friction.
		▷	Explained why friction is needed to wash hands.
		•	Washed fingers with 10 circular motions.
		•	Washed fingers while interlaced using friction and circular motions.
		•	Rinsed well (keeping hands lower than elbows).
		•	Washed wrists and forearms using friction and circular motions.
		•	Cleaned fingernails using manicure stick.
		•	Rinsed arms and hands.

51

Trial 1	Trial 2	Point Value	Performance Standards
		•	Repeated handwashing procedure (if necessary).
		•	Dried hands gently and thoroughly.
		▷	Stated the reason for drying hands gently and thoroughly.
		•	Turned off faucets using paper towel.
		•	Did not touch sink area with bare hands.
		▷	Explained the reason for not touching sink area with bare hands.
		■	Demonstrated critical thiknking skills.
		★	Completed the procedure within 5 minutes.
			Totals

Evaluation of Student Performance

EVALUATION CRITERIA			COMMENTS
Symbol	**Category**	**Point Value**	
★	Critical Step	16 points	
•	Essential Step	6 points	
■	Affective Competency	6 points	
▷	Theory Question	2 points	

Score calculation: 100 points

− ____ points missed

____ Score

Satisfactory score: 85 or above

CAAHEP Competencies Achieved

Psychomotor (Skills)
☑ III. 3. Perform handwashing.

Affective (Behavior)
☑ A. 1. Demonstrate critical thinking skills.

ABHES Competencies Achieved

☑ 4. f. Comply with federal, state, and local health laws and regulations as they relate to health care settings.
☑ 9. a. Practice standard precautions and perform disinfection/sterilization techniques.

Procedure 2-2: Applying an Alcohol-Based Hand Sanitizer

Name: _____   Date: _____

Evaluated by: _____   Score: _____

Performance Objective

Outcome:	Apply an alcohol-based hand sanitizer.
Conditions:	Given an alcohol-based hand sanitizer.
Standards:	Time: 2 minutes. Student completed procedure in _____ minutes.
	Accuracy: Satisfactory score on the Performance Evaluation Checklist.

Performance Evaluation Checklist

Trial 1	Trial 2	Point Value	Performance Standards
		•	Inspected the hands to make sure they are not visibly soiled.
		▷	Stated the procedure to follow if the hands are visibly soiled.
		•	Removed watch or pushed it up on the forearm.
		•	Removed rings.
			Applied the alcohol-based hand sanitizer to the palm of one hand as follows:
		•	*Gel:* Applied an amount of gel or lotion approximately equal to the size of a dime.
		•	*Foam:* Applied an amount of foam approximately equal to the size of a walnut.
		▷	Explained why it is important not to use more than the recommended amount of hand sanitizer.
		•	Thoroughly spread the hand sanitizer over the surface of both hands up to $\frac{1}{2}$ inch above the wrist.
		•	Spread the hand sanitizer around and under the fingernails.
		▷	Explained why it is important to cover the entire surface of the hands.
		•	Rubbed the hands together until they were dry.
		•	Did not touch anything until the hands were dry.
		■	Demonstrated critical thinking skills.
		★	Completed the procedure within 2 minutes.
			Totals

Evaluation of Student Performance

EVALUATION CRITERIA			COMMENTS
Symbol	**Category**	**Point Value**	
★	Critical Step	16 points	
•	Essential Step	6 points	
■	Affective Competency	6 points	
▷	Theory Question	2 points	

Score calculation:

100 points

− _____ points missed

_____ Score

Satisfactory score: 85 or above

CAAHEP Competencies Achieved

Psychomotor (Skills)
☑ III. 3. Perform handwashing.

Affective (Behavior)
☑ A. 1. Demonstrate critical thinking skills.

ABHES Competencies Achieved

☑ 4. f. Comply with federal, state, and local health laws and regulations as they relate to health care settings.
☑ 8. a. Practice standard precautions and perform disinfection/sterilization techniques.

Procedure 2-A: Determination of Exam Glove Size

Name: _____   Date: _____

Evaluated by: _____   Score: _____

Performance Objective

Outcome:	Determined your correct exam glove size.
Conditions:	Given a cloth tape measure, disposable exam gloves, and an exam glove sizing chart.
Standards:	Time: 5 minutes. Student completed procedure in _____ minutes.
	Accuracy: Satisfactory score on the Performance Evaluation Checklist.

Performance Evaluation Checklist

Trial 1	Trial 2	Point Value	Performance Standards
		•	Extended your dominant hand and laid it on a flat surface with the fingers together and the hand relaxed.
		▷	Explained why the dominant hand is preferred for determining glove size.
		•	Placed a cloth tape measure around your hand just below the knuckles.
		▷	Stated why a cloth tape measure should be used.
		•	Measured the circumference in inches of the widest part of the palm of your dominant hand. *(If necessary, asked another person to perform this step.)*
		•	Determined your approximate exam glove size by rounding the measurement to the nearest whole inch.
		•	Translated the measurement number to the approximate letter size using an exam glove sizing chart.
		▷	Stated what should be done if the glove manufacturer includes a sizing chart on their glove box or website.
		•	Donned a pair of gloves in your approximate letter size determined by the hand measurement.
		•	*Performed the following assessment to determine if the gloves fit correctly:* a. The gloves were snug on your hand without restricting movements. b. The gloves were comfortable and fit like a second skin. c. Your fingers could move normally without stretching the gloves too much during movement and flexion. d. If the fit of your gloves meet these criteria, this is your correct glove size.
		•	*Performed the following assessment to determine if your gloves are too large:* a. When applying the gloves, they do not have to stretch very much to fit your hands. b. Wrinkles are observed around your palms and the rest of the glove bunches up around your wrists. c. Your fingertips do not reach the end of the gloves, leaving material dangling at the end of each finger. d. If the fit of your gloves meet one or more of these criteria, the gloves are too large. e. Obtain the next size smaller and repeat the assessment. If necessary, repeat this step until you have determined your correct glove size.

Chapter **2 Medical Asepsis and the OSHA Standard**

Trial 1	Trial 2	Point Value	Performance Standards
		•	*Performed the following assessment to determine if your gloves are too small:* a. When applying the gloves, they must stretch significantly for your hands to fit inside. b. The fingertips of your gloves press against your fingers and may even puncture through the gloves. c. The gloves are uncomfortable and movements are stifled by the gloves. d. If the fit of your gloves meet one or more of these criteria, the gloves are too small. e. Obtain the next size larger and repeat the assessment. If necessary, repeat this step until you have determined your correct glove size.
		★	Completed the procedure in 5 minutes.
			Totals

Evaluation of Student Performance

EVALUATION CRITERIA			COMMENTS
Symbol	**Category**	**Point Value**	
★	Critical Step	16 points	
•	Essential Step	6 points	
■	Affective Competency	6 points	
▷	Theory Question	2 points	

Score calculation:

100 points

− _____ points missed

_____ Score

Satisfactory score: 85 or above

CAAHEP Competencies Achieved

Psychomotor (Skills)
☑ I. 10. Perform a quality control measure.
☑ III. 2. Select appropriate barrier/personal protective equipment (PPE).

ABHES Competencies Achieved

☑ 8. a. Practice standard precautions and perform disinfection/sterilization techniques.

General Exam Glove Sizing Chart

Hand Measurement (In Inches)	Exam Glove Size
6	XS
7	S
8	M
9	L
10	XL

EVALUATION OF COMPETENCY

Procedure 2-3: Application and Removal of Clean Disposable Gloves

Name: _____   Date: _____

Evaluated by: _____   Score: _____

Performance Objective

Outcome:	Apply and remove clean disposable gloves.
Conditions:	Given the appropriate-sized clean disposable gloves.
Standards:	Time: 5 minutes. Student completed procedure in _____ minutes.
	Accuracy: Satisfactory score on the Performance Evaluation Checklist.

Performance Evaluation Checklist

Trial 1	Trial 2	Point Value	Performance Standards
			Application of Clean Gloves
		★	Determined your proper glove size.
		•	Removed all rings.
		▷	Stated why rings should be removed.
		•	Sanitized the hands.
		•	Chose the appropriate-sized gloves.
		▷	Explained what can happen if the gloves are too small or too large.
		•	Applied the gloves.
		•	Adjusted the gloves so that they fit comfortably.
		•	Inspected the gloves for tears.
		▷	Stated the procedure to follow if a glove is torn.
			Removal of Clean Gloves
		•	Grasped the outside of the left glove 1 to 2 inches from the top with the gloved right hand.
		•	Slowly pulled left glove off the hand.
		•	Pulled the left glove free, and scrunched it into a ball with the gloved right hand.
		•	Placed the index and middle fingers of the left hand on the inside of the right glove.
		•	Did not allow the clean hand to touch outside of the glove.
		•	Pulled the glove off the right hand, enclosing the balled-up left glove.
		•	Discarded both gloves in an appropriate waste container.
		▷	Stated when gloves should be discarded in a biohazardous waste container.
		•	Sanitized the hands.

Chapter **2** **Medical Asepsis and the OSHA Standard**

Trial 1	Trial 2	Point Value	Performance Standards
		▷	Stated why the hands should be sanitized after removing gloves.
		■	Demonstrated critical thinking skills.
		★	Completed the procedure in 5 minutes.
			Totals

Evaluation of Student Performance

EVALUATION CRITERIA			COMMENTS
Symbol	**Category**	**Point Value**	
★	Critical Step	16 points	
•	Essential Step	6 points	
■	Affective Competency	6 points	
▷	Theory Question	2 points	

Score calculation:

    100 points

−   points missed

    ___Score

Satisfactory score: 85 or above

CAAHEP Competencies Achieved

Psychomotor (Skills)
☑   III. 2. Select appropriate barrier/personal protective equipment (PPE).

Affective (Behavior)
☑   A. 1. Demonstrate critical thinking skills.

ABHES Competencies Achieved

☑   4. f. Comply with federal, state, and local health laws and regulations as they relate to health care settings.
☑   8. a. Practice standard precautions and perform disinfection/sterilization techniques.

Procedure 2-B: Proper Use of a Sharps Container

Name: _____   Date: _____

Evaluated by: _____   Score: _____

Performance Objective

Outcome:	Demonstrate the proper use of a sharps container.
Conditions:	Given the following: Sharps container and a contaminated sharp.
Standards:	Time: 3 minutes.　　　Student completed procedure in _____ minutes.
	Accuracy: Satisfactory score on the Performance Evaluation Checklist.

Performance Evaluation Checklist

Trial 1	Trial 2	Point Value	Performance Standards
		•	Ensured that the sharps container met the following OSHA Standards: a. Was closable b. Was puncture resistant c. Was leakproof d. Was labeled with a biohazard warning label e. Was color-coded in red
		•	Located the sharps container as close as possible to the area of use.
		▷	Stated why the sharps container should be located close to the area of use.
		•	Made sure the sharps container was maintained in an upright position.
		•	Immediately after use, placed the contaminated sharp in the sharps container.
		•	Dropped the contaminated sharp into the container without touching the sides of the container.
		•	Stated examples of items that must be discarded in a sharps container.
		•	Did not reach into the sharps container with the hands.
		•	Replaced the sharps container on a regular basis and did not allow it to overfill.
		▷	Stated when a sharps container should be replaced.
		■	Demonstrated critical thinking skills.
		★	Completed the procedure within 5 minutes.
			Totals

Evaluation of Student Performance

EVALUATION CRITERIA			COMMENTS
Symbol	**Category**	**Point Value**	
★	Critical Step	16 points	
•	Essential Step	6 points	
■	Affective Competency	6 points	
▷	Theory Question	2 points	

Score calculation:

100 points

−   points missed

___Score

Satisfactory score: 85 or above

CAAHEP Competencies Achieved

Psychomotor (Skills)

☑ III. 1. Participate in bloodborne pathogen training.
☑ III.10. Demonstrate proper disposal of biohazardous material
    a. Sharps
    b. Regulated waste

Affective (Behavior)

☑ Demonstrate critical thinking skills.

ABHES Competencies Achieved

☑ 4. f. Comply with federal, state, and local health laws and regulations as they relate to health care settings.
☑ 8. a. Practice standard precautions and perform disinfection/sterilization techniques.
☑ 9. c. Dispose of biohazardous materials.

Procedure 2-C: Disposal of Hazardous Material

Name: _____   Date: _____

Evaluated by: _____   Score: _____

Performance Objective

Outcome:	Handle and prepare regulated medical waste for pickup by a medical waste service.
Conditions:	Given the following: disposable gloves, biohazard sharps container, biohazards bags, cardboard box with biohazard labels, packing tape, tracking record.
Standards:	Time: 5 minutes. Student completed procedure in _____ minutes.
	Accuracy: Satisfactory score on the Performance Evaluation Checklist.

Performance Evaluation Checklist

Trial 1	Trial 2	Point Value	Performance Standards
			Handling regulated waste
		•	Sanitized hands and applied gloves.
		•	Closed and locked the lid of the full sharps container before removing it from the examining room.
		▷	Stated the reason for closing the lid of the sharps container before removing it from the examining room.
		•	Did not open, empty, or clean the sharps container.
		•	If the sharps container was leaking, placed it in a second container that is closable, leakproof, and appropriately labeled.
		•	Securely closed the full biohazard bag before removing it from an examining room.
	•	•	If required by the medical office policy, double-bag by placing the primary bag inside a second biohazard bag.
		•	Transported the biohazard containers to a secure area away from the general public.
			Preparing regulated waste for pickup by a medical waste service
		•	Placed sharps containers and biohazard bags into a cardboard box provided by the medical waste service.
		•	Removed gloves and sanitized the hands.
		•	Securely sealed the box with packing tape.
		•	Made sure that a biohazard warning label appeared on two opposite sides of the box.
		•	Stored the biohazard box in a labeled locked room inside the facility or in a labeled locked collection container outside the facility.
		▷	Stated why biohazard boxes awaiting pickup must be stored in a locked storage area.
		•	Completed a tracking record, if required by your state.

Chapter **2 Medical Asepsis and the OSHA Standard**

Trial 1	Trial 2	Point Value	Performance Standards
		▷	Stated what information is included on a tracking record.
		■	Demonstrated critical thinking skills.
		★	Completed the procedure within 5 minutes.
			Totals

Evaluation of Student Performance

EVALUATION CRITERIA			COMMENTS
Symbol	**Category**	**Point Value**	
★	Critical Step	16 points	
•	Essential Step	6 points	
▷	Affective Competency	6 points	
■	Theory Question	2 points	

Score calculation: 100 points

       −   points missed

       ___Score

Satisfactory score: 85 or above

CAAHEP Competencies Achieved

Psychomotor (Skills)
☑ III. 1. Participate in bloodborne pathogen training.
☑ III.10. Demonstrate proper disposal of biohazardous material
    c. Sharps
    d. Regulated waste

Affective (Behavior)
☑ A. 1. Demonstrate critical thinking skills.

ABHES Competencies Achieved

☑ 4. f. Comply with federal, state, and local health laws and regulations as they relate to health care settings.
☑ 8. a. Practice standard precautions and perform disinfection/sterilization techniques.
☑ 9. c. Dispose of biohazardous materials.

Sterilization and Disinfection

CHAPTER ASSIGNMENTS

√ After Completing	Date Due	Study Guide Pages	STUDY GUIDE ASSIGNMENTS (CTA = Critical Thinking Activity)	Possible Points	Points You Earned
		67	?☰ Pretest	10	
		68	Term Key Term Assessment	15	
		68-74	Evaluation of Learning questions	56	
		74-75	CTA A: Safety Data Sheet	15	
		75-77	CTA B: Obtaining a Safety Data Sheet	18	
		77-78	CTA C: Sanitization	8	
		78	CTA D: Storage of a Chemical Disinfectant	4	
		78	CTA E: Sterilization	10	
			Evolve: What Happens Now? (Record points earned)		
			Evolve: Quiz Show (Record points earned)		
			Evolve: Apply Your Knowledge questions (Record points earned)	10	
			Evolve: Video Evaluation	36	
		67	?☰ Posttest	10	
			ADDITIONAL ASSIGNMENTS		
			Total points		

√ When Assigned by Your Instructor	Study Guide Pages	Practices Required	LABORATORY ASSIGNMENTS (Procedure Number and Name)	Score*
	81	3	**Practice for Competency** 3-1: Sanitization of Instruments	
	83-85		**Evaluation of Competency** 3-1: Sanitization of Instruments	
	81	3	**Practice for Competency** 3-2: Wrapping Instruments Using Sterilization Paper	
	87-88		**Evaluation of Competency** 3-2: Wrapping Instruments Using Sterilization Paper	*
	81	3	**Practice for Competency** 3-3: Wrapping Instruments Using a Pouch	
	89-90		**Evaluation of Competency** 3-3: Wrapping Instruments Using a Pouch	*
	81	3	**Practice for Competency** 3-4: Sterilizing Items in an Autoclave	
	91-92		**Evaluation of Competency** 3-4: Sterilizing Items in an Autoclave	*
			ADDITIONAL ASSIGNMENTS	

Notes

Name: _____ Date: _____

True or False

_____ 1. A bacterial spore consists of a hard, thick-walled capsule that can resist adverse conditions.

_____ 2. The purpose of sanitization is to remove all microorganisms and spores from a contaminated article.

_____ 3. According to OSHA, gloves do not need to be worn during the sanitization process.

_____ 4. Glutaraldehyde (Cidex) is a high-level disinfectant.

_____ 5. High-level disinfection kills all microorganisms but not spores.

_____ 6. Sterilization is the process of destroying all forms of microbial life except for bacterial spores.

_____ 7. Autoclave tape indicates whether an autoclaved item is sterile.

_____ 8. The wrapper used to autoclave articles should prevent contaminants from getting in during handling and storage.

_____ 9. Tap water should be used in the autoclave.

_____ 10. The outside of the autoclave should be wiped every day with a damp cloth and a mild detergent.

? POSTTEST

True or False

_____ 1. The agent used to destroy microorganisms on an article depends on the size of the article.

_____ 2. The purpose of the Hazard Communication Standard is to ensure that employees avoid hazardous chemicals in the workplace.

_____ 3. The Hazard Communication Standard requires that the label of a hazardous chemical include hazard pictograms.

_____ 4. Stethoscopes must be decontaminated using a high-level disinfectant.

_____ 5. The autoclave must be operated at a pressure of at least 15 pounds of pressure per square inch and a temperature of at least 212° F.

_____ 6. A sterilization strip should be positioned in the center of a wrapped pack.

_____ 7. The best means of determining the effectiveness of the sterilization process are biologic indicators.

_____ 8. The proper time for sterilizing an article in the autoclave depends on what is being autoclaved.

_____ 9. A pack that has been in the storage cupboard for 4 weeks should be resterilized.

_____ 10. Ethylene oxide gas is used by medical manufacturers to sterilize disposable items.

Directions: Match each key term with its definition.

_____ 1. Autoclave

_____ 2. Critical item

_____ 3. Detergent

_____ 4. Disinfectant

_____ 5. Hazardous chemical

_____ 6. Health hazard

_____ 7. Incubate

_____ 8. Load

_____ 9. Noncritical item

_____ 10. Physical hazard

_____ 11. Safety Data Sheet

_____ 12. Sanitization

_____ 13. Semicritical item

_____ 14. Spore

_____ 15. Sterilization

A. To provide proper conditions for growth and development

B. The potential of a chemical to catch fire, explode, or react with other chemicals.

C. An item that comes in contact with intact skin but not mucous membranes

D. A hard, thick-walled capsule formed by some bacteria that contains only the essential parts of the protoplasm of the bacterial cell

E. An item that comes in contact with sterile tissue or the vascular system

F. An apparatus for the sterilization of materials, using steam under pressure

G. An agent that cleanses by emulsifying dirt and oil

H. An item that comes into contact with nonintact skin or intact mucous membranes

I. The items that are being sterilized

J. An agent used to destroy pathogenic microorganisms but not their spores (usually applied to inanimate objects)

K. A document that provides detailed information regarding a chemical and its hazards, and measures to take to prevent injury and illness when handling the chemical

L. A series of steps designed to remove debris from an item and to reduce the number of microorganisms to a safe level.

M. The process of destroying all forms of microbial life, including spores

N. Any chemical that is classified as a health or physical hazard

O. The potential of a chemical to cause acute toxicity, skin corrosion or irritation, serious eye damage or irritation, respiratory or skin sensitization, germ cell mutagenicity, cancer or reproductive toxicity, or is an aspiration hazard.

EVALUATION OF LEARNING

Directions: Fill in each blank with the correct answer.

1. How does one determine what type of physical or chemical agent to use to destroy microorganisms on an article?

_____

_____

2. List two diseases that are caused by bacteria that produce spores.

_____

_____

3. What are the characteristics of bacterial spores?

_____

_____

4. What is the purpose of the Hazard Communication Standard?

_____

_____

5. What is the difference between a health hazard and a physical hazard?

_____

_____

6. What is the purpose of the Globally Harmonized System of Classification and Labeling of Chemicals (GHS)?

_____

_____

_____

7. List four examples of hazardous chemicals that may be used in the medical office.

_____

_____

8. What information must be included on a hazardous chemical label?

_____

_____

_____

9. What is the purpose of a signal word?

_____

_____

10. What is the meaning of the following signal words?

    a. Danger: _____

    b. Warning: _____

11. What is the difference between a precautionary statement and a hazard statement?

_____

_____

_____

12. What is a GHS hazard pictogram, and what is its purpose?

_____

_____

13. List and briefly describe the information that must be included on a Safety Data Sheet.

_____

_____

_____

_____

_____

_____

_____

14. What is the purpose of sanitizing an item?

    _____

    _____

15. What is the advantage of using the ultrasound method to clean instruments?

    _____

    _____

16. Why should gloves be worn during the sanitization procedure?

    _____

    _____

17. Why should instruments be handled carefully?

    _____

18. Why should a chemical not be used past its expiration date?

    _____

19. Why must a cleaning agent with a neutral pH be used to sanitize instruments?

    _____

    _____

20. What type of brush should be used to clean the following parts of an instrument?

    a. Surface of an instrument: _____

    b. Grooves, crevices, or serrations: _____

21. How should each of the following be checked for defects and proper working condition?

    a. Blades of an instrument: _____

    b. Tips of an instrument: _____

    c. Instrument with a box lock: _____

    d. Cutting edge of a sharp instrument: _____

    e. Scissors: _____

22. What is the purpose of lubricating an instrument?

    _____

    _____

23. What is the definition of high-level disinfection?

    _____

    _____

24. List one example of an item that requires high-level disinfection. List one example of a high-level disinfectant.

_____

_____

25. List two examples of items that can be disinfected through intermediate-level disinfection. List one example of an intermediate-level disinfectant.

_____

_____

_____

26. List two examples of items that are disinfected by low-level disinfection.

_____

27. What disinfectant does OSHA recommend for the decontamination of blood spills?

_____

28. Why is it important to remove all debris from an article before it is disinfected?

_____

_____

29. Explain the difference between the shelf life and use life of a chemical disinfectant.

_____

_____

30. What is the purpose of sterilization?

_____

31. What is a critical item? List an example of a critical item.

_____

_____

32. What is the purpose of the pressure used in the autoclaving process?

_____

_____

33. How are microorganisms and spores killed during an autoclave cycle?

_____

_____

34. What is the minimum temperature and pressure that must be used to sterilize articles with the autoclave?

_____

_____

35. What information does the CDC recommend be documented in an autoclave log regarding each cycle?

_____

_____

_____

36. What is the purpose of a sterilization indicator?

_____

_____

37. What should be done if a sterilization indicator does not change properly?

_____

_____

38. How should sterilization indicators be stored? Explain the reason for this.

_____

_____

39. What are the advantages and disadvantages of autoclave tape?

_____

_____

40. How should a sterilization strip be placed in a wrapped pack?

_____

41. How often should a biologic indicator be used to monitor an autoclave?

_____

42. What is the purpose of wrapping articles to be autoclaved?

_____

_____

43. List two properties of a good wrapper for use in autoclaving.

_____

_____

44. List two examples of wrapping materials used for the autoclave and identify an advantage of each type.

_____

_____

45. Why shouldn't tap water be used to fill the water reservoir of an autoclave?

_____

_____

46. How should the following be positioned in the autoclave?

    a. Small packs: _____

    b. Large packs: _____

    c. Sterilization pouches: _____

47. Why is more time needed to autoclave a large minor office surgery pack as compared to unwrapped instruments?

_____

_____

48. What are the three different types of autoclave cycles?

_____

49. Why must a sterilized load be allowed to dry before it is removed from the autoclave?

_____

_____

50. What is event-related sterility?

_____

_____

51. How should sterilized packs be stored?

_____

_____

52. Describe the care an autoclave should receive on a daily basis.

_____

_____

_____

53. Why is a longer exposure period needed to ensure sterilization when using the dry-heat oven?

_____

_____

54. What effect does moist heat have on instruments with sharp cutting edges?

_____

55. How does the medical manufacturing industry use ethylene oxide gas sterilization?

_____

_____

_____

56. What guidelines must be followed when using cold sterilization?

_____

_____

CRITICAL THINKING ACTIVITIES

A. Safety Data Sheet

Refer to the Safety Data Sheet (SDS) in the textbook (see Fig. 3.4) and answer the following questions.

1. What is the brand name of this chemical?

_____

2. What is the recommended use of glutaraldehyde?

_____

3. What are the hazard classifications of glutaraldehyde?

_____

_____

4. What is the signal word of glutaraldehyde?

_____

5. What hazard statements are associated with glutaraldehyde?

_____

_____

_____

6. What are the first aid measures for glutaraldehyde for each of the following?

   a. Skin contact: _____

   _____

   b. Eye contact: _____

   _____

   c. Inhalation: _____

   _____

   d. Ingestion: _____

   _____

7. What should be done if glutaraldehyde is spilled?

_____

_____

8. How should glutaraldehyde be stored?

_____

9. What type of personal protective equipment should be used with glutaraldehyde?

_____

10. Describe the appearance and odor of glutaraldehyde.

_____

11. What conditions should be avoided with glutaraldehyde?

_____

12. What symptoms can occur from overexposure to glutaraldehyde for each of the following?

   a. Inhalation: _____

   b. Skin contact: _____

   c. Eye contact: _____

   d. Ingestion: _____

13. What medical conditions are aggravated by exposure to glutaraldehyde?

_____

14. Does glutaraldehyde cause cancer?

_____

15. What is the disposal method for glutaraldehyde?

_____

_____

_____

B. Obtaining a Safety Data Sheet

Obtain an SDS for one of the following hazardous chemicals and answer the questions.

   To locate an SDS on the Internet, enter the name of the chemical into a search engine with the abbreviation "SDS." (Example: Cidex SDS)

- Cidex
- MetriCide
- Cidex OPA
- CaviCide
- MadaCide
- SaniZide
- Wavicide
- Sporox II
- Envirocide
- Clorox bleach

1. What is the product name of this hazardous chemical?

_____

2. What is the brand or trade name of this chemical?

_____

75

3. Who manufactures this chemical?

_____

4. What number would you call if an emergency occurred with this chemical?

_____

5. What is the recommended use of this chemical?

_____

6. What is the hazard classification of this chemical?

_____

_____

7. What is the signal word for this chemical?

_____

8. What hazard statements are associated with this chemical?

_____

_____

9. Sketch the hazard pictograms associated with this chemical below:

10. What are the precautionary statements associated with this chemical?

_____

_____

11. What are the first aid measures for this chemical?

_____

_____

12. What should be done if this chemical is spilled?

_____

13. What are the precautions for safe handling of this chemical?

_____

_____

14. How should this chemical be stored?

_____

76

15. What type of personal protective equipment should be used with this chemical?

_____

_____

16. What are the acute health hazards associated with this chemical?

_____

_____

17. What medical conditions are aggravated by exposure to this chemical?

_____

_____

18. What is the disposal method for this chemical?

_____

_____

C. Sanitization

For each of the following situations involving sanitization, write C if the technique is correct and I if the technique is incorrect. If the situation is correct, state the principle underlying the technique. If the situation is incorrect, explain what might happen if the technique were performed in the incorrect manner.

_____ 1. A contaminated surgical instrument is left in the examination room.

_____

_____

_____ 2. The medical assistant does not wear utility and exam gloves when sanitizing surgical instruments.

_____

_____

_____ 3. The medical assistant piles instruments in a heap while preparing them for sanitization.

_____

_____

_____ 4. The medical assistant forgets to read the Safety Data Sheet before decontaminating surgical instruments in Cidex.

_____

_____

_____ 5. The medical assistant uses dishwashing detergent to sanitize surgical instruments.

_____

_____

_____ 6. Dried blood is not completely cleansed from hemostatic forceps before they are sterilized in the autoclave.

_____

_____

Chapter **3** **Sterilization and Disinfection**

_____ 7. The medical assistant inspects all instruments for defects and proper working condition before sterilizing them.

_____

_____

_____ 8. The medical assistant lubricates hemostatic forceps with a steam-penetrable lubricant before sterilizing them.

_____

_____

D. Storage of a Chemical Disinfectant

You have just received a 0.5 gallon container of Cidex Plus. You look at the label on the container and notice the following:
- Expiration date: 8/7/25
- Use life: 28 days
- Reuse life: 28 days

Based on this information, answer the following questions.

1. If the Cidex Plus is left unopened on the shelf, when would it expire and need to be discarded?

_____

2. You open and activate the Cidex Plus on 9/1/23. What date should you write on the container?

_____

3. You next fill a disinfectant container with the Cidex Plus and disinfect some articles in it. On what date would the Cidex Plus be unusable and need to be disposed?

_____

4. On what date would you need to discard the rest of the container of Cidex Plus, if it is not used?

_____

_____

E. Sterilization

For each of the following situations involving sterilization of articles in the autoclave, write C if the technique is correct, and I if the technique is incorrect. If the situation is correct, state the principle underlying the technique. If the situation is incorrect, explain what might happen if the technique were performed in the incorrect manner.

_____ 1. The medical assistant marks the autoclave tape on a wrapped pack with the date of sterilization.

_____

_____

_____ 2. The medical assistant opens a hemostat before placing it in a sterilization pouch.

_____

_____

_____ 3. Tap water is used to fill the water reservoir of the autoclave.

_____

_____

_____ 4. The medical assistant places four sterilization pouches on top of one another in the autoclave.

_____

_____

_____ 5. The medical assistant places small packs to be sterilized approximately 1 to 3 inches apart in the autoclave.

_____

_____

_____ 6. Biologic indicators are placed in the autoclave where steam will penetrate most easily.

_____

_____

_____ 7. The medical assistant uses disposable exam gloves to remove a load from the autoclave.

_____

_____

_____ 8. The medical assistant removes a load from the autoclave while it is still wet.

_____

_____

_____ 9. The medical assistant notices a tear in one of the wrappers while removing articles from the autoclave. He or she rewraps and resterilizes the article.

_____

_____

_____ 10. The medical assistant notices that a sterilized wrapped article stored on the storage shelf has opened up. He or she retapes the pack and places it back in the storage shelf.

_____

_____

Notes

Procedure 3-1: Sanitization of Instruments

Sanitize instruments. In the space provided, indicate the following:

A. Name of the disinfectant _____

B. Name of the instrument cleaner _____

C. Names of instruments sanitized _____

Procedure 3-2: Wrapping Instruments Using Paper or Muslin, and Procedure 3-3: Wrapping Instruments Using a Pouch

Wrap articles for autoclaving. In the space provided, list the information you indicated on the label of each pack which includes the contents of the pack, the date, and your initials.

Information indicated on the label of the wrapped article:

_____

_____

_____

_____

Procedure 3-4: Sterilizing Articles in the Autoclave

Sterilize articles in the autoclave. In the space provided, indicate the articles you sterilized.

_____

_____

_____

Notes

Procedure 3-1: Sanitization of Instruments

Name: _____ Date: _____

Evaluated by: _____ Score: _____

Performance Objective

Outcome:	Sanitize instruments.
Conditions:	Given the following: disposable gloves, utility gloves, contaminated instruments, chemical disinfectant and SDS, disinfectant container, instrument cleaner and SDS, basin, nylon brush, wire brush, paper towels, cloth towel, and instrument lubricant.
Standards:	Time: 10 minutes. Student completed procedure in _____ minutes.
	Accuracy: Satisfactory score on the Performance Evaluation Checklist.

Performance Evaluation Checklist

Trial 1	Trial 2	Point Value	Performance Standards
		•	Reviewed the SDS for hazardous chemicals being used.
		•	Applied gloves.
		•	Transported the contaminated instruments to the cleaning area.
		•	Applied heavy-duty utility gloves over the disposable gloves.
		▷	Stated the purpose of the utility gloves.
		•	Separated sharp instruments and delicate instruments from other instruments.
		▷	Explained why instruments should be separated.
		•	Immediately rinsed the instruments thoroughly under warm running water.
		▷	Stated why the instruments should be rinsed immediately.
			Decontamination of the Instruments
		•	Checked the expiration date of the chemical disinfectant.
		▷	Explained why an expired disinfectant should not be used.
		•	Observed all personal safety precautions listed on the label.
		•	Followed label manufacturer's instructions for proper activation, dilution, and use of the disinfectant.
		•	Labeled the disinfecting container with the name of the disinfectant and the reuse expiration date.
		•	Poured the disinfectant into the labeled container.
		•	Completely submerged the items in the disinfectant.
		•	Covered the disinfectant container.
		▷	Stated the reason for covering the container.
		•	Disinfected the items for 10 minutes.

Trial 1	Trial 2	Point Value	Performance Standards
		▷	Explained the reason for decontaminating the instruments.
			Cleaning the Instruments: Manual Method
		•	Checked the expiration date of the instrument cleaner.
		•	Observed all personal safety precautions.
		•	Followed manufacturer's directions for proper use and mixing of the instrument cleaner.
		•	Removed articles from disinfectant and placed them in the basin containing the instrument cleaner.
		•	Cleaned all surfaces of each instrument with a nylon brush.
		•	Cleaned grooves, crevices, or serrations with a wire brush.
		•	Removed stains using an instrument stain remover.
		•	Scrubbed each instruments until it was visibly clean and free from debris and stains.
		▷	Explained why all debris must be removed from each instrument.
			Cleaning the Instruments: Ultrasound Method
		•	Checked the expiration date of the ultrasonic instrument cleaner.
		•	Prepared the cleaning solution in the ultrasonic cleaner.
		•	Observed all personal safety precautions listed on label.
		•	Removed the items from the disinfectant.
		•	Separated instruments of dissimilar metals.
		•	Properly placed the instruments in the ultrasonic cleaner.
		•	Positioned hinged instruments in an open position.
		▷	Stated why hinged instruments must be in an open position.
		•	Ensured that sharp instruments did not touch other instruments.
		•	Checked to make sure all instruments were fully submerged.
		•	Placed the lid on the ultrasonic cleaner.
		•	Turned on the ultrasonic cleaner.
		•	Cleaned the instruments for the length of time recommended by the manufacturer.
		•	Removed the instruments from the machine.
			Completion of the Procedure
		•	Rinsed each instrument thoroughly with warm water for 20 to 30 seconds.
		▷	Explained why instruments should be rinsed in warm water.
		•	Dried each instrument with a paper towel.
		•	Placed instrument on a towel for additional drying.
		▷	Stated the reason for drying the instruments.

Trial 1	Trial 2	Point Value	Performance Standards
		•	Inspected each instrument for defects and proper working condition.
		•	Lubricated hinged instruments in an open position.
		•	Opened and closed the instrument to distribute the lubricant.
		•	Placed the lubricated instrument on a towel to drain.
		▷	Stated the reason for lubricating instruments.
		•	Disposed of the cleaning solution according to the manufacturer's instructions.
		•	Removed both sets of gloves and sanitized hands.
		•	Wrapped the instruments.
		•	Sterilized the instruments in the autoclave.
		★	Completed the procedure within 10 minutes.
			Totals

Evaluation of Student Performance

EVALUATION CRITERIA			COMMENTS
Symbol	**Category**	**Point Value**	
★	Critical Step	16 points	
•	Essential Step	6 points	
■	Affective Competency	6 points	
▷	Theory Question	2 points	

Score calculation: 100 points

    – _____ points missed

    _____ Score

Satisfactory score: 85 or above

CAAHEP Competency Achieved

Psychomotor (Skills)
☑ III. 4. Prepare items for autoclaving.

ABHES Competency Achieved

☑ 8. a. Practice standard precautions and perform disinfection/sterilization techniques.

Chapter **3** Sterilization and Disinfection

Notes

Procedure 3-2: Wrapping an Instrument Using Sterilization Paper

Name: _____   Date: _____

Evaluated by: _____   Score: _____

Performance Objective

Outcome:	Wrap an instrument using sterilization paper.
Conditions:	Given the following: sanitized instrument, sterilization paper, sterilization indicator strip, autoclave tape, and a permanent marker.
Standards:	Time: 5 minutes. Student completed procedure in _____ minutes.
	Accuracy: Satisfactory score on the Performance Evaluation Checklist.

Performance Evaluation Checklist

Trial 1	Trial 2	Point Value	Performance Standards
		•	Sanitized hands.
		•	Assembled equipment.
		•	Selected the appropriate-sized wrapping paper.
		•	Checked the expiration date on the sterilization indicator box.
		▷	Stated why outdated strips should not be used.
		•	Placed wrapping paper on clean, flat surface.
		•	Turned the wrap in a diagonal position to the body.
		•	Placed instrument in the center of wrapping paper.
		•	Placed instruments with movable joints in an open position.
		▷	Stated why instruments with movable joints must be placed in an open position.
		•	Placed a sterilization strip in the center of the wrap next to the instrument.
		•	Folded wrapping paper up from the bottom and doubled back a small corner.
		•	Folded over one edge of wrapping paper and doubled back the corner.
		•	Folded over the other edge of wrapping paper and doubled back the corner.
		•	Folded the wrapping paper up from the bottom, pulled the top flap down and secured it with autoclave tape.
		•	Ensured that the pack was firm enough for handling, but loose enough to permit proper circulation of steam.
		▷	Stated why instruments are wrapped for autoclaving.
		•	Labeled and dated the pack. Included initials.
		▷	Stated the purpose of dating the pack.
		★	Completed the procedure within 5 minutes.
			Totals

87

Evaluation of Student Performance

EVALUATION CRITERIA			COMMENTS
Symbol	**Category**	**Point Value**	
★	Critical Step	16 points	
•	Essential Step	6 points	
■	Affective Competency	6 points	
▷	Theory Question	2 points	

Score calculation: 100 points

− ____ points missed

____Score

Satisfactory score: 85 or above

CAAHEP Competency Achieved

Psychomotor (Skills)
☑ III. 4. Prepare items for autoclaving.

ABHES Competency Achieved

☑ 8. a. Practice standard precautions and perform disinfection/sterilization techniques.

Procedure 3-3: Wrapping Instruments Using a Pouch

Name: _____   Date: _____

Evaluated by: _____   Score: _____

Performance Objective

Outcome:	Wrap an instrument for autoclaving.
Conditions:	Given the following: sanitized instrument, sterilization pouch, and a permanent marker.
Standards:	Time: 5 minutes. Student completed procedure in _____ minutes.
	Accuracy: Satisfactory score on the Performance Evaluation Checklist.

Performance Evaluation Checklist

Trial 1	Trial 2	Point Value	Performance Standards
		•	Sanitized hands.
		•	Assembled equipment.
		•	Selected the appropriate-sized pouch.
		•	Placed the pouch on a clean, flat surface.
		•	Labeled and dated the pack. Included initials.
		•	Inserted the instrument into the open end of the pouch.
		▷	Explained how to insert an instrument with a movable joint.
		•	Sealed the pouch.
		•	Sterilized the pouch in the autoclave.
		★	Completed the procedure within 5 minutes.
		Totals	

Evaluation of Student Performance

<table>
<tr><th colspan="3">EVALUATION CRITERIA</th><th>COMMENTS</th></tr>
<tr><td>Symbol</td><td>Category</td><td>Point Value</td><td></td></tr>
<tr><td>★</td><td>Critical Step</td><td>16 points</td><td></td></tr>
<tr><td>•</td><td>Essential Step</td><td>6 points</td><td></td></tr>
<tr><td>■</td><td>Affective Competency</td><td>6 points</td><td></td></tr>
<tr><td>▷</td><td>Theory Question</td><td>2 points</td><td></td></tr>
</table>

Score calculation: 100 points

−_____ points missed

_____Score

Satisfactory score: 85 or above

CAAHEP Competency Achieved

Psychomotor (Skills)

☑ III. 4. Prepare items for autoclaving.

ABHES Competency Achieved

☑ 8. a. Practice standard precautions and perform disinfection/sterilization techniques.

Procedure 3-4: Sterilizing Items in an Autoclave

Name: _____   Date: _____

Evaluated by: _____   Score: _____

Performance Objective

Outcome:	Sterilize a load in the autoclave.
Conditions:	Using an autoclave and operating manual, distilled water, wrapped items, and heat-resistant gloves
Standards:	Time: 10 minutes. Student completed procedure in _____ minutes.
	Accuracy: Satisfactory score on the Performance Evaluation Checklist.

Performance Evaluation Checklist

Trial 1	Trial 2	Point Value	Performance Standards
		•	Assembled equipment.
		•	Checked the water level in the autoclave.
		•	Properly loaded the autoclave.
		▷	Stated how far apart to place small packs and large packs.
		▷	Explained two ways for positioning pouches in the autoclave.
		•	Did not allow the packs to touch the chamber walls.
		•	Ensured that at least 1 inch separated the autoclave trays.
		•	Closed and latched the door of the autoclave.
		•	Determined the autoclave cycle according to what is being sterilized (unwrapped items, pouches, wrapped items).
		•	Selected the desired autoclave cycle by pressing the appropriate button on the autoclave.
		•	Pressed the start button.
		▷	Explained what occurs during each of the following stages of the autoclave cycle: a. Filling b. Heating c. Sterilizing d. Sterilizing e. Venting f. Drying g. Ready
		•	Turned off the autoclave.
		•	Removed the load from the autoclave using heat-resistant gloves.
		▷	Stated the reason for using heat-resistant gloves.
		•	Inspected the packs as they were removed for damage.
		▷	Explained what should be done if a pack is torn.

Chapter **3** **Sterilization and Disinfection**

Trial 1	Trial 2	Point Value	Performance Standards
		•	Checked the autoclave tape on the outside of the packs.
		▷	Stated the use of autoclave tape.
		•	Documented monitoring information in the autoclave log.
		•	Stored the packs in a clean dust-proof area.
		•	Placed the most recently sterilized packs behind previously sterilized packs.
		•	Maintained appropriate daily care of the autoclave.
		▷	Described the care the autoclave should receive each day.
		■	Demonstrated critical thinking skills.
		★	Completed the procedure within 10 minutes.
			Totals

Evaluation of Student Performance

EVALUATION CRITERIA			COMMENTS
Symbol	**Category**	**Point Value**	
★	Critical Step	16 points	
•	Essential Step	6 points	
■	Affective Competency	6 points	
▷	Theory Question	2 points	

Score calculation: 100 points

− _____ points missed

_____ Score

Satisfactory score: 85 or above

CAAHEP Competencies Achieved

Psychomotor (Skills)
☑ III. 5. Perform sterilization procedures.
☑ VI. 8. Perform routine maintenance of administrative or clinical equipment.

Affective (Behavior)
☑ A. 1. Demonstrate critical thinking skills.

ABHES Competency Achieved

☑ 4. f. Comply with federal, state, and local health laws and regulations as they relate to health care settings.
☑ 8. a. Practice standard precautions and perform disinfection/sterilization techniques.

4 Vital Signs

√ After Completing	Date Due	Study Guide Pages	STUDY GUIDE ASSIGNMENTS (CTA = Critical Thinking Activity)	Possible Points	Points You Earned
		97	[?] Pretest	10	
		98-100	[Term] Key Term Assessment A. Definitions B. Word Parts (Add 1 point for each key term)	56 30	
		101-109	Evaluation of Learning questions	97	
		110-111	CTA A: Measurement of Body Temperature	18	
		112	CTA B: Alterations in Body Temperature	5	
		112	CTA C: Pulse Sites	6	
		112-113	CTA D: Pulse and Respiratory Rates	3	
		113-114	CTA E: Pulse Oximetry	8	
		114	CTA F: Blood Pressure Measurement	10	
		114-115	CTA G: Proper BP Cuff Selection	8	
		115	CTA H: Reading Blood Pressure Values	24	
			Evolve: Under Pressure (Record points earned)		
		116	CTA I: Interpreting Blood Pressure Readings	10	
		116-117	CTA J: Hypertension Risks	20	
		118-119	CTA K: Crossword Puzzle	26	
			Evolve: Road to Recovery Game: Vital Signs Terminology (Record points earned)		
			Evolve: Apply Your Knowledge questions (Record points earned)	11	

√ After Completing	Date Due	Study Guide Pages	STUDY GUIDE ASSIGNMENTS (CTA = Critical Thinking Activity)	Possible Points	Points You Earned
			Evolve: Video Evaluation	86	
		97	?≡ Posttest	10	
			ADDITIONAL ASSIGNMENTS		
			Total points		

√ When Assigned by Your Instructor	Study Guide Pages	Practices Required	LABORATORY ASSIGNMENTS: (Procedure Number and Name	Score*
	121	5	**Practice for Competency** 4-1: Measuring Oral Body Temperature—Electronic Thermometer	
	123-125		**Evaluation of Competency** 4-1: Measuring Oral Body Temperature—Electronic Thermometer	*
	121	3	**Practice for Competency** 4-2: Measuring Axillary Body Temperature—Electronic Thermometer	
	127-128		**Evaluation of Competency** 4-2: Measuring Axillary Body Temperature—Electronic Thermometer	*
	121	3	**Practice for Competency** 4-3: Measuring Rectal Body Temperature—Electronic Thermometer	
	129-131		**Evaluation of Competency** 4-3: Measuring Rectal Body Temperature—Electronic Thermometer	*
	121	5	**Practice for Competency** 4-4: Measuring Aural Body Temperature	
	133-135		**Evaluation of Competency** 4-4: Measuring Aural Body Temperature	*
	121	5	**Practice for Competency** 4-5: Measuring Temporal Artery Body Temperature	
	137-139		**Evaluation of Competency** 4-5: Measuring Temporal Artery Body Temperature	*
	122	10	**Practice for Competency** 4-6: Measuring Pulse and Respiration	
	141-143		**Evaluation of Competency** 4-6: Measuring Pulse and Respiration	*
	122	5	**Practice for Competency** 4-7: Measuring Apical Pulse	
	145-146		**Evaluation of Competency** 4-7: Measuring Apical Pulse	*

√ When Assigned by Your Instructor	Study Guide Pages	Practices Required	LABORATORY ASSIGNMENTS: (Procedure Number and Name	Score*
	122	5	**Practice for Competency** 4-8: Performing Pulse Oximetry	
	147-149		**Evaluation of Competency** 4-8: Performing Pulse Oximetry	*
	122	10	**Practice for Competency** 4-9: Measuring Blood Pressure	
	151-153		**Evaluation of Competency** 4-9: Measuring Blood Pressure	*
	122	5	**Practice for Competency** 4-10: Determining Systolic Pressure by Palpation	
	155-156		**Evaluation of Competency** 4-10: Determining Systolic Pressure by Palpation	*
	122	10	**Practice for Competency** 4-11: Measuring Blood Pressure: Automatic Method	
	157-159		**Evaluation of Competency** 4-11: Measuring Blood Pressure: Automatic Method	*
			ADDITIONAL ASSIGNMENTS	

Name: _____   Date: _____

True or False

_____ 1. The heat-regulating center of the body is the medulla.

_____ 2. A vague sense of body discomfort, weakness, and fatigue that often marks the onset of a disease is known as "the blahs."

_____ 3. If an axillary temperature of 100° F was taken orally, it would register as 101° F.

_____ 4. If the sensor lens of a tympanic membrane thermometer is dirty, the reading may be falsely low.

_____ 5. The most common site for measuring pulse is the apical site.

_____ 6. The femoral pulse site can be used to assess circulation to the foot.

_____ 7. The term used to describe an irregularity in the heart's rhythm is dysrhythmia.

_____ 8. Pulse oximetry provides the provider with information on the amount of oxygen being delivered to the tissues.

_____ 9. Blood pressure measures the contraction and relaxation of the heart.

_____ 10. When taking blood pressure, the stethoscope is placed over the brachial artery.

? POSTTEST

True or False

_____ 1. A temperature of 100° F is classified as a low-grade fever.

_____ 2. The rectal site should not be used to take the temperature of a newborn.

_____ 3. A tympanic membrane thermometer should not be used to measure temperature on a child younger than 6 years of age.

_____ 4. There are two types of temporal artery thermometers: contact and non-contact.

_____ 5. Excessive pressure should not be applied when measuring a pulse because it could obstruct the pulse.

_____ 6. A child has a faster pulse rate than an adult.

_____ 7. The normal respiratory rate of an adult ranges between 10 and 18 respirations per minute.

_____ 8. The term used to describe a bluish discoloration of the skin due to a lack of oxygen is hypoxia.

_____ 9. The oxygen saturation level of a healthy individual falls between 85% and 90%.

_____ 10. When measuring blood pressure, the patient's arm should be positioned above the level of the heart.

A. Definitions

Temperature

Directions: Match each key term with its definition.

_____ 1. Afebrile	A. An extremely high fever
_____ 2. Antipyretic	B. A vague sense of body discomfort, weakness, and fatigue often marking the onset of a disease and continuing through the course of the illness
_____ 3. Axilla	C. A body temperature that is below normal
_____ 4. Celsius scale	D. The armpit
_____ 5. Conduction	E. The transfer of energy, such as heat, through air currents
_____ 6. Convection	F. A body temperature that is above normal (pyrexia)
_____ 7. Crisis	G. An agent that reduces fever
_____ 8. Cross-contamination	H. A temperature scale on which the freezing point of water is 32° and the boiling point of water is 212°
_____ 9. Fahrenheit scale	I. The transfer of energy, such as heat, in the form of waves
_____ 10. Febrile	J. A temperature scale on which the freezing point of water is 0° and the boiling point is 100°
_____ 11. Fever	K. The midline fold that connects the undersurface of the tongue with the floor of the mouth
_____ 12. Frenulum linguae	L. Pertaining to fever
_____ 13. Hyperpyrexia	M. The transfer of energy from one object to another by direct contact
_____ 14. Hypothermia	N. A sudden falling of an elevated body temperature to normal
_____ 15. Malaise	O. Without fever; the body temperature is normal
_____ 16. Radiation	P. The process by which 24 microorganisms are unintentionally transferred from one person, object, or place to another.

Pulse

Directions: Match each key term with its definition.

_____ 1. Antecubital space	A. Between the ribs
_____ 2. Aorta	B. A pulse with an increased volume that feels very strong and full
_____ 3. Bounding pulse	C. The strength of the heartbeat
_____ 4. Bradycardia	D. The space located at the front of the elbow
_____ 5. Dysrhythmia	E. An abnormally fast heart rate (more than 100 beats per minute)
_____ 6. Intercostal	F. The major trunk of the arterial system of the body
_____ 7. Pulse rhythm	G. The time interval between heartbeats
_____ 8. Pulse volume	H. A pulse with a decreased volume that feels weak and thin
_____ 9. Tachycardia	I. An irregular rhythm
_____ 10. Thready pulse	J. An abnormally slow heart rate (less than 60 beats per minute)

Respiration and Pulse Oximetry

Directions: Match each key term with its definition.

_____ 1. Alveolus

_____ 2. Apnea

_____ 3. Bradypnea

_____ 4. Cyanosis

_____ 5. Dyspnea

_____ 6. Eupnea

_____ 7. Exhalation

_____ 8. Hyperpnea

_____ 9. Hyperventilation

_____ 10. Hypopnea

_____ 11. Hypoxemia

_____ 12. Hypoxia

_____ 13. Inhalation

_____ 14. Orthopnea

_____ 15. Pulse oximeter

_____ 16. Pulse oximetry

_____ 17. SaO_2

_____ 18. SpO_2

_____ 19. Tachypnea

A. The act of breathing out
B. A reduction in the oxygen supply to the tissues of the body
C. A decrease in the oxygen saturation of the blood; may lead to hypoxia
D. The temporary cessation of breathing
E. An abnormal increase in the respiratory rate of more than 20 respirations per minute
F. A device used to measure the oxygen saturation of arterial blood
G. An abnormal decrease in the rate and depth of respiration
H. A thin-walled air sac of the lungs in which the exchange of oxygen and carbon dioxide takes place
I. The use of a pulse oximeter to measure the oxygen saturation of arterial blood
J. The act of breathing in
K. A bluish discoloration of the skin and mucous membranes first observed in the nail beds and lips
L. Abbreviation for the percentage of hemoglobin that is saturated with oxygen in arterial blood
M. The condition in which breathing is easier when an individual is in a standing or sitting position
N. Shortness of breath or difficulty in breathing
O. Abbreviation for the percentage of hemoglobin that is saturated with oxygen in arterial blood as measured by a pulse oximeter
P. Normal respiration
Q. An abnormally fast and deep type of breathing usually associated with acute anxiety conditions
R. An abnormal decrease in the respiratory rate of less than 10 respirations per minute
S. An abnormal increase in the rate and depth of respiration

Blood Pressure

Directions: Match each key term with its definition.

_____ 1. Blood pressure

_____ 2. Diastole

_____ 3. Diastolic pressure

_____ 4. Hypertension

_____ 5. Hypotension

_____ 6. Korotkoff sounds

_____ 7. Pulse pressure

_____ 8. Sphygmomanometer

_____ 9. Stethoscope

_____ 10. Systole

_____ 11. Systolic pressure

A. High blood pressure
B. The point of maximum pressure on the arterial walls
C. The phase in the cardiac cycle in which the heart relaxes between contractions
D. An instrument for measuring arterial blood pressure
E. The point of lesser pressure on the arterial walls
F. Low blood pressure
G. The phase in the cardiac cycle in which the ventricles contract, sending blood out of the heart and into the aorta and pulmonary aorta
H. An instrument for amplifying and hearing sounds produced by the body
I. The difference between the systolic and diastolic pressures
J. Sounds heard during the measurement of blood pressure that are used to determine the systolic and diastolic blood pressure readings
K. The pressure or force exerted by the circulating blood on the walls of the arteries

B. Word Parts

Directions: Indicate the meaning of each word part in the space provided. List as many medical terms as possible that incorporate the word part in the space provided.

Word Part	Meaning of Word Part	Medical Terms That Incorporate Word Part
1. anti-		
2. pyr/o		
3. -ic		
4. -pnea		
5. brady-		
6. cardi/o		
7. -ia		
8. a-		
9. cyan/o		
10. -osis		
11. dys-		
12. eu-		
13. ex-		
14. hyper-		
15. hypo-		
16. -tension		
17. therm/o		
18. ox/i		
19. in-		
20. inter-		
21. cost/o		
22. -al		
23. -mal		
24. -meter		
25. orth/o		
26. -metry		
27. sphygm/o		
28. steth/o		
29. -scope		
30. tachy-		

Temperature

Directions: Fill in each blank with the correct answer.

1. Define a vital sign.

   _____

   _____

2. What are the four vital signs?

   _____

   _____

3. What general guidelines should be followed when measuring vital signs?

   _____

   _____

4. List four ways in which heat is produced in the body.

   _____

   _____

5. List four ways in which heat is lost from the body.

   _____

   _____

6. What is the normal body temperature range? What is the average body temperature?

   _____

7. What is a fever?

   _____

   _____

8. How do diurnal variations affect body temperature?

   _____

   _____

9. How do emotional states affect body temperature?

   _____

   _____

10. How does vigorous physical exercise affect body temperature?

   _____

11. What symptoms occur during the course of a fever?

_____

_____

12. Describe the following fever patterns:

a. Continuous fever

_____

_____

b. Intermittent fever

_____

_____

c. Remittent fever

_____

_____

13. What occurs during the subsiding stage of a fever?

_____

14. What five sites are used for taking body temperature?

_____

15. List three instances in which the axillary site for taking body temperature would be preferred over the oral site.

_____

_____

16. Why does the rectal method for taking body temperature provide a very accurate temperature measurement?

_____

_____

17. When can the rectal method be used to take body temperature?

_____

_____

18. When can the aural method be used to take body temperature?

_____

_____

19. How does a temperature taken through the rectal and axillary methods compare (in terms of degrees) with a temperature taken through the oral method?

_____

_____

20. List and describe the three types of thermometers available for taking body temperature.

_____

_____

21. Explain how a tympanic membrane thermometer measures body temperature.

_____

_____

22. What are the two types of temporal artery thermometers?

_____

23. How can sweating of the forehead cause an inaccurate temporal artery temperature reading?

_____

Pulse
Directions: Fill in each blank with the correct answer.

1. What causes the pulse to occur?

_____

_____

2. What is the unit of measurement for pulse rate?

_____

3. How does physical activity affect the pulse rate?

_____

4. What is the most common site for taking the pulse?

_____

5. List two reasons for taking the pulse at the apical pulse site.

_____

_____

6. Where is the apex of the heart located?

_____

_____

7. When is the brachial artery used as a pulse site?

_____

8. When is the carotid artery used as a pulse site?

_____

9. When is the femoral artery used as a pulse site?

_____

103

10. What two pulse sites can be used to assess circulation to the foot?

_____

11. List two reasons for measuring the pulse rate.

_____

_____

12. State the normal range for a pulse rate for an adult.

_____

13. What is the normal pulse range for the following age groups:

    a. Infant: _____

    b. Toddler: _____

    c. Preschooler: _____

    d. School-age: _____

    e. Adult after age 60 years: _____

14. What is the normal pulse range for a well-trained athlete?

_____

15. What may cause tachycardia?

_____

16. How is an apical-radial pulse taken?

_____

17. What is a pulse deficit?

_____

Respiration

Directions: Fill in each blank with the correct answer.

1. What is the purpose of respiration?

_____

_____

2. What is the purpose of inhalation?

_____

_____

3. What is the purpose of exhalation?

_____

_____

4. What is included in one complete respiration?

_____

_____

5. The exchange of oxygen and carbon dioxide between the body cells and blood is known as:

_____

6. What is the name of the control center for involuntary respiration?

_____

7. Why must respiration be measured without the patient's awareness?

_____

8. What is the normal respiratory rate (range) for a normal adult?

_____

9. What is the ratio of respirations to pulse beats?

_____

10. List two factors that can increase the respiratory rate.

_____

_____

11. Describe a normal rhythm for respiration.

_____

_____

12. What can cause hyperventilation?

_____

13. What type of patient may experience hypopnea?

_____

14. Where is cyanosis first observed?

_____

_____

15. What conditions can cause cyanosis?

_____

16. What are two conditions in which dyspnea may occur?

_____

_____

17. Describe the character of normal breath sounds.

_____

_____

18. Describe the characteristics of the following abnormal breath sounds:

   a. Crackles:

   _____

   _____

   b. Rhonchi:

   _____

   _____

   c. Wheezes:

   _____

   _____

Pulse Oximetry

Directions: Fill in each blank with the correct answer.

1. What is the purpose of pulse oximetry?

   _____

   _____

2. What is the function of hemoglobin?

   _____

3. What is the oxygen saturation level of a healthy individual?

   _____

4. What can occur if the oxygen saturation level falls between 85% and 90%?

   _____

   _____

5. List three patient conditions that can cause a decreased SpO_2 value.

   _____

   _____

6. When can pulse oximetry be used for the short-term continuous monitoring of a patient?

   _____

   _____

7. What is the purpose of the pulse oximeter power-on self-test (POST)?

   _____

   _____

8. What type of site must be used for applying a pulse oximeter probe?

_____

9. How can dark fingernail polish cause a falsely low SpO_2 reading?

_____

10. How can patient movement cause an inaccurate SpO_2 reading?

_____

_____

11. What types of patients may make it difficult to properly align the oximeter probe?

_____

_____

12. List three conditions that can cause poor peripheral blood flow.

_____

_____

13. Why must a reusable oximeter probe be free of all dirt and grime before it is used?

_____

_____

Blood Pressure

Directions: Fill in each blank with the correct answer.

1. What does blood pressure measure?

_____

_____

2. Why is the diastolic pressure lower than the systolic pressure?

_____

_____

3. What are the two types of sphygmomanometers?

_____

4. What is considered normal healthy blood pressure for an adult?

_____

5. State the blood pressure range for each of the following:

   a. Elevated: _____

   b. Hypertension, stage 1: _____

   c. Hypertension, stage 2: _____

6. How do diurnal variations affect blood pressure?

_____

_____

7. What are some examples of emotional states that increase the blood pressure?

_____

8. How does the diastolic pressure of a patient in a sitting position compare with his or her diastolic pressure in a lying position?

_____

9. How does a full bladder affect the blood pressure?

_____

10. What is pulse pressure and what is the normal range for pulse pressure?

_____

_____

11. Hypertension increases the risk of developing what conditions?

_____

_____

12. Why is hypertension known as a "silent killer"?

_____

_____

13. What is primary hypertension?

_____

14. How does age affect blood pressure?

_____

15. What are the controllable factors that increase the risk for primary hypertension?

_____

_____

16. What is secondary hypertension?

_____

17. What conditions may cause hypotension?

_____

18. What is orthostatic hypotension? What is the most common cause of orthostatic hypotension?

_____

_____

19. What are the two types of stethoscope chest pieces and the use of each?

_____

_____

20. What are the parts of an aneroid sphygmomanometer?

_____

_____

21. How often should an aneroid sphygmomanometer be recalibrated?

_____

22. When would each of the following cuffs be used to measure blood pressure?

a. Small adult: _____

b. Adult: _____

c. Adult thigh: _____

23. What may occur if blood pressure is taken using a cuff that is too small or too large?

_____

_____

24. Describe how the blood pressure cuff size can be determined using the following methods:

a. Assessment of bladder length and width: _____

_____

b. Determination of arm circumference:_____

_____

c. Assessment of range and index lines: _____

_____

25. List the five phases included in the Korotkoff sounds and describe what type of sound is heard during each phase.

_____

_____

_____

_____

_____

26. List five advantages of an automated blood pressure monitor.

_____

_____

_____

_____

A. Measurement of Body Temperature

For each of the following situations involving the measurement of body temperature, write C if the technique is correct and I if the technique is incorrect. If the situation is correct, state the principle underlying the technique. If the situation is incorrect, explain what might happen if the technique were performed in the incorrect manner.

Electronic Thermometer

_____ 1. The medical assistant takes a patient's oral temperature immediately after the patient has consumed a cup of coffee.

_____

_____

_____ 2. The medical assistant instructs the patient not to talk while his or her oral temperature is being measured.

_____

_____

_____ 3. The medical assistant's bare fingers accidentally touch a used oral probe cover while discarding it.

_____

_____

_____ 4. An axillary temperature reading is documented as follows: 102.2° F.

_____

_____

_____ 5. The medical assistant forgets to lubricate the rectal probe before taking a patient's rectal temperature.

_____

_____

_____ 6. The medical assistant discards a used rectal probe in a regular waste container.

_____

_____

Tympanic Membrane Thermometer

_____ 1. A thermometer with a dirty sensor lens is used to take the temperature.

_____

_____

_____ 2. A cover is placed on the probe before taking the temperature.

_____

_____

_____ 3. The ear canal is straightened before taking the temperature.

_____

_____

_____ 4. The medical assistant does not seal the opening of the ear canal with the probe when taking the temperature.

_____

_____

_____ 5. The probe is positioned toward the opposite temple when taking the temperature.

_____

_____

_____ 6. The medical assistant cleans the temporal artery thermometer by immersing it in warm, sudsy water.

_____

_____

Temporal Artery Thermometer

_____ 1. The medical assistant checks to make sure the sensor lens is clean and intact before taking temperature.

_____

_____

_____ 2. The medical assistant brushes hair away from the patient's forehead before taking temperature.

_____

_____

_____ 3. The medical assistant positions the probe of a contact temporal artery thermometer close to the patient's hairline.

_____

_____

_____ 4. The medical assistant positions the probe of a non-contact temporal artery thermometer 4 inches away from the center of the patient's forehead.

_____

_____

_____ 5. The medical assistant slides the probe of a contact temporal artery thermometer across the patient's forehead while continually depressing the scan button.

_____

_____

_____ 6. After scanning the forehead with a contact temporal artery thermometer, the medical assistant releases the scan button and documents the patient's temperature reading.

_____

_____

B. Alterations in Body Temperature

Label the following diagram with the terms that describe the body temperature alteration.

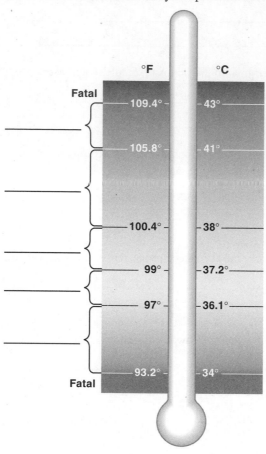

C. Pulse Sites

Locate the pulse at the following sites, and document the pulse rates below:

1. Brachial pulse _____

2. Temporal pulse _____

3. Carotid pulse _____

4. Femoral pulse _____

5. Popliteal pulse _____

6. Dorsalis pedis pulse _____

D. Pulse and Respiratory Rates

Take the pulse and respiration of a person before and after vigorous exercise, and document the results.

1. Before vigorous exercise

_____

_____

2. After vigorous exercise

_____

_____

3. Compare the results, and explain how exercise affects the pulse and respiratory rates.

_____

_____

E. Pulse Oximetry

Your provider asks you to measure the oxygen saturation level of the patients listed. For each situation, answer the following questions:

    a. What occurs with the situation?

    b. What should be done to prevent an inaccurate pulse oximetry reading?

1. Keysha Brown, a patient with chronic bronchitis, is wearing navy blue nail polish.

    a. _____

    b. _____

2. Akeno Peng has Parkinson's disease and is having difficulty controlling tremors in his hands.

    a. _____

    b. _____

3. Nicole Lowe has returned to the office for a recheck of her viral pneumonia. You are getting ready to measure her oxygen saturation and notice that bright sunlight is coming through the window where she is seated and shining on her hand.

    a. _____

    b. _____

4. Juana Garcia has come to the office because she has been experiencing dyspnea. Her hands are very cold, and it is interfering with the pulse oximetry procedure.

    a. _____

    b. _____

5. Susan Boone, a patient with asthma, is wearing artificial fingernails.

    a. _____

    b. _____

6. Carlos Perez, a patient with congestive heart failure, is at the office to have a mole removed from his back. There are bright overhead lights in the room, and they cannot be turned off because the provider needs to have good lighting to perform the surgery.

    a. _____

    b. _____

7. Ning Wu is having a sebaceous cyst removed from her chest and has been sedated for the procedure. You have applied an automatic blood pressure cuff to her right arm. The provider asks you to apply an oximeter to Ning's finger to continuously monitor her oxygen saturation level and pulse rate during the procedure.

    a. _____

    b. _____

8. Which control, indicator, or display is involved when the following occurs?

   a. The oximeter is turned on. _____

   b. The oximeter is portraying the strength of the pulse. _____

   c. The oximeter displays the oxygen saturation level. _____

   d. The oximeter displays the pulse rate. _____

   e. The battery is low. _____

F. Blood Pressure Measurement

Using the principles outlined in your textbook, explain what happens under the following circumstances:

1. The blood pressure is taken on a patient who has just undergone vigorous physical exercise.

   _____

2. The blood pressure is taken on a patient with tight sleeves.

   _____

3. The blood pressure is taken on an apprehensive patient.

   _____

4. An adult cuff is used to measure blood pressure on a young child.

   _____

5. The blood pressure is taken over clothing.

   _____

6. The arm is below heart level during blood pressure measurement.

   _____

7. The patient's legs are crossed during blood pressure measurement.

   _____

8. The rubber bladder is not centered over the brachial artery.

   _____

9. The cuff is placed $1/2$ inch above the bend in the elbows.

   _____

10. The manometer is viewed from a distance of 4 feet.

   _____

G. Proper BP Cuff Selection

Measurements of the arm circumference (in centimeters) are given for various patients. Using Table 4.7 in your textbook, indicate what size of blood pressure cuff (small adult, adult, large adult, or adult thigh) should be used with each of these patients.

1. 47 cm: _____

2. 22 cm: _____

114

3. 32 cm: _____

4. 25 cm: _____

5. 38 cm: _____

6. 27 cm: _____

7. 52 cm: _____

8. 43 cm: _____

Measure the arm circumference of four classmates with a centimeter tape measure, and document the values below. Next to each value, indicate what size blood pressure cuff should be used with each of these individuals.

1. _____

2. _____

3. _____

4. _____

H. Reading Blood Pressure Values

Read and document the following blood pressure measurements in the space provided.

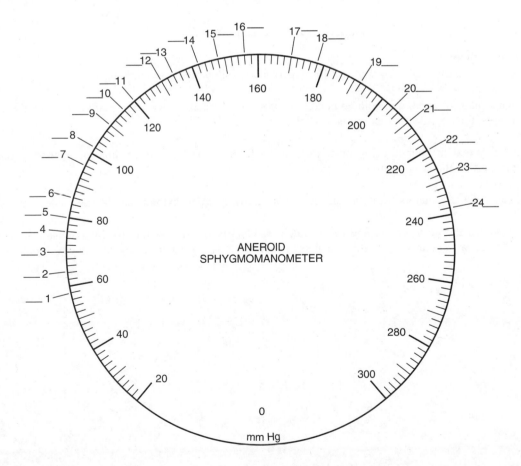

I. Interpreting Blood Pressure Readings

Classify each of the following blood pressure readings into its appropriate category. The readings are based on the average of two or more properly measured and seated blood pressure readings taken at each of two or more visits.

Normal
Elevated
Hypertension: Stage 1
Hypertension: Stage 2

1. 90/66: _____

2. 126/76: _____

3. 138/88: _____

4. 122/78: _____

5. 118/66: _____

6. 158/102: _____

7. 128/78: _____

8. 180/106: _____

9. 104/60: _____

10. 134/82: _____

J. Hypertension Risks

Create a profile of an individual who is at risk for hypertension following these guidelines:

1. Using a blank piece of paper and colored pencils, crayons, or markers, draw a figure of an individual exhibiting risk factors for hypertension. Be as creative as possible.

2. Do not use any text in your drawing other than to label items you have drawn in your picture (e.g., cigarettes). A picture is worth a thousand words!

3. Include at least six risk factors for hypertension in your drawing. Your textbook can be used as a reference source.

4. In the classroom, choose a partner and trade drawings. Identify the risk factors for hypertension in your partner's drawing. Discuss with your partner what this person could do to lower his or her chances of developing hypertension.

K. Crossword Puzzle: Vital Signs

Directions: Complete the crossword puzzle using the clues provided.

Across

6 Fever reducer
7 Fever increases this by 7% (for each ° F)
8 220 minus your age
11 Cools body
12 Invented the stethoscope
15 High BP might cause this
16 BP less than 90/60
18 Pulse range for exercising
19 Body temperature increaser
21 Drug to help COPD
23 Fever causer
24 What hypertension is known as
25 BP position for patient's arm
26 Biggest risk factor for high BP

Down

1 Diaphragm or bell
2 Lowers pulse rate over time
3 2300 mg or less per day
4 Above 130/80
5 Profuse perspiration
9 Fever that occurs with the flu
10 Asthma breath sounds
13 Center BP cuff over this
14 Leading cause of COPD
17 COPD example
20 BP sounds
22 Treatment for hypertension

Notes

PRACTICE FOR COMPETENCY

Measuring Body Temperature

Measure body temperature with each of the following types of thermometers, and document the results in the chart provided.

Procedures 4-1, 4-2, and 4-3: Electronic Thermometer (Oral, Axillary, and Rectal)
Procedure 4-4: Tympanic Membrane Thermometer (Aural)
Procedure 4-5: Temporal Artery Thermometer (Contact and Non-Contact)

CHART	
Date	

Procedure 4-6: Pulse and Respiration

Measure the radial pulse and respiration. Describe the rhythm and volume of the pulse. Describe the rhythm and depth of the respirations. Document the results in the chart provided.

Procedure 4-7: Apical Pulse

Measure apical pulse. Describe the rhythm and volume of the pulse. Document the results in the chart provided.

Procedure 4-8: Pulse Oximetry

Measure the oxygen saturation level and document the results in the chart provided.

Procedure 4-9: Manual Blood Pressure Measurement

Measure blood pressure through the manual method. Document the results in the chart provided.

Procedure 4-10: Determining Systolic Pressure by Palpation

Determine systolic pressure by palpation.

Procedure 4-11: Automatic Blood Pressure Measurement

Measure blood pressure through the automatic method. Document the results in the chart provided.

CHART	
Date	

Procedure 4-1: Measuring Oral Body Temperature—Electronic Thermometer

Name: _____   Date: _____

Evaluated by: _____   Score: _____

Performance Objective

Outcome:	Measure oral body temperature.
Conditions:	Given the following: electronic thermometer and oral probe, probe cover, and a waste container.
Standards:	Time: 5 minutes. Student completed procedure in _____ minutes.
	Accuracy: Satisfactory score on the Performance Evaluation Checklist.

Performance Evaluation Checklist

Trial 1	Trial 2	Point Value	Performance Standards
		•	Sanitized hands.
		•	Assembled equipment.
		•	Removed thermometer from its storage base.
		•	Attached oral probe to thermometer unit.
		•	Inserted probe into the thermometer.
		•	Greeted the patient and introduced yourself.
		•	Identified the patient and explained the procedure.
		•	Asked the patient whether he or she has ingested hot or cold beverages.
		▷	Explained what to do if the patient has recently ingested a hot or cold beverage.
		•	Removed probe from the thermometer.
		▷	Explained what occurs when probe is removed from the thermometer.
		•	Attached probe cover to probe.
		▷	Stated the purpose of the probe cover.
		•	Correctly inserted the probe in patient's mouth.
		•	Instructed the patient to keep the mouth closed.
		▷	Explained why the mouth should be kept closed.
		•	Held probe in place until an audible tone was heard.
		•	Noted patient's temperature reading on display screen.
		•	Removed probe from patient's mouth.
		•	Discarded probe cover in a regular waste container.
		•	Did not allow fingers to come in contact with cover.
		•	Returned probe to the thermometer unit.
		▷	Stated what occurs when probe is returned to the thermometer.

Trial 1	Trial 2	Point Value	Performance Standards
		•	Returned the thermometer unit to its storage base.
		•	Sanitized hands.
		•	Documented the results correctly.
		★	The results were identical to the reading on the display screen.
		▷	Stated the normal body temperature range for an adult (97° F to 99° F).
		■	Demonstrated critical thinking skills.
		★	Completed the procedure within 5 minutes.
			Totals

CHART

Date	

Evaluation of Student Performance

EVALUATION CRITERIA			COMMENTS
Symbol	**Category**	**Point Value**	
★	Critical Step	16 points	
•	Essential Step	6 points	
■	Affective Competency	6 points	
▷	Theory Question	2 points	

Score calculation: 100 points

− _____ points missed

_____ Score

Satisfactory score: 85 or above

CAAHEP Competencies Achieved

Psychomotor (Skills)
☑ I. 1. b. Accurately measure and record temperature.

Affective (Behavior)
☑ A. 1. Demonstrate critical thinking skills.

ABHES Competency Achieved

☑ 8. b. Obtain and document chief complaint, patient history, and vital signs.

Notes

Procedure 4-2: Measuring Axillary Body Temperature—Electronic Thermometer

Name: _____ Date: _____

Evaluated by: _____ Score: _____

Performance Objective

Outcome:	Measure axillary body temperature.
Conditions:	Given the following: electronic thermometer and oral probe, probe cover, and a waste container.
Standards:	Time: 5 minutes. Student completed procedure in _____ minutes.
	Accuracy: Satisfactory score on the Performance Evaluation Checklist.

Performance Evaluation Checklist

Trial 1	Trial 2	Point Value	Performance Standards
		•	Sanitized hands.
		•	Assembled equipment.
		•	Removed thermometer from its storage base.
		•	Attached oral probe to thermometer unit.
		•	Inserted probe into the thermometer.
		•	Greeted the patient and introduced yourself.
		•	Identified the patient and explained the procedure.
		•	Removed clothing from patient's shoulder and arm.
		•	Made sure that the axilla was dry.
		•	Removed probe from the thermometer.
		•	Attached probe cover to probe.
		•	Placed probe in the center of the patient's axilla.
		•	Ensured that the arm was held close to the body.
		▷	Explained why the arm must be held close to the body.
		•	Held probe in place until an audible tone was heard.
		•	Removed probe from patient's axilla.
		•	Noted patient's temperature reading on display screen.
		•	Discarded probe cover in a regular waste container.
		•	Did not allow fingers to come in contact with cover.
		•	Returned probe to the thermometer unit.
		•	Returned the thermometer unit to its storage base.
		•	Sanitized hands.

Trial 1	Trial 2	Point Value	Performance Standards
		•	Documented the results correctly.
		★	The results were identical to the reading on the display screen.
		■	Demonstrated critical thinking skills.
		★	Completed the procedure within 5 minutes.
			Totals

CHART

Date	

Evaluation of Student Performance

EVALUATION CRITERIA			COMMENTS
Symbol	**Category**	**Point Value**	
★	Critical Step	16 points	
•	Essential Step	6 points	
■	Affective Competency	6 points	
▷	Theory Question	2 points	

Score calculation: 100 points

− _____ points missed

_____Score

Satisfactory score: 85 or above

CAAHEP Competencies Achieved

Psychomotor (Skills)
☑ I. 1. b. Accurately measure and record temperature.

Affective (Behavior)
☑ A. 1. Demonstrate critical thinking skills.

ABHES Competency Achieved

☑ 8. b. Obtain and document chief complaint, patient history, and vital signs.

Procedure 4-3: Measuring Rectal Body Temperature—Electronic Thermometer

Name: _____   Date: _____

Evaluated by: _____   Score: _____

Performance Objective

Outcome:	Measure rectal body temperature.
Conditions:	Given the following: electronic thermometer, rectal probe, probe cover, lubricant, disposable gloves, tissues, and a waste container.
Standards:	Time: 5 minutes. Student completed procedure in _____ minutes.
	Accuracy: Satisfactory score on the Performance Evaluation Checklist.

Performance Evaluation Checklist

Trial 1	Trial 2	Point Value	Performance Standards
		•	Sanitized hands.
		•	Assembled equipment.
		•	Removed thermometer from its storage base.
		•	Attached rectal probe to thermometer unit.
		•	Inserted probe into the thermometer.
		•	Greeted the patient and introduced yourself.
		•	Identified the patient and explained the procedure.
		•	Applied gloves.
		▷	Stated the reason for applying gloves.
		•	Positioned and draped the patient.
		▷	Explained how to position an adult and an infant.
		•	Removed probe from the thermometer.
		•	Attached probe cover to probe.
		•	Applied lubricant up to a level of 1 inch.
		▷	Stated the purpose of the lubricant.
		•	Instructed patient to lie still.
		•	Separated the buttocks and properly inserted the thermometer.
		▷	Stated how far the thermometer should be inserted for adults, children, and infants.
		•	Held probe in place until an audible tone was heard.
		•	Removed the probe in the same direction as it was inserted.
		•	Noted patient's temperature reading on display screen.
		•	Discarded probe cover in a regular waste container.

Trial 1	Trial 2	Point Value	Performance Standards
		▷	Explained why the cover can be discarded in a regular waste container.
		•	Returned probe to the thermometer unit.
		•	Returned the thermometer unit to its storage base.
		•	Wiped the anal area with tissues.
		•	Removed gloves and sanitized hands.
		•	Documented the results correctly.
		★	The results were identical to the reading on the display screen.
		■	Demonstrated critical thinking skills.
		★	Completed the procedure within 5 minutes.
			Totals

CHART	
Date	

Evaluation of Student Performance

EVALUATION CRITERIA			COMMENTS
Symbol	**Category**	**Point Value**	
★	Critical Step	16 points	
•	Essential Step	6 points	
■	Affective Competency	6 points	
▷	Theory Question	2 points	

Score calculation: 100 points

     −   points missed

     ___Score

Satisfactory score: 85 or above

CAAHEP Competencies Achieved

Psychomotor (Skills)

☑ I. 1. b. Accurately measure and record temperature.

Affective (Behavior)

☑ A. 1. Demonstrate critical thinking skills.

ABHES Competency Achieved

☑ 8. b. Obtain and document chief complaint, patient history, and vital signs.

Notes

Procedure 4-4: Measuring Aural Body Temperature

Name: _____ Date: _____

Evaluated by: _____ Score: _____

Performance Objective

Outcome:	Measure aural body temperature.
Conditions:	Given the following: tympanic membrane thermometer, probe cover, and a waste container.
Standards:	Time: 5 minutes.　　　Student completed procedure in _____ minutes.
	Accuracy: Satisfactory score on the Performance Evaluation Checklist.

Performance Evaluation Checklist

Trial 1	Trial 2	Point Value	Performance Standards
		•	Sanitized hands.
		•	Assembled equipment.
		•	Greeted the patient and introduced yourself.
		•	Identified the patient and explained the procedure.
		•	Removed thermometer from its storage base.
		•	Checked to make sure the sensor lens was clean and intact.
		▷	Stated what might occur if the sensor lens is dirty.
		•	Attached a cover on the probe.
		▷	Explained the purpose of the probe cover.
		•	Observed the screen to determine if the thermometer is ready to use.
		•	Held the thermometer in the dominant hand.
		•	Straightened the patient's ear canal with the nondominant hand.
		▷	Explained the purpose of straightening the ear canal.
		•	Inserted the probe into the patient's ear canal and sealed the opening without causing the patient discomfort.
		•	Pointed the tip of the probe toward the opposite temple.
		▷	Stated the reason for pointing the probe toward the opposite temple.
		•	Asked the patient to remain still.
		•	Depressed the activation button for 1 full second or until an audible tone is heard.
		•	Removed the thermometer from the ear canal and noted the patient's temperature on the display screen.
		▷	Stated what should be done if the temperature seems too low.
		•	Disposed of the probe cover in a waste container. Wiped the sensor lens with an antiseptic.

Trial 1	Trial 2	Point Value	Performance Standards
		•	Replaced the thermometer in its storage base.
		▷	Explained the reason for storing the thermometer in its base.
		•	Sanitized hands.
		•	Documented the results correctly.
		★	The results were identical to the reading on the display screen.
		■	Demonstrated critical thinking skills.
		★	Completed the procedure within 5 minutes.
			Totals

CHART

Date	

Evaluation of Student Performance

EVALUATION CRITERIA			COMMENTS
Symbol	**Category**	**Point Value**	
★	Critical Step	16 points	
•	Essential Step	6 points	
■	Affective Competency	6 points	
▷	Theory Question	2 points	

Score calculation: 100 points

   −   points missed

     ___Score

Satisfactory score: 85 or above

CAAHEP Competencies Achieved

Psychomotor (Skills)

☑ I. 1. b. Accurately measure and record temperature.

Affective (Behavior)

☑ A. 1. Demonstrate critical thinking skills.

ABHES Competency Achieved
☑ 8. b. Obtain and document chief complaint, patient history, and vital signs.

Notes

Procedure 4-5: Measuring Temporal Artery Body Temperature

Name: _____   Date: _____

Evaluated by: _____   Score: _____

Performance Objective

Outcome:	Measure temporal artery body temperature.
Conditions:	Given the following: contact temporal artery thermometer and a disposable probe cover, contact temporal artery thermometer, antiseptic wipe or cotton swab moistened with alcohol, and a waste container.
Standards:	Time: 5 minutes. Student completed procedure in _____ minutes.
	Accuracy: Satisfactory score on the Performance Evaluation Checklist.

Performance Evaluation Checklist

Trial 1	Trial 2	Point Value	Performance Standards
		•	Sanitized the hands and assembled equipment.
		•	Greeted the patient and introduced yourself.
		•	Identified the patient and explained the procedure.
		•	Checked to make sure the sensor lens is clean and intact.
		▷	Stated why the sensor lens should be clean and intact.
		•	Placed a disposable cover onto the probe or cleaned the probe with an antiseptic and allowed it to dry.
			Contact temporal artery thermometer measurement:
		•	Selected an appropriate site (right or left side of the forehead).
		▷	Stated the location of the temporal artery.
		•	Brushed away any hair that is covering the scanning sites (forehead and area behind the earlobe).
		▷	Explained why hair must be brushed away.
		•	Held the thermometer in the dominant hand with the thumb on the scan button.
		•	Gently positioned the probe of the thermometer on the center of the patient's forehead midway between the eyebrow and hairline.
		•	Depressed the scan button and kept it depressed for the entire measurement.
		▷	Stated why the scan button must be continually depressed.
		•	Slowly and gently slid the probe straight across one side of the forehead midway between the eyebrow and the upper hairline.
		•	Continued until the hairline was reached, making sure to keep the probe flush against the forehead.

Trial 1	Trial 2	Point Value	Performance Standards
		•	Keeping the button depressed, lifted the probe from the forehead and placed it behind the earlobe for 1 to 2 seconds.
		▷	Stated why the temperature is measured behind the earlobe when using a contact tympanic membrane thermometer.
		•	Released the scan button and noted the temperature on the display screen.
		▷	Stated what should be done if the temperature needs to be taken again.
		•	Disposed of the probe cover in a regular waste container.
		•	Wiped the sensor lens with an antiseptic.
			Non-contact temporal artery thermometer measurement:
		•	Prepared the patient by brushing away any hair that is covering the forehead.
		•	If sweat is present, wiped the patient's forehead with a soft cloth.
		▷	Stated why sweat must be wiped from the patient's forehead.
		•	Held the thermometer in the dominant hand and positioned the probe 2 inches away from the center of the patient's forehead between the eyebrows).
		▷	Stated what may occur if the thermometer is positioned more than 2 inches away from the forehead.
		•	Held the thermometer steady and pressed the scan button until an audible tone is heard.
		•	Released the scan button and noted the temperature on the display screen.
		•	Wiped the sensor lens with an antiseptic.
			Complete both procedures as follows:
		•	Sanitized hands.
		•	Documented the results correctly.
		★	The results were identical to the reading on the display screen.
		•	Stored the thermometer in a clean, dry area.
		■	Demonstrated critical thinking skills.
		★	Completed the procedure within 5 minutes.
			Totals

CHART

Date	

Evaluation of Student Performance

EVALUATION CRITERIA			COMMENTS
Symbol	**Category**	**Point Value**	
★	Critical Step	16 points	
•	Essential Step	6 points	
■	Affective Competency	6 points	
▷	Theory Question	2 points	

Score calculation: 100 points

− _____ points missed

___Score

Satisfactory score: 85 or above

CAAHEP Competencies Achieved

Psychomotor (Skills)
☑ I. 1. b. Accurately measure and record temperature.

Affective (Behavior)
☑ A. 1. Demonstrate critical thinking skills.

ABHES Competencies Achieved

☑ 8. b. Obtain and document chief complaint, patient history, and vital signs.

Notes

Procedure 4-6: Measuring Pulse and Respiration

Name: _____ Date: _____

Evaluated by: _____ Score: _____

Performance Objective

Outcome:	Measure radial pulse and respiration.
Conditions:	Using a watch with a second hand.
Standards:	Time: 5 minutes. Student completed procedure in _____ minutes.
	Accuracy: Satisfactory score on the Performance Evaluation Checklist.

Performance Evaluation Checklist

Trial 1	Trial 2	Point Value	Performance Standards
		•	Sanitized hands.
		•	Greeted the patient and introduced yourself.
		•	Identified the patient and explained the procedure.
		•	Observed patient for any signs that might affect the pulse rate or respiratory rate.
		▷	Stated two factors that would increase the pulse rate.
		•	Positioned the patient in a comfortable seated position.
		•	Placed three middle fingertips over the radial pulse site.
		▷	Explained why the pulse should not be taken with the thumb.
		•	Applied moderate, gentle pressure until the pulse was felt.
		▷	Stated what will occur if too much pressure is applied over the radial artery.
		•	Counted the pulse for 30 seconds and made a mental note of the number.
		•	Determined the rhythm and volume of the pulse.
		▷	Stated when the pulse should be measured for a full minute.
		•	Continued to hold the fingers on the patient's wrist.
		▷	Explained why respirations should be taken without the patient's awareness.
		•	Observed the rise and fall of patient's chest.
		•	Counted the number of respirations for 30 seconds and made a mental note of the number.
		▷	Stated what makes up one respiration.
		•	Determined the rhythm and depth of the respirations.
		•	Observed the patient's color.
		•	Sanitized hands.

Trial 1	Trial 2	Point Value	Performance Standards
		•	Multiplied the pulse and respiration values by 2.
		•	Documented the results correctly.
		★	The results were within ±2 beats of the evaluator's results.
		★	The respiratory rate was within 1 respiration of the evaluator's measurement.
		▷	Stated the normal adult range for the pulse rate (60–100 beats/min).
		▷	Stated the normal adult range for the respiratory rate (12–20 respirations/minute).
		■	Demonstrated critical thinking skills.
		★	Completed the procedure within 5 minutes.
			Totals

CHART

Date	

Evaluation of Student Performance

EVALUATION CRITERIA			COMMENTS
Symbol	**Category**	**Point Value**	
★	Critical Step	16 points	
•	Essential Step	6 points	
■	Affective Competency	6 points	
▷	Theory Question	2 points	

Score calculation: 100 points

     –   points missed

       ___Score

Satisfactory score: 85 or above

Psychomotor (Skills)
☑   I. 1. c. Accurately measure and record pulse.
☑   I. 1. d. Accurately measure and record respirations.

Affective (Behavior)
☑   A. 1. Demonstrate critical thinking skills.

ABHES Competency Achieved

☑   8. b. Obtain and document chief complaint, patient history, and vital signs.

Notes

Procedure 4-7: Measuring Apical Pulse

Name: _____   Date: _____

Evaluated by: _____   Score: _____

Performance Objective

Outcome:	Measure apical pulse.
Conditions:	Given the following: stethoscope and antiseptic wipe.
Standards:	Using a watch with a second hand.
	Time: 5 minutes. Student completed procedure in _____ minutes.
	Accuracy: Satisfactory score on the Performance Evaluation Checklist.

Performance Evaluation Checklist

Trial 1	Trial 2	Point Value	Performance Standards
		•	Sanitized hands.
		•	Greeted the patient and introduced yourself.
		•	Identified the patient and explained the procedure.
		•	Observed the patient for any signs that might affect the pulse rate.
		•	Assembled equipment.
		•	Rotated the chest piece to the bell position.
		•	Cleaned earpieces and chest piece with antiseptic wipe.
		▷	Stated the reason for cleaning stethoscope with an antiseptic.
		•	Asked the patient to unbutton or remove his or her shirt.
		•	Positioned patient in a sitting or lying position.
		•	Warmed chest piece of the stethoscope.
		▷	Explained the reason for warming chest piece.
		•	Inserted earpieces of stethoscope in a forward position in the ears.
		▷	Explained why the earpieces must be directed forward.
		•	Placed the chest piece over the apex of the heart.
		▷	Described the location of the apex of the heart.
		•	Counted the number of heartbeats for 30 seconds and multiplied by 2.
		★	The results were within ±2 beats of the evaluator's results.
		•	Sanitized hands.
		•	Documented the results correctly.
		•	Cleaned earpieces and chest piece with an antiseptic wipe.
		■	Demonstrated critical thinking skills.

Trial 1	Trial 2	Point Value	Performance Standards
		★	Completed the procedure within 5 minutes.
			Totals

CHART

Date	

Evaluation of Student Performance

EVALUATION CRITERIA			COMMENTS
Symbol	**Category**	**Point Value**	
★	Critical Step	16 points	
•	Essential Step	6 points	
■	Affective Competency	6 points	
▷	Theory Question	2 points	

Score calculation: 100 points

    −   points missed

    ___Score

Satisfactory score: 85 or above

CAAHEP Competencies Achieved

Psychomotor (Skills)
☑ I. 1. c. Accurately measure and record pulse.

Affective (Behavior)
☑ A. 1. Demonstrate critical thinking skills.

ABHES Competency Achieved

☑ 8. b. Obtain and document chief complaint, patient history, and vital signs.

Procedure 4-8: Performing Pulse Oximetry

Name: _____   Date: _____

Evaluated by: _____   Score: _____

Performance Objective

Outcome:	Perform pulse oximetry.
Conditions:	Given the following: handheld pulse oximeter, and an antiseptic wipe.
Standards:	Time: 5 minutes. Student completed procedure in _____ minutes.
	Accuracy: Satisfactory score on the Performance Evaluation Checklist.

Performance Evaluation Checklist

Trial 1	Trial 2	Point Value	Performance Standards
		•	Sanitized hands and assembled equipment.
		•	Ensured the probe opened and closed smoothly and that the windows were clean.
		•	Disinfected the probe windows and platforms and allowed them to dry.
		▷	Stated the purpose of disinfecting the probe windows.
		•	Greeted the patient and introduced yourself.
		•	Identified the patient and explained the procedure.
		•	Seated the patient in a chair with the lower arm supported just below heart level and the palm facing down.
		▷	Explained why the arm should be supported.
		•	Selected an appropriate finger to apply the probe.
		•	Observed the patient's finger to make sure it is free of dark fingernail polish or an artificial nail.
		•	Checked to make sure the patient's fingertip is clean.
		•	Checked to make sure the patient's finger is not cold.
		▷	Explained what to do if the patient's finger is cold.
		•	Made sure that ambient light will not interfere with the measurement.
		▷	Explained why ambient light should be avoided.
		•	Positioned the probe securely on the fingertip with the fleshy tip of the finger covering the window and the tip of the finger touching the end of the probe stop.
		•	Ensured that the LED and the light sensor are aligned opposite to each other.
		•	Instructed the patient to keep his or her finger stationary and to breathe normally.
		▷	Stated why the patient must remain still.
		•	Turned on the oximeter.
		•	Waited while the oximeter went through its power-on self-test (POST).

147

Trial 1	Trial 2	Point Value	Performance Standards
		▷	Explained the purpose of the POST.
		•	Allowed several seconds for the oximeter to detect the pulse and calculate the oxygen saturation.
		•	Ensured that the pulse strength indicator fluctuates with each pulsation and that the pulse signal is strong.
		▷	Stated what should be done if the oximeter is unable to locate a pulse.
		•	Left the probe in place until the oximeter displayed a reading.
		•	Noted the oxygen saturation value and pulse rate.
		★	The results were identical to the evaluator's results.
		▷	Stated the normal oxygen saturation level of a healthy adult (95–99%).
		▷	Stated what should be done if the oxygen saturation is less than 95%.
		•	Removed the probe from the patient's finger.
		•	Sanitized hands.
		•	Documented the results correctly.
		•	Disinfected the probe with an antiseptic wipe.
		•	Properly stored the monitor in a clean, dry area.
		■	Demonstrated critical thinking skills.
		★	Completed the procedure within 5 minutes.
			Totals

CHART

Date	

Evaluation of Student Performance

EVALUATION CRITERIA			COMMENTS
Symbol	**Category**	**Point Value**	
★	Critical Step	16 points	
•	Essential Step	6 points	
■	Affective Competency	6 points	
▷	Theory Question	2 points	

Score calculation: 100 points

−_____ points missed

_____Score

Satisfactory score: 85 or above

CAAHEP Competencies Achieved

Psychomotor (Skills)
☑ I. 1. i. Accurately measure and record oxygen saturation.

Affective (Behavior)
☑ A. 1. Demonstrate critical thinking skills.

ABHES Competency Achieved

☑ 8. b. Obtain and document chief complaint, patient history, and vital signs.

Notes

Procedure 4-9: Measuring Blood Pressure

Name: _____   Date: _____

Evaluated by: _____   Score: _____

Performance Objective

Outcome:	Measure blood pressure.
Conditions:	Given the following: stethoscope, sphygmomanometer, and an antiseptic wipe.
Standards:	Time: 5 minutes. Student completed procedure in _____ minutes.
	Accuracy: Satisfactory score on the Performance Evaluation Checklist.

Performance Evaluation Checklist

Trial 1	Trial 2	Point Value	Performance Standards
		•	Sanitized hands.
		•	Assembled equipment.
		•	Rotated the chest piece to the diaphragm position.
		•	Cleaned earpieces and chest piece of stethoscope with an antiseptic wipe.
		•	Greeted the patient and introduced yourself.
		•	Identified the patient and explained the procedure.
		•	Observed patient for any signs that might influence the blood pressure reading.
		▷	Stated signs that would influence the blood pressure reading.
		•	Determined how high to pump the cuff (palpated systolic pressure or checked the patient's medical record).
		•	Positioned patient in a sitting position with the legs uncrossed and feet flat on the floor.
		•	Allowed the patient to relax in a sitting position for at least 5 minutes.
		•	Made sure that the patient's arm was uncovered.
		▷	Explained why blood pressure should not be taken over clothing.
		•	Positioned patient's arm at heart level with the palm facing up.
		•	Determined the proper cuff size.
		▷	Explained how to determine the proper cuff size.
		▷	Made sure the cuff was completely deflated and there was no residual air in the cuff.
		•	Located the brachial pulse with the fingertips.
		▷	Stated the location of the brachial pulse.
		•	Centered bladder over the brachial pulse site.
		▷	Explained why the bladder should be centered over the brachial pulse site.
		•	Placed cuff on patient's arm 1 to 2 inches above bend in elbow.

151

Trial 1	Trial 2	Point Value	Performance Standards
		•	Wrapped cuff smoothly and snugly around patient's arm and secured it.
		•	Assess the appropriate tightness of the cuff by ensuring that one finger can be slipped easily under the cuff.
		•	Positioned self and/or manometer for direct viewing and at a distance of no more than 3 feet.
		•	Instructed the patient to relax and not to talk.
		•	Inserted earpieces of stethoscope in a slightly forward position in the ears.
		•	Located the brachial pulse again.
		•	Placed diaphragm of the stethoscope over the brachial pulse site to make a tight seal.
		▷	Explained why there should be good contact of the diaphragm with the skin.
		•	Made sure the diaphragm was not touching cuff.
		▷	Explained why the diaphragm should not touch the cuff.
		•	Closed valve on bulb by turning thumbscrew to the right.
		•	Rapidly pumped air into cuff up to a level approximately 30 mm Hg above the palpated or previously measured systolic pressure.
		•	Did not overinflate the cuff.
		▷	Explained why the cuff should not be overinflated.
		•	Released pressure at a moderate, steady rate by turning thumbscrew to the left.
		▷	Stated what could occur if the pressure is released too slowly.
		•	Heard and noted the first clear tapping sound (systolic pressure).
		•	Heard and noted the point on the scale at which the sounds ceased (diastolic pressure).
		•	Continued to deflate the cuff for another 10 mm Hg.
		•	Quickly and completely deflated cuff to zero and removed earpieces from ears.
		▷	Stated how long to wait before taking the blood pressure again on the same arm.
		•	Carefully removed cuff from patient's arm.
		•	Sanitized hands.
		•	Calculated an average of the readings if two or more blood pressure readings were taken.
		•	Documented the results correctly.
		★	The results were within ±2 mm Hg of the evaluator's results.
		▷	Stated the normal blood pressure for an adult (less than 120/80 mm Hg).
		•	Cleaned earpieces and chest piece with an antiseptic wipe.
		■	Demonstrated critical thinking skills.
		★	Completed the procedure within 5 minutes.

Trial 1	Trial 2	Point Value	Performance Standards
			Totals

CHART	
Date	

Evaluation of Student Performance

EVALUATION CRITERIA			COMMENTS
Symbol	**Category**	**Point Value**	
★	Critical Step	16 points	
•	Essential Step	6 points	
■	Affective Competency	6 points	
▷	Theory Question	2 points	

Score calculation: 100 points

— ___ points missed

___ Score

Satisfactory score: 85 or above

CAAHEP Competencies Achieved

Psychomotor (Skills)
☑ I. 1. a. Accurately measure and record blood pressure.

Affective (Behavior)
☑ A. 1. Demonstrate critical thinking skills.

ABHES Competency Achieved

☑ 8. b. Obtain and document chief complaint, patient history, and vital signs.

Notes

Procedure 4-10: Determining Systolic Pressure by Palpation

Name: _____   Date: _____

Evaluated by: _____   Score: _____

Performance Objective

Outcome:	Determine systolic pressure by palpation.
Conditions:	Given the following: stethoscope, sphygmomanometer, and an antiseptic wipe.
Standards:	Time: 5 minutes. Student completed procedure in _____ minutes.
	Accuracy: Satisfactory score on the Performance Evaluation Checklist.

Performance Evaluation Checklist

Trial 1	Trial 2	Point Value	Performance Standards
		•	Sanitized hands.
		•	Assembled equipment.
		•	Located the brachial pulse with the fingertips.
		•	Placed the cuff on the patient's arm so that the inner bladder was centered over the brachial pulse site.
		•	Wrapped the cuff smoothly and snugly around the patient's arm and secured the end of it.
		•	Positioned the manometer for direct viewing and at a distance of no more than 3 feet.
		•	Located the radial pulse with your fingertips.
		•	Closed the valve on the bulb and pumped air into the cuff until the pulsation ceased.
		•	Released the valve at a moderate rate of 2 to 3 mm Hg per heartbeat while palpating the artery with the fingertips.
		•	Documented the point at which the pulsation reappears as the palpated systolic pressure.
		★	The results was within ±2 mm Hg of the evaluator's results.
		•	Deflated the cuff completely and wait 15 to 30 seconds before measuring the blood pressure.
		■	Demonstrated critical thinking skills.
		★	Completed the procedure within 5 minutes.
			Totals

CHART	
Date	

155

Evaluation of Student Performance

EVALUATION CRITERIA			COMMENTS
Symbol	**Category**	**Point Value**	
★	Critical Step	16 points	
•	Essential Step	6 points	
■	Affective Competency	6 points	
▷	Theory Question	2 points	

Score calculation: 100 points

－   points missed

_____ Score

Satisfactory score: 85 or above

CAAHEP Competencies Achieved

Psychomotor (Skills)
☑   I. 1. a. Accurately measure and record blood pressure

Affective (Behavior)
☑   A. 1. Demonstrate critical thinking skills.

ABHES Competency Achieved

☑   8. b. Obtain and document chief complaint, patient history, and vital signs.

Procedure 4-11: Measuring Blood Pressure: Automatic Method

Name: _____   Date: _____

Evaluated by: _____   Score: _____

Performance Objective

Outcome:	Measure blood pressure using an automatic blood pressure monitor.
Conditions:	Given the following: automatic blood pressure monitor
Standards:	Time: 5 minutes. Student completed procedure in _____ minutes.
	Accuracy: Satisfactory score on the Performance Evaluation Checklist.

Performance Evaluation Checklist

Trial 1	Trial 2	Point Value	Performance Standards
		•	Sanitized hands.
		•	Assembled equipment.
		•	Connected the air tube to the monitor.
		•	Greeted the patient and introduced yourself.
		•	Identified the patient and explained the procedure.
		•	Observed patient for any signs that might influence the blood pressure reading.
		▷	Stated what should be done if it was not possible to reduce or eliminate signs that might influence the blood pressure reading.
		•	Positioned patient in a sitting position with the legs uncrossed and feet flat on the floor.
		•	Allowed the patient to relax in a sitting position for at least 5 minutes.
		•	Made sure that the patient's arm was uncovered.
		•	Positioned patient's arm at heart level with the palm facing upward.
		•	Determined the correct cuff size.
		•	Located the brachial pulse with the fingertips.
		•	Centered bladder over the brachial pulse site.
		•	Placed cuff on patient's arm approximately 1 inch above bend in elbow with the artery position indicator placed above the brachial pulse site.
		•	Wrapped cuff smoothly and snugly around patient's arm and secured it.
		•	The cuff was snug but not too tight.
		•	Assessed the tightness of the cuff by ensuring sure one finger slipped easily under the cuff.
		•	Positioned the digital display screen for direct viewing at a distance of no more than 3 feet.
		•	Instructed the patient not to relax and not to talk.

157

Trial 1	Trial 2	Point Value	Performance Standards
		•	Made sure the patient's arm does not rest on the air tube.
		▷	Stated what can occur if the patient talks or moves.
		▷	Explained what can occur if the patient's arm rests on the air tube.
		•	Pressed the START/STOP button.
		•	Made a mental note of the systolic and diastolic pressures and the pulse rate on the display screen.
		•	Sanitized hands.
		•	Documented the results correctly.
		★	The results were identical to the readings on the display screen.
		■	Demonstrated critical thinking skills.
		▷	Completed the procedure within 5 minutes.
			Totals

CHART	
Date	

Evaluation of Student Performance

EVALUATION CRITERIA			COMMENTS
Symbol	**Category**	**Point Value**	
★	Critical Step	16 points	
•	Essential Step	6 points	
■	Affective Competency	6 points	
▷	Theory Question	2 points	

Score calculation: 100 points

−   points missed

_____Score

Satisfactory score: 85 or above

5   The Physical Examination

√ After Completing	Date Due	Study Guide Pages	STUDY GUIDE ASSIGNMENTS (CTA = Critical Thinking Activity)	Possible Points	Points You Earned
		165	?▦ Pretest	10	
			⚷ Term Key Term Assessment		
		166	A. Definitions	17	
		166	B. Word Parts	9	
			(Add 1 point for each key term)		
		167-170	▦ Evaluation of Learning questions	33	
		170-171	CTA A: Preparation of the Examining Room	10	
		171	CTA B: Reading Weight Measurements	15	
			Evolve: By the Pound (Record points earned)		
		172	CTA C: Reading Height Measurements	11	
			Evolve: Feet and Inches (Record points earned)		
		173	CTA D: Calculating BMI	12	
		173	CTA E: Patient Positions	10	
			Evolve: Let's Get Physical (Record points earned)		
		174	CTA F: Examination Techniques	10	
		175	CTA G: Crossword Puzzle	26	
			Evolve: Apply Your Knowledge questions	10	
			Evolve: Video Evaluation	54	
		165	?▦ Posttest	10	

√ After Completing	Date Due	Study Guide Pages	STUDY GUIDE ASSIGNMENTS (CTA = Critical Thinking Activity)	Possible Points	Points You Earned
			ADDITIONAL ASSIGNMENTS		
			Total points		

√ When Assigned By Your Instructor	Study Guide Pages	Practices Required	LABORATORY ASSIGNMENTS (Procedure Number and Name)	Score*
	177-178	5	**Practice for Competency** 5-1: Measuring Weight and Height	
	179-181		**Evaluation of Competency** 5-1: Measuring Weight and Height	*
	177-178	3	**Practice for Competency** 5-A: Body Mechanics	
	183-185		**Evaluation of Competency** 5-A: Body Mechanics	*
	177-178	3	**Practice for Competency** 5-2: Sitting Position	
	187-188		**Evaluation of Competency** 5-2: Sitting Position	*
	177-178	3	**Practice for Competency** 5-3: Supine Position	
	189-190		**Evaluation of Competency** 5-3: Supine Position	*
	177-178	3	**Practice for Competency** 5-4: Prone Position	
	191-192		**Evaluation of Competency** 5-4: Prone Position	*
	177-178	3	**Practice for Competency** 5-5: Dorsal Recumbent Position	
	193-194		**Evaluation of Competency** 5-5: Dorsal Recumbent Position	*
	177-178	3	**Practice for Competency** 5-6: Lithotomy Position	
	195-197		**Evaluation of Competency** 5-6: Lithotomy Position	*
	177-178	3	**Practice for Competency** 5-7: Modified Left Lateral Recumbent Position	
	199-200		**Evaluation of Competency** 5-7: Modified Left Lateral Recumbent Position	*
	177-178	3	**Practice for Competency** 5-8: Knee-Chest Position	
	201-203		**Evaluation of Competency** 5-8: Knee-Chest Position	*

163

√ When Assigned By Your Instructor	Study Guide Pages	Practices Required	LABORATORY ASSIGNMENTS (Procedure Number and Name)	Score*
	177-178	3	**Practice for Competency** 5-9: Fowler's Position	
	205-206		**Evaluation of Competency** 5-9: Fowler's Position	*
	177-178	3	**Practice for Competency** 5-10: Wheelchair Transfer	
	207-210		**Evaluation of Competency** 5-10: Wheelchair Transfer	*
	177-178	3	**Practice for Competency** 5-11: Assisting with the Physical Examination	
	211-214		**Evaluation of Competency** 5-11: Assisting with the Physical Examination	*
			ADDITIONAL ASSIGNMENTS	

Name: _____   Date: _____

True or False

_____ 1. A complete patient examination consists of a physical examination and laboratory tests.

_____ 2. Arthritis is an example of a chronic illness.

_____ 3. An otoscope is used to examine the eyes.

_____ 4. A patient should be identified by name and date of birth.

_____ 5. The reason for weighing a prenatal patient is to determine the baby's due date.

_____ 6. The height of an adult is measured during every office visit.

_____ 7. The lithotomy position is used to examine the vagina.

_____ 8. Inspection involves the observation of the patient for any signs of disease.

_____ 9. Measuring blood pressure is an example of auscultation.

_____10. The supine position is used to examine the back.

? POSTTEST

True or False

_____ 1. The prognosis is what is wrong with the patient.

_____ 2. A risk factor means that a patient will develop a certain disease.

_____ 3. Electrocardiography is an example of a therapeutic procedure.

_____ 4. The function of a speculum is to open a body orifice for viewing.

_____ 5. The process of measuring the patient is known as mensuration.

_____ 6. A reason for weighing a child is to determine drug dosage.

_____ 7. The purpose of draping a patient is to make it easier for the provider to examine the patient.

_____ 8. The modified left lateral recumbent position is used for flexible sigmoidoscopy.

_____ 9. Measuring pulse is an example of percussion.

_____10. BMI is the acronym for *body mass index.*

A. Definitions

Directions: Match each key term with its definition.

_____ 1. Audiometer

_____ 2. Auscultation

_____ 3. Bariatrics

_____ 4. Body mechanics

_____ 5. Clinical diagnosis

_____ 6. Diagnosis

_____ 7. Differential diagnosis

_____ 8. Inspection

_____ 9. Mensuration

_____ 10. Ophthalmoscope

_____ 11. Otoscope

_____ 12. Palpation

_____ 13. Percussion

_____ 14. Percussion hammer

_____ 15. Prognosis

_____ 16. Speculum

_____ 17. Symptom

A. A lighted instrument with a lens for examining the interior of the eye

B. A tentative diagnosis of a patient's condition obtained through the evaluation of the health history and the physical examination, without the benefit of laboratory or diagnostic tests

C. An instrument for opening a body orifice or cavity for viewing

D. An instrument used to measure hearing

E. The process of measuring a patient

F. The scientific method for determining and identifying a patient's condition

G. The process of tapping the body to detect signs of disease

H. The process of observing a patient to detect signs of disease

I. Any change in the body or its functioning that indicates that a disease might be present

J. The process of listening to the sounds produced within the body to detect signs of disease

K. A determination of which of two or more diseases with similar symptoms is producing a patient's symptoms

L. A lighted instrument with a lens for examining the external ear canal and tympanic membrane

M. The process of feeling with the hands to detect signs of disease

N. An instrument with a rubber head, used for testing reflexes

O. The probable course and outcome of a patient's condition and the patient's prospects for recovery

P. The branch of medicine that deals with the treatment and control of obesity and diseases associated with obesity

Q. Use of the correct muscles to maintain proper balance, posture, and body alignment to accomplish a task safely and efficiently.

B Word Parts

Directions: Indicate the meaning of each word part in the space provided. List as many medical terms as possible that incorporate the word part in the space provided.

Word Part	Meaning of Word Part	Medical Terms That Incorporate Word Part
1. audi/o		
2. -meter		
3. bar/o		
4. -iatrics		
5. dia-		
6. -gnosis		
7. ophthalm/o		
8. -scope		
9. ot/o		

Directions: Fill in each blank with the correct answer.

1. What are the three parts of a complete patient examination?

   _____

   _____

2. List two functions of a patient examination.

   _____

   _____

3. What is the purpose of establishing a final diagnosis?

   _____

   _____

4. Why is there a space for indicating the clinical diagnosis on the laboratory request form?

   _____

   _____

5. What is a risk factor?

   _____

   _____

6. What is a screening test?

   _____

   _____

7. What is an acute illness? List two examples of acute illnesses.

   _____

   _____

8. What is a chronic illness? List two examples of chronic illnesses.

   _____

   _____

9. Explain the difference between a therapeutic procedure and a diagnostic procedure and provide examples of each.

   _____

   _____

   _____

10. How should a patient be identified?

   _____

   _____

11. Why is it important to properly identify the patient?

_____

_____

12. How can patient apprehension be reduced during a physical examination?

_____

_____

13. Why should patients be asked if they need to void before the physical examination?

_____

_____

14. What is the purpose of measuring weight?

_____

_____

15. Describe the two types of scales commonly used in the medical office to measure weight.

_____

_____

_____

16. What is the purpose of determining body mass index?

_____

_____

17. Why is it important to use proper body mechanics?

_____

_____

18. What are the four curvatures of the vertebral column, and what is their purpose?

_____

_____

19. What body mechanics principles should be followed for each of the following?

   a. Physical condition of the body

   _____

   _____

   b. Reaching for something

   _____

   _____

   c. Working height

   _____

   _____

d. Storing heavy and lighter items on shelves

_____

_____

e. Retrieving an item from an overhead shelf

_____

_____

f. Lifting an object

_____

_____

g. Transferring a patient

_____

_____

h. Patient who starts to fall

_____

_____

i. You are unsure about your ability to lift a heavy object

_____

_____

20. What is the purpose of positioning and draping?

_____

_____

_____

21. Indicate three types of examinations for which the supine position is used.

_____

_____

22. Indicate two types of examinations for which the lithotomy position is used.

_____

_____

23. Indicate one type of examination for which the knee-chest position is used.

_____

_____

24. What is the purpose of a wheelchair?

_____

_____

25. What is the purpose of a transfer belt for both the patient and the medical assistant?

_____

_____

26. What should the medical assistant do if he or she does not think it is possible to transfer a patient from a wheelchair to the examining table?

_____

_____

27. What is performed during a complete physical examination?

_____

_____

28. What is the advantage of using EHR software to document the results of a physical examination?

_____

_____

29. What are four types of assessments that can be made through inspection?

_____

_____

30. What are four types of assessments that can be made through palpation?

_____

_____

31. What can be assessed through the use of percussion?

_____

_____

32. What type of assessments can be made using auscultation?

_____

_____

33. What type of stethoscope chest piece should be used to assess the heart?

_____

CRITICAL THINKING ACTIVITIES

A. Preparation of the Examining Room

For each of the following examining room preparation guidelines, indicate the problems that may result if the guideline is not followed.

	Preparation	Problems If Not Performed
1.	Ensure the examining room is well lit.	
2.	Restock supplies that are getting low.	
3.	Empty waste containers frequently.	
4.	Replace biohazard containers as necessary.	
5.	Make sure room is well ventilated.	
6.	Maintain room temperature that is comfortable for the patient.	

170

	Preparation	Problems If Not Performed
7.	Clean and disinfect examining table daily.	
8.	Change the examining table paper after each patient.	
9.	Check equipment and instruments to make sure they are in proper working condition.	
10.	Know how to operate and care for each piece of equipment and instrument.	

B. Reading Weight Measurements

The diagram is an illustration of a portion of the calibration bar of an upright balance beam scale. In the spaces provided, document the weight measurements indicated on the calibration bar. In all cases, assume that the lower weight is resting in the 100-lb notched groove.

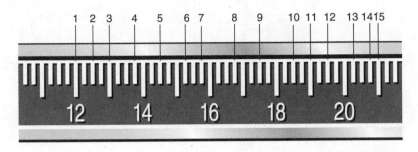

1. _____

2. _____

3. _____

4. _____

5. _____

6. _____

7. _____

8. _____

9. _____

10. _____

11. _____

12. _____

13. _____

14. _____

15. _____

C. Reading Height Measurements

The diagram is an illustration of a portion of the calibration rod of an upright balance beam scale. In the spaces provided, indicate the height measurements in feet and inches indicated on the calibration rod.

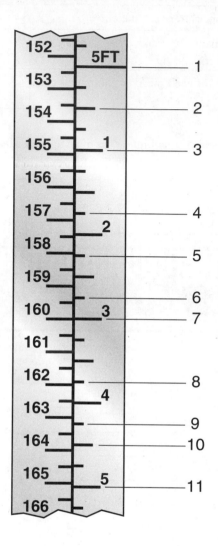

1. _____

2. _____

3. _____

4. _____

5. _____

6. _____

7. _____

8. _____

9. _____

10. _____

11. _____

D. Calculating Body Mass Index (using a BMI calculator on the internet)

1. Using a BMI calculator website or the "Highlight on Body Mass Index" box on pages 152-153 of your textbook, determine your BMI. Interpret your BMI using Table 5-2: Interpretation of Body Mass Index in your textbook. Document the results below.

_____

2. Determine the BMI of the following individuals and document the value in the space provided. Interpret each BMI value according to the information indicated in Table 5-2 in your textbook.

	Weight	Height	BMI	Interpretation of BMI
1.	146	5 ft 5 in		
2.	175	5 ft 6 in		
3.	106	5 ft 9 in		
4.	122	5 ft 1 in		
5.	260	6 ft		
6.	180	6 ft 8 in		
7.	330	5 ft 11 in		
8.	150	5 ft 4 in		
9.	170	5 ft 2 in		
10.	151	6 ft 4 in		

3. List the diseases that an individual with an above-normal BMI has an increased chance of developing.

_____

_____

_____

_____

E. Patient Positions
In which position would you place the patient for the following examinations or procedures?

1. Measurement of rectal temperature of an adult _____

2. Examination of the back _____

3. Measurement of vital signs _____

4. Pelvic examination _____

5. Examination of the upper extremities _____

6. Examination of the eyes, ears, nose, and throat _____

7. Examination of the breasts _____

8. Flexible sigmoidoscopy _____

9. Administration of an enema _____

10. Examination of the upper body of a patient with emphysema _____

173

F. Examination Techniques

List the examination technique (e.g., inspection, palpation, percussion, auscultation) that is used in each of the following situations.

1. A patient with a stutter _____

2. Taking the radial pulse _____

3. Finding the location of the apical pulse _____

4. Taking the apical pulse _____

5. Taking respiration (may be two answers, depending on method) _____

6. A patient with cracked lips _____

7. Checking for lumps in the breast

8. Checking reflexes _____

9. Obtaining the fetal heart rate _____

10. A patient with a fever (may be several methods) _____

G. Crossword Puzzle: The Physical Examination

Directions: Complete the crossword puzzle using the clues provided.

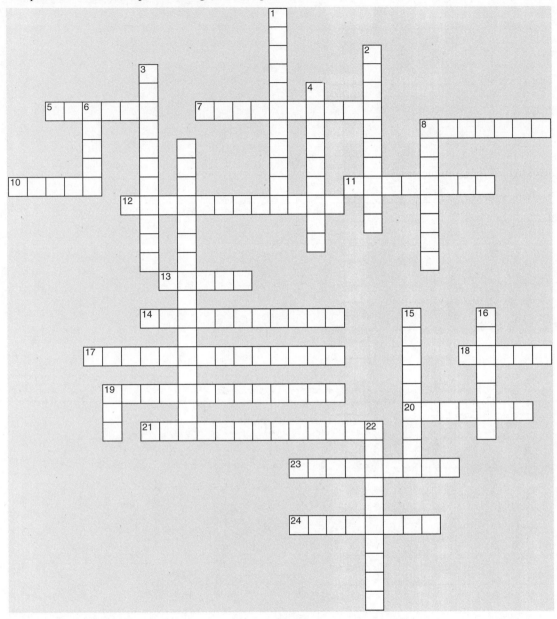

Across

- **5** Face up
- **7** BMI: 25 to 29.9
- **8** "Listen to heart" position
- **10** Severe and intense condition
- **11** Ear examiner
- **12** I am listening
- **13** Five feet in inches
- **14** Measuring the patient
- **17** Eye examiner
- **18** Provides warmth and modesty
- **19** How to accomplish a task safely
- **20** Can cause premature death
- **21** Early detection of a condition
- **23** What is the probable outcome?
- **24** Metric unit of weight

Down

- **1** BMI: 16 to 18.49
- **2** Metric unit of height
- **3** Curative procedure
- **4** GYN position
- **6** Face down
- **8** Orifice opener
- **9** Reflex tester
- **15** What is wrong with you?
- **16** Long-time illness
- **19** Correlates with total body fat
- **22** Hearing tester

Notes

Procedure 5-1: Weight and Height.
Take weight and height measurements. Document results in the chart provided.

Procedure 5-A: Body Mechanics.
Demonstrate proper body mechanics while standing, sitting, and lifting an object.

Procedures 5-2 to 5-9: Positioning and Draping.
Position and drape an individual in each of the following positions: sitting, supine, prone, dorsal recumbent, lithotomy, modified left lateral recumbent, knee-chest, and Fowler's.

Procedure 5-10: Wheelchair Transfer.
Transfer a patient from a wheelchair to the examining table and from the examining table to a wheelchair.

Procedure 5-11: Assisting with the Physical Examination.
Prepare the patient and assist, with a physical examination. In the chart provided, document the results of the procedures you performed while assisting with the examination (e.g., vital signs, height, and weight).

CHART	
Date	

CHART	
Date	

Procedure 5-1: Measuring Weight and Height

Name: _____   Date: _____

Evaluated by: _____   Score: _____

Performance Objective

Outcome:	Measure weight and height using an upright balance scale.
Conditions:	Given a paper towel.
	Using an upright balance scale.
Standards:	Time: 5 minutes. Student completed procedure in _____ minutes.
	Accuracy: Satisfactory score on the performance evaluation checklist.

Performance Evaluation Checklist

Trial 1	Trial 2	Point Value	Performance Standards
			Weight
		•	Sanitized hands.
			Checked the balance scale for accuracy
		•	Made sure that the upper and lower weights were on zero.
		•	Looked at the indicator point to make sure the scale is balanced.
		▷	Stated what is observed if the scale is balanced.
		▷	Explained what to do if the indicator point rests below the center.
		▷	Explained what to do if the indicator point rests above the center.
		▷	Stated what occurs if the scale is not balanced.
		•	Greeted the patient and introduced yourself.
		•	Identified the patient and explained the procedure.
		•	Instructed patient to remove shoes and heavy outer clothing.
		•	Assisted patient onto the scale.
		•	Instructed patient not to move.
			Balanced the scale
		•	Moved the lower weight to the groove that did not cause the indicator point to drop to the bottom of the balance area.
		▷	Stated why the lower weight should be seated firmly in its groove.
		•	Slid the upper weight slowly until the indicator point came to a rest at the center of the balance area.

179

Trial 1	Trial 2	Point Value	Performance Standards
		•	Read the results to the nearest quarter pound. Jotted down this value or made a mental note of it.
		★	The reading was identical to the evaluator's reading.
		•	Asked the patient to step off the scale.
			Height
		•	Slid the calibration rod until it was above the patient's height.
		•	Opened the measuring bar to its horizontal position.
		•	Instructed the patient to step onto the scale platform with his or her back to the scale.
		•	Instructed patient to stand erect and to look straight ahead.
		•	Carefully lowered the measuring bar until it rested gently on top of the patient's head.
		•	Made sure that the bar was in a horizontal position.
		•	Instructed the patient to step down and put on his or her shoes.
		•	Read the marking to the nearest quarter inch. Jotted down this value or made a mental note of it.
		★	The reading was identical to the evaluator's reading.
		•	Returned the measuring bar to its vertical position.
		•	Slid the calibration rod to its lowest position.
		•	Returned the weights to zero.
		•	Sanitized hands.
		•	Documented the results correctly.
		■	Demonstrated active listening.
		▲	Recognized personal boundaries.
		★	Completed the procedure within 5 minutes.
			TOTALS
CHART			
Date			

Evaluation of Student Performance

<table>
<tr><th colspan="3">EVALUATION CRITERIA</th><th>COMMENTS</th></tr>
<tr><td>**Symbol**</td><td>**Category**</td><td>**Point Value**</td><td></td></tr>
<tr><td>★</td><td>Critical Step</td><td>16 points</td><td></td></tr>
<tr><td>•</td><td>Essential Step</td><td>6 points</td><td></td></tr>
<tr><td>■</td><td>Affective Competency</td><td>6 points</td><td></td></tr>
<tr><td>◆</td><td>Theory Question</td><td>2 points</td><td></td></tr>
<tr><td colspan="3">**Score calculation:** 100 points
       –   points missed
          ___Score
Satisfactory score: 85 or above</td><td></td></tr>
</table>

CAAHEP Competencies Achieved

Psychomotor (Skills)

☑ I. 1. e. Accurately measure and record height.
☑ I. 1. f. Accurately measure and record weight.

Affective (Behavior)

☑ A. 4. Demonstrate active listening.
☑ A. 6. Recognize personal boundaries.

ABHES Competencies Achieved

☑ 7. g. Display professionalism through written and verbal communication.
☑ 8. c. Assist provider with general/physical examination.

Notes

Procedure 5-A: Body Mechanics

Name: _____ Date: _____

Evaluated by: _____ Score: _____

Performance Objective

Outcome:	Demonstrate proper body mechanics while standing, sitting, and lifting an object.
Conditions:	Given the following: object for lifting.
	Using a chair.
Standards:	Time: 10 minutes. Student completed procedure in _____ minutes.
	Accuracy: Satisfactory score on the performance evaluation checklist.

Performance Evaluation Checklist

Trial 1	Trial 2	Point Value	Performance Standards
			Standing
		•	Wore comfortable low-heeled shoes that provide good support.
		•	Held the head erect at the midline of the body.
		•	Maintained the back as straight as possible with the pelvis tucked inward.
		•	The chest is forward with the shoulders back and the abdomen drawn in and kept flat.
		▷	Stated the purpose of standing correctly.
		•	Knees are slightly flexed.
		•	Feet are pointing forward and parallel to each other about 3 inches apart.
		▷	Explained the reason for proper positioning of the feet.
		•	Arms are positioned comfortably at the side.
		•	Weight of the body is evenly distributed over both feet.
			Sitting
		•	Sat in a chair with a firm back.
		•	Back and buttocks are supported against the back of the chair.
		•	Body weight is evenly distributed over the buttocks and thighs.
		•	A small pillow or rolled towel is used.
		▷	Stated the use of the pillow or rolled towel.
		•	Feet are flat on the floor.
		•	Knees are level with the hips.
		▷	Explained what to do if prolonged sitting is required.

Trial 1	Trial 2	Point Value	Performance Standards
			Lifting
		•	Determined the weight of the object.
		▷	Stated the purpose of determining the weight of an object before lifting it.
		•	Stood in front of the object with the feet 6 to 8 inches apart.
		•	The toes are pointed outward and one foot is slightly forward.
		•	Tightened the stomach and gluteal muscles in preparation for the lift.
		•	Bent the body at the knees and hips.
		▷	Stated the purpose of bending the body at the knees and hips.
		•	Grasped the object firmly with both hands.
		•	Lifted the object smoothly with the leg muscles while keeping the back straight.
		▷	Stated why the leg muscles and not the back muscles should be used to lift the object.
		•	Held the object as close to the body as possible at waist level.
		▷	Stated why the object should not be lifted higher than the chest.
		•	Turned by pivoting the whole body.
		•	Made sure the area of transport of the object is dry and free of clutter.
		•	Lowered the object slowly while bending from the knees.
		★	Completed the procedures within 10 minutes.
			TOTALS

Evaluation of Student Performance

EVALUATION CRITERIA			COMMENTS
Symbol	**Category**	**Point Value**	
★	Critical Step	16 points	
•	Essential Step	6 points	
■	Affective Competency	6 points	
▷	Theory Question	2 points	

Score calculation: 100 points

−   points missed

_____Score

Satisfactory score: 85 or above

CAAHEP Competency Achieved
Psychomotor (Skills)
☑ XII. 3. Use proper body mechanics.

ABHES Competency Achieved
☑ 4. e. Perform risk management procedures.

Notes

Procedure 5-2: Sitting Position

Name: _____   Date: _____

Evaluated by: _____   Score: _____

Performance Objective

Outcome:	Position and drape an individual in the sitting position.
Conditions:	Given the following: a patient gown and a drape.
	Using an examining table.
Standards:	Time: 5 minutes. Student completed procedure in _____ minutes.
	Accuracy: Satisfactory score on the performance evaluation checklist.

Performance Evaluation Checklist

Trial 1	Trial 2	Point Value	Performance Standards
		•	Sanitized hands.
		•	Greeted the patient and introduced yourself.
		•	Identified the patient.
		•	Explained what type of examination or procedure will be performed.
		•	Provided patient with a patient gown.
		•	Instructed patient to remove clothing and to put on a patient gown with the opening in front.
		•	Pulled out the footrest and assisted the patient into a sitting position.
		•	The patient's buttocks and thighs were firmly supported on the edge of the table.
		•	Placed a drape over the patient's thighs and legs.
		•	Assisted the patient off the table after the examination.
		•	Returned the footrest to its normal position.
		•	Instructed the patient to get dressed.
		•	Discarded the gown and drape in a waste container.
		▷	Stated one use of the sitting position.
		■	Recognized persona boundaries.
		*	Completed the procedure within 5 minutes.
			TOTALS

Evaluation of Student Performance

<table>
<tr><th colspan="3">EVALUATION CRITERIA</th><th>COMMENTS</th></tr>
<tr><th>Symbol</th><th>Category</th><th>Point Value</th><th></th></tr>
<tr><td>*</td><td>Critical Step</td><td>16 points</td><td></td></tr>
<tr><td>•</td><td>Essential Step</td><td>6 points</td><td></td></tr>
<tr><td>■</td><td>Affective Competency</td><td>6 points</td><td></td></tr>
<tr><td>▷</td><td>Theory Question</td><td>2 points</td><td></td></tr>
</table>

Score calculation: 100 points

— _____ points missed

_____ Score

Satisfactory score: 85 or above

CAAHEP Competencies Achieved

Psychomotor (Skills)

☑ I. 8. Instruct and prepare a patient for a procedure or a treatment.
☑ XII. 3. Use proper body mechanics.

Affective (Behavior)

☑ A. 1. Recognize personal boundaries.

ABHES Competency Achieved

☑ 8. c. Assist provider with general/physical examination.

EVALUATION OF COMPETENCY

Procedure 5-3: Supine Position

Name: _____   Date: _____

Evaluated by: _____   Score: _____

Performance Objective

Outcome:	Position and drape an individual in the supine position.
Conditions:	Given the following: a patient gown and a drape.
	Using an examining table.
Standards:	Time: 5 minutes. Student completed procedure in _____ minutes.
	Accuracy: Satisfactory score on the performance evaluation checklist.

Performance Evaluation Checklist

Trial 1	Trial 2	Point Value	Performance Standards
		•	Sanitized hands.
		•	Greeted the patient and introduced yourself.
		•	Identified the patient.
		•	Explained what type of examination or procedure will be performed.
		•	Provided patient with a patient gown.
		•	Instructed patient to remove clothing and to put on a patient gown with the opening in front.
		•	Pulled out the footrest and assisted the patient into a sitting position.
		•	Placed a drape over the patient's thighs and legs.
		•	Asked the patient to move back on the table.
		•	Pulled out the table extension while supporting the patient's lower legs.
		•	Asked the patient to lie down on his or her back with the legs together.
		•	Placed the patient's arms above the head or alongside the body.
		•	Positioned the drape lengthwise over the patient.
		▷	Stated the purpose of the drape.
		•	Moved the drape according to the body parts being examined.
		•	Assisted the patient back into a sitting position after the examination.
		•	Slid the table extension back into place while supporting the patient's lower legs.
		•	Assisted the patient from the examining table.
		•	Returned the footrest to its normal position.

Trial 1	Trial 2	Point Value	Performance Standards
		•	Instructed the patient to get dressed.
		•	Discarded the gown and drape in a waste container.
		▷	Stated one use of the supine position.
		■	Recognized personal boundaries.
		*	Completed the procedure within 5 minutes.
			TOTALS

Evaluation of Student Performance

EVALUATION CRITERIA			COMMENTS
Symbol	**Category**	**Point Value**	
★	Critical Step	16 points	
•	Essential Step	6 points	
■	Affective Competency	6 points	
▷	Theory Question	2 points	

Score calculation: 100 points

    −   points missed

      ___Score

Satisfactory score: 85 or above

CAAHEP Competencies Achieved

Psychomotor (Skills)

☑ I. 8. Instruct and prepare a patient for a procedure or a treatment.
☑ XII. 3. Use proper body mechanics.

Affective (Behavior)

☑ A. 6. Recognize personal boundaries.

ABHES Competency Achieved

☑ 8. c. Assist provider with general/physical examination.

Procedure 5-4: Prone Position

Name: _____   Date: _____

Evaluated by: _____   Score: _____

Performance Objective

Outcome:	Position and drape an individual in the prone position.
Conditions:	Given the following: a patient gown and a drape.
	Using an examining table.
Standards:	Time: 5 minutes. Student completed procedure in _____ minutes.
	Accuracy: Satisfactory score on the performance evaluation checklist.

Performance Evaluation Checklist

Trial 1	Trial 2	Point Value	Performance Standards
		•	Sanitized hands.
		•	Greeted the patient and introduced yourself.
		•	Identified the patient.
		•	Explained what type of examination or procedure will be performed.
		•	Provided patient with a patient gown.
		•	Instructed patient to remove clothing and to put on a patient gown with the opening in back.
		•	Pulled out the footrest and assisted the patient into a sitting position.
		•	Placed a drape over the patient's thighs and legs.
		•	Asked the patient to move back on the table.
		•	Pulled out the table extension while supporting the patient's lower legs.
		•	Asked the patient to lie down on his or her back.
		•	Positioned the drape lengthwise over the patient.
		•	Asked the patient to turn onto his or her stomach by rolling toward you.
		•	Provided assistance.
		▷	Stated the reason for providing assistance.
		•	Positioned the patient with his or her legs together and the head turned to one side.
		•	Placed the patient's arms above the head or alongside the body.
		•	Adjusted the drape as needed so that it is positioned lengthwise.
		•	Moved the drape according to the body parts being examined.
		•	After completion of the examination, asked the patient to turn back over by rolling towards you.

Trial 1	Trial 2	Point Value	Performance Standards
		•	Assisted the patient into the supine position after the examination.
		•	Assisted the patient into a sitting position.
		•	Slid the table extension back into place while supporting the patient's lower legs.
		•	Assisted the patient from the examining table.
		•	Returned the footrest to its normal position.
		•	Instructed the patient to get dressed.
		•	Discarded the gown and drape in a waste container.
		▷	Stated one use of the prone position.
		■	Recognized personal boundaries.
		★	Completed the procedure within 5 minutes.
			TOTALS

Evaluation of Student Performance

EVALUATION CRITERIA			COMMENTS
Symbol	**Category**	**Point Value**	
★	Critical Step	16 points	
•	Essential Step	6 points	
■	Affective Competency	6 points	
▷	Theory Question	2 points	

Score calculation: 100 points

− ___ points missed

___ Score

Satisfactory score: 85 or above

CAAHEP Competencies Achieved

Psychomotor (Skills)

☑ I. 8. Instruct and prepare a patient for a procedure or a treatment.
☑ XII. 3. Use proper body mechanics.

Affective (Behavior)

☑ A. 6. Recognize personal boundaries.

ABHES Competency Achieved

☑ 8. c. Assist provider with general/physical examination.

Procedure 5-5: Dorsal Recumbent Position

Name: _____   Date: _____

Evaluated by: _____   Score: _____

Performance Objective

Outcome:	Position and drape an individual in the dorsal recumbent position.
Conditions:	Given the following: a patient gown and a drape.
	Using an examining table.
Standards:	Time: 5 minutes. Student completed procedure in _____ minutes.
	Accuracy: Satisfactory score on the performance evaluation checklist.

Performance Evaluation Checklist

Trial 1	Trial 2	Point Value	Performance Standards
		•	Sanitized hands.
		•	Greeted the patient and introduced yourself.
		•	Identified the patient.
		•	Explained what type of examination or procedure will be performed.
		•	Provided patient with a patient gown.
		•	Instructed patient to remove clothing and to put on a patient gown with the opening in front.
		•	Pulled out the footrest and assisted the patient into a sitting position.
		•	Placed a drape over the patient's thighs and legs.
		•	Asked the patient to move back on the table.
		•	Pulled out the table extension while supporting the patient's lower legs.
		•	Asked the patient to lie down on his or her back.
		•	Placed the patient's arms above their head or alongside the body.
		•	Positioned the drape diagonally over the patient.
		•	Asked the patient to bend the knees and place each foot at the edge of the table with the soles of the feet flat on the table.
		•	Provided assistance.
		•	Pushed in the table extension and the footrest.
		•	Adjusted the drape as needed.
		•	Folded back the center corner of the drape when the provider was ready to examine the patient.

193

Trial 1	Trial 2	Point Value	Performance Standards
		•	Pulled out the footrest and the table extension after the examination.
		•	Assisted the patient back into a supine position and then into a sitting position.
		•	Slid the table extension back into place while supporting the patient's lower legs.
		•	Assisted the patient from the examining table.
		•	Returned the footrest to its normal position.
		•	Instructed the patient to get dressed.
		•	Discarded the gown and drape in a waste container.
		▷	Stated one use of the dorsal recumbent position.
		■	Recognized personal boundaries.
		★	Completed the procedure within 5 minutes.
			TOTALS

Evaluation of Student Performance

EVALUATION CRITERIA			COMMENTS
Symbol	**Category**	**Point Value**	
★	Critical Step	16 points	
•	Essential Step	6 points	
■	Affective Competency	6 points	
▷	Theory Question	2 points	

Score calculation: 100 points

− _____ points missed

_____ Score

Satisfactory score: 85 or above

CAAHEP Competencies Achieved

Psychomotor (Skills)

☑ I. 8. Instruct and prepare a patient for a procedure or a treatment.
☑ XII. 3. Use proper body mechanics.

Affective (Behavior)

☑ A. 6. Recognize personal boundaries.

ABHES Competency Achieved

☑ 8. c. Assist provider with general/physical examination.

EVALUATION OF COMPETENCY

Procedure 5-6: Lithotomy Position

Name: _____   Date: _____

Evaluated by: _____   Score: _____

Performance Objective

Outcome:	Position and drape an individual in the lithotomy position.
Conditions:	Given the following: a patient gown and a drape.
	Using an examining table.
Standards:	Time: 5 minutes. Student completed procedure in _____ minutes.
	Accuracy: Satisfactory score on the performance evaluation checklist.

Performance Evaluation Checklist

Trial 1	Trial 2	Point Value	Performance Standards
		•	Sanitized hands.
		•	Greeted the patient and introduced yourself.
		•	Identified the patient.
		•	Explained what type of examination or procedure will be performed.
		•	Provided patient with a patient gown.
		•	Instructed patient to remove clothing and to put on a patient gown with the opening in front.
		•	Pulled out the footrest and assisted the patient into a sitting position.
		•	Placed a drape over the patient's thighs and legs.
		•	Asked the patient to move back on the table.
		•	Pulled out the table extension while supporting the patient's lower legs.
		•	Asked the patient to lie down on his or her back.
		•	Placed the patient's arms above head or alongside body.
		•	Positioned the drape diagonally over the patient.
		•	Pulled out the stirrups and positioned them at an angle.
		•	Positioned the stirrups so that they were level with the examining table and pulled out approximately 1 foot from the edge of the table.
		•	Asked the patient to bend the knees and place each foot into a stirrup.
		•	Provided assistance.
		•	Pushed in the table extension and the footrest.

Trial 1	Trial 2	Point Value	Performance Standards
		•	Instructed the patient to slide buttocks to the edge of the table and to rotate thighs outward as far as is comfortable.
		•	Repositioned the drape as needed.
		•	Folded back the center corner of the drape when the provider was ready to examine the genital area.
		•	After completion of the examination, pulled out the footrest and the table extension.
		•	Asked the patient to slide the buttocks back from the end of the table.
		•	Lifted the patient's legs out of the stirrups at the same time and placed them on the table extension.
		▷	Stated why both legs should be lifted at the same time.
		•	Returned stirrups to the normal position.
		•	Assisted the patient back into a sitting position.
		•	Slid the table extension back into place while supporting the patient's lower legs.
		•	Assisted the patient from the examining table.
		•	Returned the footrest to its normal position.
		•	Instructed the patient to get dressed.
		•	Discarded the gown and drape in a waste container.
		▷	Stated one use of the lithotomy position.
		■	Recognized personal boundaries.
		★	Completed the procedure within 5 minutes.
			TOTALS

Evaluation of Student Performance

EVALUATION CRITERIA			COMMENTS
Symbol	**Category**	**Point Value**	
★	Critical Step	16 points	
•	Essential Step	6 points	
■	Affective Competency	6 points	
▷	Theory Question	2 points	

Score calculation: 100 points

− _____ points missed

____ Score

Satisfactory score: 85 or above

CAAHEP Competencies Achieved

Psychomotor (Skills)

☑   I. 8. Instruct and prepare a patient for a procedure or a treatment.
☑   XII. 3. Use proper body mechanics.

Affective (Behavior)

☑   A. 6. Recognize personal boundaries.

ABHES Competency Achieved

☑   8. c. Assist provider with general/physical examination.

Notes

Procedure 5-7: Modified Left Lateral Recumbent Position

Name: _____   Date: _____

Evaluated by: _____   Score: _____

Performance Objective

Outcome:	Position and drape an individual in the modified left lateral recumbent position.
Conditions:	Given the following: a patient gown and a drape.
	Using an examining table.
Standards:	Time: 5 minutes. Student completed procedure in _____ minutes.
	Accuracy: Satisfactory score on the performance evaluation checklist.

Performance Evaluation Checklist

Trial 1	Trial 2	Point Value	Performance Standards
		•	Sanitized hands.
		•	Greeted the patient and introduced yourself.
		•	Identified the patient.
		•	Explained what type of examination or procedure will be performed.
		•	Provided patient with a patient gown.
		•	Instructed patient to remove clothing and to put on a patient gown with the opening in back.
		•	Pulled out the footrest and assisted the patient into a sitting position.
		•	Placed a drape over the patient's thighs and legs.
		•	Asked the patient to move back on the table.
		•	Pulled out the table extension while supporting the patient's lower legs.
		•	Asked the patient to lie down on his or her back.
		•	Positioned the drape lengthwise over the patient.
		•	Asked the patient to turn onto the left side.
		•	Provided assistance.
		•	Positioned the left arm behind the body and the right arm forward with the elbow bent.
		•	Assisted the patient in flexing the legs with the right leg flexed sharply and the left leg flexed slightly.
		•	Adjusted the drape by folding back the drape to expose the anal area when the provider was ready to examine the patient.
		•	Assisted the patient into a supine position and then into a sitting position following the examination.

Trial 1	Trial 2	Point Value	Performance Standards
		•	Slid the table extension back into place while supporting the patient's lower legs.
		•	Assisted the patient from the examining table.
		•	Returned the footrest to its normal position.
		•	Instructed the patient to get dressed.
		•	Discarded the gown and drape in a waste container.
		▷	Stated one use of the modified left lateral recumbent position.
		■	Recognized personal boundaries.
		★	Completed the procedure within 5 minutes.
			TOTALS

Evaluation of Student Performance

EVALUATION CRITERIA			COMMENTS
Symbol	**Category**	**Point Value**	
★	Critical Step	16 points	
•	Essential Step	6 points	
■	Affective Competency	6 points	
▷	Theory Question	2 points	

Score calculation: 100 points

    −   points missed

     ___Score

Satisfactory score: 85 or above

CAAHEP Competencies Achieved
Psychomotor (Skills)
☑ I. 8. Instruct and prepare a patient for a procedure or a treatment. ☑ XII. 3. Use proper body mechanics.
Affective (Behavior)
☑ A. 6. Recognize personal boundaries.

ABHES Competency Achieved
☑ 8. c. Assist provider with general/physical examination.

Procedure 5-8: Knee-Chest Position

Name: _____   Date: _____

Evaluated by: _____   Score: _____

Performance Objective

Outcome:	Position and drape an individual in the knee-chest position.
Conditions:	Given the following: a patient gown and a drape.
	Using an examining table.
Standards:	Time: 5 minutes. Student completed procedure in _____ minutes.
	Accuracy: Satisfactory score on the performance evaluation checklist.

Performance Evaluation Checklist

Trial 1	Trial 2	Point Value	Performance Standards
		•	Sanitized hands.
		•	Greeted the patient and introduced yourself.
		•	Identified the patient.
		•	Explained what type of examination or procedure will be performed.
		•	Provided patient with a patient gown.
		•	Instructed patient to remove clothing and to put on a patient gown with the opening in back.
		•	Pulled out the footrest and assisted the patient into a sitting position.
		•	Placed a drape over the patient's thighs and legs.
		•	Asked the patient to move back on the table.
		•	Pulled out the table extension while supporting the patient's lower legs.
		•	Assisted the patient into the supine position and then into the prone position.
		•	Positioned the drape diagonally over the patient.
		•	Asked the patient to bend the arms at the elbows and rest them alongside the head.
		•	Asked the patient to elevate the buttocks while keeping the back straight.
		•	Turned the patient's head to one side, with the weight of the body supported by the chest.
		•	Used a pillow for additional support, if needed.
		•	Separated the knees and lower legs approximately 12 inches.
		•	Adjusted the drape diagonally as needed.

Trial 1	Trial 2	Point Value	Performance Standards
		•	Folded back a small portion of the drape to expose the anal area when the provider was ready to examine the patient.
		•	Assisted the patient into a prone position and then into a supine position after the examination.
		•	Allowed the patient to rest in a supine position before sitting up.
		▷	Stated why the patient should be allowed to rest.
		•	Assisted the patient into a sitting position
		•	Slid the table extension back into place while supporting the patient's lower legs.
		•	Assisted the patient from the examining table.
		•	Returned the footrest to its normal position.
		•	Instructed the patient to get dressed.
		•	Discarded the gown and drape in a waste container.
		▷	Stated one use of the knee-chest position.
		■	Recognized personal boundaries.
		★	Completed the procedure within 5 minutes.
			TOTALS

Evaluation of Student Performance

EVALUATION CRITERIA			COMMENTS
Symbol	**Category**	**Point Value**	
★	Critical Step	16 points	
•	Essential Step	6 points	
■	Affective Competency	6 points	
▷	Theory Question	2 points	

Score calculation: 100 points

− _____ points missed

_____ Score

Satisfactory score: 85 or above

CAAHEP Competencies Achieved
Psychomotor (Skills)
☑ I. 8. Instruct and prepare a patient for a procedure or a treatment.
☑ XII. 3. Use proper body mechanics.
Affective (Behavior)
☑ A. 6. Recognize personal boundaries.

ABHES Competency Achieved
☑ 8. c. Assist provider with general/physical examination.

Notes

Procedure 5-9: Fowler's Position

Name: _____   Date: _____

Evaluated by: _____   Score: _____

Performance Objective

Outcome:	Position and drape an individual in the Fowler's position.
Conditions:	Given the following: a patient gown and a drape.
	Using an examining table.
Standards:	Time: 5 minutes. Student completed procedure in _____ minutes.
	Accuracy: Satisfactory score on the performance evaluation checklist.

Performance Evaluation Checklist

Trial 1	Trial 2	Point Value	Performance Standards
		•	Sanitized hands.
		•	Greeted the patient and introduced yourself.
		•	Identified the patient.
		•	Explained what type of examination or procedure will be performed.
		•	Provided patient with a patient gown.
		•	Instructed patient to remove clothing and to put on a patient gown with the opening in front.
		•	Positioned the head of the table at a 45-degree angle for a -semi-Fowler's position or at a 90-degree angle for a full Fowler's position.
		•	Pulled out the footrest and assisted the patient into a sitting position.
		•	Placed a drape over the patient's thighs and legs.
		•	Pulled out the table extension while supporting the patient's lower legs.
		•	Asked the patient to lean back against the table head.
		•	Provided assistance.
		•	Positioned the drape lengthwise over the patient.
		•	Moved the drape according to the body parts being examined.
		•	Assisted the patient into a sitting position after the examination.
		•	Slid the table extension back into place while supporting the patient's lower legs.
		•	Assisted the patient from the examining table.
		•	Instructed the patient to get dressed.
		•	Returned the head of the table and the footrest to their normal positions.
		•	Discarded the gown and drape in a waste container.

Trial 1	Trial 2	Point Value	Performance Standards
		▷	Stated one use of the Fowler's position.
		■	Recognized personal boundaries.
		★	Completed the procedure within 5 minutes.
			TOTALS

Evaluation of Student Performance

EVALUATION CRITERIA			COMMENTS
Symbol	**Category**	**Point Value**	
★	Critical Step	16 points	
•	Essential Step	6 points	
■	Affective Competency	6 points	
▷	Theory Question	2 points	

Score calculation: 100 points

− _____ points missed

_____ Score

Satisfactory score: 85 or above

CAAHEP Competencies Achieved

Psychomotor (Skills)

☑ I. 8. Instruct and prepare a patient for a procedure or a treatment.
☑ XII. 3. Use proper body mechanics.

Affective (Behavior)

☑ A. 6. Recognize personal boundaries.

ABHES Competency Achieved

☑ 8. c. Assist provider with general/physical examination.

Procedure 5-10: Wheelchair Transfer

Name: _____   Date: _____

Evaluated by: _____   Score: _____

Performance Objective

Outcome:	Transfer a patient from a wheelchair to the examining table and from the examining table to a wheelchair.
Conditions:	Given the following: transfer belt.
	Using an examining table and a wheelchair.
Standards:	Time: 10 minutes. Student completed procedure in _____ minutes.
	Accuracy: Satisfactory score on the performance evaluation checklist.

Performance Evaluation Checklist

Trial 1	Trial 2	Point Value	Performance Standards
			Transferring to the examining table:
		•	Sanitized hands.
		•	Greeted the patient and introduced yourself.
		•	Identified the patient and explained the procedure.
		•	Determined whether the patient has the mental and physical capability to perform the transfer.
		•	Estimated the weight of the patient and whether he or she can assist in the transfer.
		•	Assessed your ability to safely make the transfer.
		•	Wrapped the transfer belt around the patient's waist and fastened it.
		•	The belt was snug with just enough space to allow the fingers to be inserted comfortably.
		▷	Stated why the belt should be snug.
		•	With the patient's stronger side next to the table, positioned the wheelchair at a 45-degree angle to the end of the examining table.
		•	If the table is height-adjustable, adjusted it to the same height as the wheelchair or slightly lower.
		•	If the table is not height-adjustable, pulled out the footrest.
		•	Locked the brakes of the wheelchair.

207

Trial 1	Trial 2	Point Value	Performance Standards
		▷	Stated why the brakes should be locked.
		•	Folded back the wheelchair footrests.
		•	Informed the patient what to do during the transfer.
		•	Made sure the patient's feet were flat on the floor.
		•	Stood in front of the patient with the feet 6 to 8 inches apart, with one foot slightly forward and the knees bent.
		•	Asked the patient to place his or her hands on the armrests of the wheelchair and to lean forward.
		•	Grasped the transfer belt on either side of the patient's waist using an underhand grasp.
		▷	Stated the purpose of the transfer belt.
		•	Instructed the patient to push off the armrests and into a standing position on the count of 3.
		•	Straightened the knees and assisted the patient to a standing position by pulling upward on the transfer belt.
		•	Kept the back straight lifted with the knees, arms, and legs, and not the back.
		•	Pivoted and positioned the patient's buttocks and back of the legs toward the examining table.
		•	Instructed the patient to step backward onto the footrest, one foot at a time.
		•	Gradually lowered the patient into a sitting position on the examining table.
		•	Removed the transfer belt.
		•	Unlocked the wheelchair and moved it out of the way.
		•	Pushed in the footrest of the examining table.
		•	Stayed with the patient to prevent falls.
			Transferring to the wheelchair:
		•	Wrapped the transfer belt snugly around the patient's waist and fastened it.
		•	Positioned the wheelchair at a 45-degree angle to the end of the examining table.
		•	If the table is height-adjustable, adjusted it to the same height as the wheelchair or slightly lower.
		•	If the table is not height-adjustable, pulled out the footrest.
		•	Locked the wheelchair in place and folded back the footrests, if needed.
		•	Informed the patient what to do during the transfer.

Trial 1	Trial 2	Point Value	Performance Standards
		•	Stood in front of the patient with the feet 6 to 8 inches apart, with one foot slightly forward and the knees bent.
		•	Asked the patient to place his or her arms on your shoulders.
		•	Did not allow the patient to place his or her arms around your neck.
		•	Grasped the transfer belt on either side of the patient's waist using an underhand grasp.
		•	Instructed the patient to stand on the count of 3.
		•	Straightened your knees and assisted the patient to a standing position by pulling upward on the transfer belt.
		•	Instructed the patient to step down from the footrest, one foot at a time.
		•	Pivoted the patient until the back of the legs are against the seat of the wheelchair.
		•	Asked the patient to grasp the armrests of the wheelchair.
		•	Gradually lowered the patient into the wheelchair by bending at the knees.
		•	Removed the transfer belt and made sure the patient was -comfortable.
		•	Repositioned the wheelchair footrests and assisted the patient in placing his or her feet in them.
		•	Unlocked the wheelchair.
		•	Pushed in the footrest of the examining table.
		■	Recognized personal boundaries.
		★	Completed the procedure within 10 minutes.
			TOTALS

Evaluation of Student Performance

EVALUATION CRITERIA			COMMENTS
Symbol	**Category**	**Point Value**	
★	Critical Step	16 points	
•	Essential Step	6 points	
■	Affective Competency	6 points	
▷	Theory Question	2 points	

Score calculation; 100 points

− ____ points missed

____Score

Satisfactory score: 85 or above

CAAHEP Competencies Achieved

Psychomotor (Skills)

☑ I. 8. Instruct and prepare a patient for a procedure or a treatment.
☑ XII. 3. Use proper body mechanics.

Affective (Behavior)

☑ A. 6. Recognize personal boundaries.

ABHES Competencies Achieved

☑ 8. c. Assist provider with general/physical examination.
☑ 8. j. Accommodate patients with special needs.

Procedure 5-11: Assisting with the Physical Examination

Name: _____   Date: _____

Evaluated by: _____   Score: _____

Performance Objective

Outcome:	Prepare the patient and assist with a physical examination.
Conditions:	Given the following: equipment for the type of examination to be performed, patient examination gown, and drapes.
	Using an examining table.
Standards:	Time: 20 minutes. Student completed procedure in _____ minutes.
	Accuracy: Satisfactory score on the performance evaluation checklist.

Performance Evaluation Checklist

Trial 1	Trial 2	Point Value	Performance Standards
		•	Prepared examination room.
		•	Sanitized hands.
		•	Assembled all necessary equipment.
		•	Arranged instruments in a neat and orderly manner.
		•	Obtained the patient's medical record.
		•	Went to the waiting room, and asked the patient to come back.
		•	Escorted the patient to the examination room.
		•	Asked the patient to be seated.
		•	Greeted the patient and introduced yourself.
		•	Identified the patient by full name and date of birth.
		▷	Stated why a calm and friendly manner should be used.
		•	Seated yourself facing the patient at a distance of 3 to 4 feet.
		•	Obtained and documented essential patient information on patient allergies, current medications, and patient symptoms.
		•	Measured vital signs and documented results.
		▷	Stated the adult normal range for temperature (97° F to 99° F), pulse (60 to 100 beats/min), respiration (12 to 20 breaths/min), and blood pressure (<120/80 mm Hg).
		•	Measured weight and height, and documented results.
		•	Determined the patient's BMI and documented it in the patient's medical record.
		•	Asked patient if he or she needs to void.

211

Trial 1	Trial 2	Point Value	Performance Standards
		▷	Stated why the patient should be asked to void.
		•	Instructed patient to remove all clothing and put on an examining gown.
		•	Left the room to provide patient with privacy.
		•	Made patient's medical record available to the provider (if using a PPR).
		•	Checked to make sure patient is ready to be seen.
		•	Informed provider that the patient is ready.
			Assisted the provider:
		•	Ensured the patient was in a sitting position on examination table.
		•	Handed the ophthalmoscope to the provider when requested.
		•	Dimmed the lights when the provider was ready to use the ophthalmoscope.
		▷	Stated why the lights are dimmed.
		▷	Stated the proper use of the ophthalmoscope.
		•	Handed the otoscope to the examiner when requested.
		▷	Stated the proper use of the otoscope.
		•	Is able to change the speculum and bulb in the otoscope.
		•	Handed the tongue depressor to the examiner when requested.
		•	Offered reassurance to patient as needed.
		•	Positioned patient as required for examination of the remaining body systems.
			Assisted and instructed patient:
		•	Allowed patient to rest in a sitting position before getting off the examining table.
		▷	Stated why the patient should be allowed to rest before getting off the table.
		•	Assisted patient off the examining table.
		•	Instructed patient to get dressed.
		•	Provided patient with any necessary instructions.
		▷	Stated what type of instructions may need to be relayed to the patient.
		•	Sanitized hands and documented any instructions given to the patient.
		•	Escorted the patient to the reception area.
			Cleaned the examination room:
		•	Discarded paper on the examining table.
		•	Applied gloves and cleaned and disinfected the table.
		•	Unrolled a fresh length of paper on the table.

Trial 1	Trial 2	Point Value	Performance Standards
		•	Discarded all disposable supplies into an appropriate waste container.
		•	Checked to make sure ample supplies are available.
		•	Removed reusable equipment for sanitization, sterilization, or disinfection.
		■	Demonstrated critical thinking skills.
		■	Reassured patients.
		■	Demonstrated empathy for patients' concerns.
		■	Demonstrated active listening.
		■	Respected diversity.
		■	Recognized personal boundaries.
		★	Completed the procedure within 20 minutes.
			TOTALS

CHART

Date	

Evaluation of Student Performance

EVALUATION CRITERIA			COMMENTS
Symbol	**Category**	**Point Value**	
★	Critical Step	16 points	
•	Essential Step	6 points	
■	Affective Competency	6 points	
▷	Theory Question	2 points	

Score calculation: 100 points

− _____ points missed

_____ Score

Satisfactory score: 85 or above

CAAHEP Competencies Achieved

Psychomotor (Skills)

☑ I. 3. Perform patient screening following established protocols.
☑ I. 8. Instruct and prepare a patient for a procedure or a treatment.
☑ I. 9. Assist provider with a patient exam.
☑ Respond to nonverbal communication.
☑ V. 2. Correctly use and pronounce medical terminology in health care interactions.
☑ V. 3. Coach patients regarding: a. office policies b. medical encounters.
☑ VI. 3. Input data using an electronic system.
☑ X. 2. Apply HIPAA rules in regard to (a) privacy (b) release of information.
☑ X. 3. Document patient care accurately in the medical record.
☑ XII. 3. Use proper body mechanics.

Affective (Behavior)

☑ A. 1. Demonstrate critical thinking skills.
☑ A. 2. Reassure patients.
☑ A. 3. Demonstrate empathy for patients' concerns.
☑ A. 4. Demonstrate active listening.
☑ A. 5. Respect diversity.
☑ A. 6. Recognize personal boundaries.

ABHES Competencies Achieved

☑ 4. a. Follow documentation guidelines.
☑ 5. e. Analyze the effect of hereditary, cultural, and environmental influences on behavior.
☑ 7. f. Maintain inventory of equipment and supplies.
☑ 7. g. Display professionalism through written and verbal communications.
☑ 8. b. Obtain and document chief complaint, patient history, and vital signs.
☑ 8. c. Assist provider with general/physical examination.
☑ 8. h. Teach self-examination, disease management and health promotion.
☑ 8. i. Identify community resources and Complementary and Alternative Medicine practices (CAM).

Eye and Ear Assessment and Procedures

CHAPTER ASSIGNMENTS

√ After Completing	Date Due	Study Guide Pages	STUDY GUIDE ASSIGNMENTS (CTA = Critical Thinking Activity)	Possible Points	Points You Earned
		219	Pretest	10	
		220	Key Term Assessment A. Definitions B. Word Parts (Add 1 point for each key term)	14 11	
		221-224	Evaluation of Learning questions	47	
		224	CTA A: Measuring Distance Visual Acuity	6	
		225	CTA B: Interpreting Visual Acuity Results	4	
		225	CTA C: Documenting Visual Acuity Results	4	
		226	CTA D: Ear Procedures	8	
		227	CTA E: Dear Gabby	10	
		228	CTA F: Crossword Puzzle	23	
		229	CTA G: Eye and Ear Conditions	40	
			Evolve: Can You Hear Me Now? (Record points earned)		
			Evolve: Eye-dentify (Record points earned)		
			Evolve: Apply Your Knowledge questions	10	
			Evolve: Video Evaluation	69	
		219	Posttest	10	

√ After Completing	Date Due	Study Guide Pages	STUDY GUIDE ASSIGNMENTS (CTA = Critical Thinking Activity)	Possible Points	Points You Earned
			ADDITIONAL ASSIGNMENTS		
			Total points		

√ When Assigned by Your Instructor	Study Guide Pages	Practices Required	LABORATORY ASSIGNMENTS (Procedure Number and Name)	Score*
	231	5	**Practice for Competency** 6-1: Assessing Distance Visual Acuity—Snellen Chart	
	233-235		**Evaluation of Competency** 6-1: Assessing Distance Visual Acuity—Snellen Chart	*
	231-232	3	**Practice for Competency** 6-2: Assessing Color Vision: Ishihara Test	
	237-239		**Evaluation of Competency** 6-2: Assessing Color Vision: Ishihara Test	*
	231	3	**Practice for Competency** 6-3: Performing an Eye Irrigation	
	241-243		**Evaluation of Competency** 6-3: Performing an Eye Irrigation	*
	231	3	**Practice for Competency** 6-4: Performing an Eye Instillation	
	245-247		**Evaluation of Competency** 6-4: Performing an Eye Instillation	*
	231	3	**Practice for Competency** 6-5: Performing an Ear Irrigation	
	249-251		**Evaluation of Competency** 6-5: Performing an Ear Irrigation	*
	231	3	**Practice for Competency** 6-6: Performing an Ear Instillation	
	253-255		**Evaluation of Competency** 6-6: Performing an Ear Instillation	*
			ADDITIONAL ASSIGNMENTS	

Notes

Name: _____   Date: _____

True or False

_____ 1. Refraction refers to the bending of light rays so that they can be focused on the retina.

_____ 2. A person who is farsighted has a condition known as myopia.

_____ 3. An optometrist can perform eye surgery.

_____ 4. The Snellen eye test is conducted at a distance of 20 feet.

_____ 5. The Snellen eye chart should be positioned at the medical assistant's eye level.

_____ 6. An instillation of antibiotic eye drops may be performed to treat an eye infection.

_____ 7. Conjunctivitis caused by a bacterium is not contagious.

_____ 8. The most specific type of hearing test is the tuning fork test.

_____ 9. Serous otitis media can result in a conductive hearing loss.

_____ 10. An ear instillation may be performed to treat an ear infection.

?≡ **POSTTEST**

True or False

_____ 1. A person who cannot see objects close up has a condition known as amblyopia.

_____ 2. Visual acuity refers to sharpness of vision.

_____ 3. Presbyopia is a decrease in the elasticity of the lens due to the aging process.

_____ 4. An optician fills prescriptions for eyeglasses.

_____ 5. The Snellen Big E chart is used with school-aged children.

_____ 6. The most common color vision defects are congenital in nature.

_____ 7. The external auditory canal of an adult is straightened by pulling the ear downward and backward.

_____ 8. The range of frequencies for normal speech is 300 to 4000 Hz.

_____ 9. Intense noise can result in a sensorineural hearing loss.

_____ 10. Tympanometry is used to diagnose patients with auditory nerve damage.

A. Definitions

Directions: Match each key term with its definition.

_____ 1. Astigmatism

_____ 2. Audiometer

_____ 3. Canthus

_____ 4. Cerumen

_____ 5. Hyperopia

_____ 6. Impacted cerumen

_____ 7. Instillation

_____ 8. Irrigation

_____ 9. Myopia

_____10. Otoscope

_____11. Presbyopia

_____12. Refraction

_____13. Tympanic membrane

_____14. Visual acuity

A. The washing of a body canal with a flowing solution
B. A decrease in the elasticity of the lens that occurs with aging, resulting in a decreased ability to focus on close objects
C. A refractive error in which the light rays are brought to a focus behind the retina resulting in difficulty viewing objects at a reading or working distance.
D. The deflection or bending of light rays by a lens
E. The junction of the eyelids at either corner of the eye
F. A refractive error in which the light rays are brought to a focus in front of the retina resulting in difficulty viewing objects at a distance.
G. The dropping of a liquid into a body cavity
H. An instrument used to examine the external ear canal and tympanic membrane
I. A yellowish waxy substance secreted by the glands in the ear canal.
J. An instrument used to quantitatively measure hearing acuity for the various frequencies of sound waves
K. A thin, semitransparent membrane located between the external ear canal and the middle ear that receives and transmits sound waves
L. A refractive error that causes distorted and blurred vision for both near and far objects due to a cornea that is oval shaped
M. Cerumen that is wedged firmly together in the ear canal so as to be immovable.
N. Acuteness or sharpness of vision.

B. Word Parts

Directions: Indicate the meaning of each word part in the space provided. List as many medical terms as possible that incorporate the word part in the space provided.

Word Part	Meaning of Word Part	Medical Terms That Incorporate Word Part
1. a-		
2. stigm/a		
3. -ism		
4. audi/o		
5. -meter		
6. hyper-		
7. -opia		
8. ot/o		
9. -scope		
10. tympan/o		
11. -ic		

Directions: Fill in each blank with the correct answer.

1. What is the name of the tough white outer layer of the eye?

   _____

2. What is the function of the following structures that make up the choroid?

   a. Blood vessels: _____

   b. Pigment: _____

3. What is the function of the muscles making up the ciliary body?

   _____

4. What is the function of the lens?

   _____

5. What is the function of the iris?

   _____

6. What is the function of the retina?

   _____

7. What parts of the eye are covered with conjunctiva?

   _____

8. What is visual acuity?

   _____

9. What type of vision does a person with normal visual acuity have?

   _____

10. What is an error of refraction?

   _____

11. How does myopia cause an error of refraction?

   _____

12. What type of symptoms might be experienced with myopia?

   _____

   _____

13. How does hyperopia cause an error of refraction?

   _____

14. What methods can be used to correct myopia?

   _____

15. What causes an individual with astigmatism to have distorted and blurred vision?

_____

16. What is presbyopia and when does it begin to occur?

_____

_____

17. Describe what each of the following eye specialists is qualified to perform.

a. Ophthalmologist

_____

_____

b. Optometrist

_____

_____

c. Optician

_____

_____

18. What condition can be detected by measuring distance visual acuity?

_____

19. What type of patient would warrant use of the Snellen Big E eye chart? (Give two examples.)

_____

20. Explain the significance of number above the line and the number below the line next to each line of letters on the Snellen eye chart.

Above the line: _____

Below the line: _____

21. List two conditions that can be detected by measuring near visual acuity.

_____

22. What does the line marked 20/20 indicate on the Snellen eye chart?

_____

23. Explain the difference between congenital and acquired color vision defects.

_____

_____

24. What is a polychromatic plate?

_____

_____

25. List three reasons for performing eye irrigation.

_____

_____

26. List three reasons for performing eye instillation.

_____

_____

27. What are the three divisions of the ear?

_____

28. What is the function of the ear auricle?

_____

_____

29. What is the function of cerumen?

_____

30. Explain why the external auditory canal must be straightened when viewing it with an otoscope.

_____

31. What is the normal appearance of the tympanic membrane?

_____

32. What are the names of the three small bones located in the middle ear?

_____

33. What is the purpose of the eustachian tube?

_____

34. What is the function of the semicircular canals?

_____

35. What is the range of frequencies for normal speech?

_____

36. What causes conductive hearing loss?

_____

37. List five conditions that may cause conductive hearing loss.

_____

_____

38. What causes sensorineural hearing loss?

_____

Chapter 6 Eye and Ear Assessment and Procedures

39. List four conditions that may result in sensorineural hearing loss.

_____

_____

40. What are the two types of hearing tests that can be performed with tuning forks?

_____

41. What information is obtained through audiometry?

_____

42. What information is obtained through tympanometry?

_____

_____

43. List three reasons for performing ear irrigation.

_____

_____

44. When should an ear irrigation not be performed and why?

_____

45. Explain how impacted cerumen is removed from the ear.

_____

_____

46. List three reasons for performing ear instillation.

_____

_____

47. Explain how to straighten the external auditory canal in an adult and in children 3 years old or younger.

Adult: _____

Children (3 years old or younger): _____

CRITICAL THINKING ACTIVITIES

A. Measuring Distance Visual Acuity

For each of the following situations, write **C** if the technique is correct and **I** if the technique is incorrect.

_____ 1. The patient is not given an opportunity to study the Snellen chart before beginning the test.

_____ 2. The Snellen chart is positioned at the medical assistant's eye level.

_____ 3. The patient is instructed to use his or her hand to cover the eye that is not being tested.

_____ 4. The medical assistant instructs the patient to close the eye that is not being tested.

_____ 5. The first line that the medical assistant asks the patient to identify is the 20/20 line.

_____ 6. The medical assistant observes the patient for signs of squinting or leaning forward during the test.

224

B. Interpreting Visual Acuity Results

1. A patient has a distance visual acuity reading of 20/30 in the right eye. Using this information, answer the following questions:

   a. How far was the patient from the eye chart?

   _____

   b. At what distance would a person with normal acuity be able to read this line?

   _____

2. A patient has a distance visual acuity reading of 20/10 in the left eye. Using this information, answer the following questions:

   a. How far was the patient from the eye chart?

   _____

   b. At what distance would a person with normal acuity be able to read this line?

   _____

C. Documenting Visual Acuity Results

Properly document the distance visual acuity results in the spaces provided. In all cases, the line indicated is the smallest line the patient could read at a distance of 20 feet.

1. The patient read the line marked 20/30 with the right eye with two errors; with the left eye, the patient read the line marked 20/30 with one error. The patient was wearing corrective lenses.

   _____

   _____

2. The patient read the line marked 20/20 with the right eye with one error; with the left eye, the patient read the line marked 20/20 with no errors. The patient was wearing corrective lenses.

   _____

   _____

3. The patient read the line marked 20/40 with the right eye with two errors; with the left eye, the patient read the line marked 20/30 with one error. The patient exhibited squinting and frowning during the test. The patient was not wearing corrective lenses.

   _____

   _____

4. The patient read the line marked 20/15 with the right eye with no errors; with the left eye, the patient read the line marked 20/20 with one error. The patient was not wearing corrective lenses.

   _____

   _____

D. Ear Procedures

Explain the principle for each of the following procedures.

Ear Irrigation

1. Positioning the patient's head so that it is tilted toward the affected ear

   _____

   _____

2. Cleansing the outer ear before irrigating

   _____

   _____

3. Straightening the external auditory canal

   _____

   _____

4. Injecting the irrigating solution toward the roof of the ear canal

   _____

   _____

5. Making sure not to obstruct the canal opening

   _____

   _____

Ear Instillation

6. Positioning the patient's head so that it is tilted toward the unaffected ear

   _____

   _____

7. Instructing the patient to lie on the unaffected side after the instillation

   _____

   _____

8. Placing a cotton wick in the patient's ear

   _____

   _____

E. Dear Gabby

Gabby has a middle ear infection and is not feeling well. She wants you to fill in for her. In the space provided, respond to the following letter.

Dear Gabby:

I am dating the sweetest and dearest man. "Mike" has only one flaw. He likes loud music. He had a powerful stereo sound system installed in his car. When we drive somewhere in his car, he blasts the music. Sometimes, when we are driving down a street, people even turn around to see where the loud music is coming from. The music hurts my ears, and I cannot think straight. My ears even start ringing when we go on a trip. When I am talking to Mike, he says I mumble, and I have to speak extra loud around him. I keep telling Mike that the loud music is going to damage our hearing, but he says that we are way too young for that and that only old people have trouble hearing. Please help me, Gabby, because I love going on trips with Mike, but not if my ears hurt afterward.

Signed, Ears Are Ringing

_____
_____
_____
_____
_____
_____
_____
_____
_____
_____

F. Crossword Puzzle: Eye and Ear

Directions: Complete the crossword puzzle using the clues provided.

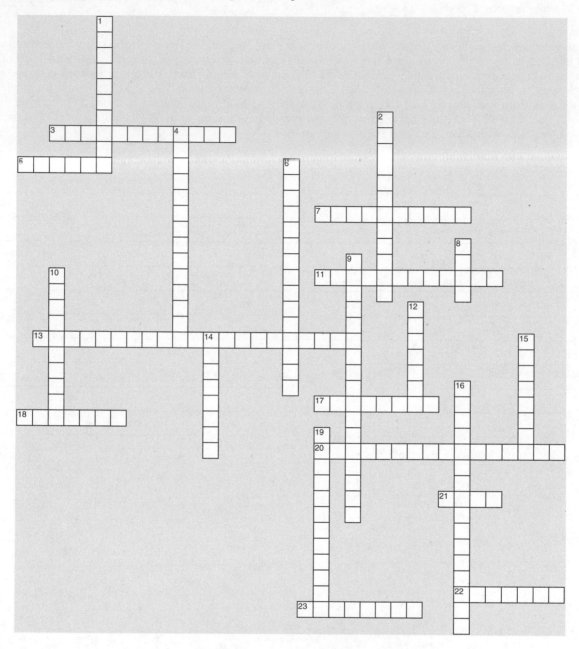

Across

3 Assessment of mobility of eardrum
5 Cannot see far away
7 Caught it!
11 Normal DVA
13 Impacted cerumen may cause this
17 Fills eyeglasses prescriptions
18 Earwax
20 Drum in your ear
21 Eye chart for preschoolers
22 Loudness of sound measurement
23 Color blindness test

Down

1 Decreased lens elasticity
2 Sharpness of vision
4 Stabilizes ear pressure
6 Physician who diagnoses and treats eye disorders
8 Focuses light rays on retina
9 Fluid in middle ear
10 Instrument that measures hearing
12 Organ of hearing
14 Straighten this before ear irrigation
15 A cause of pink eye
16 Middle ear infection
19 Fixed stapes

G. Eye and Ear Conditions

1. You and your classmates work at a large clinic. It is National Eye and Ear Week. The providers at your clinic ask you and your classmates to develop and design informative, creative, and colorful brochures about eye and ear conditions. Each student should select a different condition from the list below. On a separate sheet of paper, write 5 true or false questions related to the information in your brochure.

2. Present your brochure to the class. After all the brochures have been presented, each student should ask their questions to the class to see how well they understand eye and ear conditions. (*Note:* You can take notes during the presentations and refer to them when answering the questions.)

Eye
1. Amblyopia (lazy eye)
2. Age-related macular degeneration
3. Astigmatism
4. Blepharitis
5. Cataracts
6. CMV retinitis
7. Corneal ulcer
8. Corneal abrasion
9. Strabismus (cross-eyed)
10. Diabetic retinopathy
11. Drooping eyelids (ptosis)
12. Dry eyes
13. Floaters and spots
14. Glaucoma
15. Keratoconus
16. Ocular hypertension
17. Retinal detachment
18. Retinitis pigmentosa
19. Stye

Ear
1. Acute mastoiditis
2. External otitis
3. Meniere's disease
4. Noise-induced hearing loss
5. Presbycusis
6. Serous otitis media

Notes

Eye Assessment and Procedures

Procedure 6-1: Distance Visual Acuity

Assess distance visual acuity using a Snellen eye chart, and document results in the chart provided. Circle any readings that indicate distance visual acuity above or below average.

Procedure 6-2: Color Vision

Assess color vision, and document results in the Ishihara charting grid provided. Circle any abnormal results.

Procedure 6-3: Eye Irrigation

Perform an eye irrigation, and document the procedure in the chart provided.

Procedure 6-4: Eye Instillation

Perform an eye instillation, and document the procedure in the chart provided.

Ear Procedures

Procedure 6-5: Ear Irrigation

Perform an ear irrigation, and document the procedure in the chart provided.

Procedure 6-6: Ear Instillation

Perform an ear instillation, and document the procedure in the chart provided.

Chart	
Date	

DOCUMENTATION GRID FOR THE ISHIHARA TEST

Plate No.	Normal Person	Results
1	12	
2	8	
3	5	
4	29	
5	74	
6	7	
7	45	
8	2	
9	X	
10	16	
11	Traceable	
Date:		
Evaluated by:		

DOCUMENTATION GRID FOR THE ISHIHARA TEST

Plate No.	Normal Person	Results
1	12	
2	8	
3	5	
4	29	
5	74	
6	7	
7	45	
8	2	
9	X	
10	16	
11	Traceable	
Date:		
Evaluated by:		

Procedure 6-1: Assessing Distance Visual Acuity—Snellen Chart

Name: _____ Date: _____

Evaluated by: _____ Score: _____

Performance Objective

Outcome:	Assess distance visual acuity.
Conditions:	Given the following: Snellen eye chart, eye occluder, and an antiseptic wipe.
Standards:	Time: 5 minutes. Student completed procedure in _____ minutes.
	Accuracy: Satisfactory score on the Performance Evaluation Checklist.

Performance Evaluation Checklist

Trial 1	Trial 2	Point Value	Performance Standards
		•	Sanitized hands.
		•	Assembled equipment.
		•	Disinfected the eye occluder with an antiseptic wipe.
		•	Greeted the patient and introduced yourself.
		•	Identified the patient and explained the procedure.
		•	Determined whether the patient wears corrective lenses and instructed patient to leave them on during the test.
		•	Positioned patient 20 feet from the eye chart.
		•	Positioned the center of the eye chart at patient's eye level.
		•	Instructed patient to cover the left eye with the occluder and to keep the left eye open.
		▷	Stated how the occluder should be positioned if the patient wears glasses.
		▷	Explained why the patient's left eye should remain open.
		•	Instructed patient not to squint during the test.
		▷	Explained why the patient should not squint during the test.
		•	Asked patient to identify the 20/70 line, using the right eye.
		▷	Stated why the test should begin with a line that is above the 20/20 line.
		•	Proceeded down the chart if the patient identified the 20/70 line or proceeded up the chart if the patient was unable to identify the 20/70 line.
		•	Continued until the smallest line of letters that the patient could read was reached.
		•	Observed patient for any unusual symptoms.
		•	Jotted down the numbers next to the smallest line read by the patient.
		•	Asked patient to cover the right eye and to keep the right eye open.
		•	Measured visual acuity in the left eye.

233

Trial 1	Trial 2	Point Value	Performance Standards
		•	Jotted down the numbers next to the smallest line read by the patient.
		★	The visual acuity measurements were identical to the evaluator's measurements.
		•	Documented the results correctly.
		•	Disinfected the occluder with an antiseptic wipe.
		•	Sanitized hands.
		■	Demonstrated critical thinking skills.
		★	Completed the procedure within 5 minutes.
			Totals

CHART

Date	

Evaluation of Student Performance

EVALUATION CRITERIA			COMMENTS
Symbol	**Category**	**Point Value**	
★	Critical Step	16 points	
•	Essential Step	6 points	
■	Affective Competency	6 points	
▷	Theory Question	2 points	

Score calculation: 100 points

− ___ points missed

___ Score

Satisfactory score: 85 or above

CAAHEP Competencies Achieved

Psychomotor (Skills)
☑ I. 8. Instruct and prepare a patient for a procedure or a treatment.

Affective (Behavior)
☑ A. 1. Demonstrated critical thinking skills.

ABHES Competencies Achieved

☑ 4. a. Follow documentation guidelines.
☑ 8. e. Perform specialty procedures, including but not limited to pediatric care, minor surgery, cardiac, respiratory, OB-GYN, neurological, and gastroenterology.

Notes

Procedure 6-2: Assessing Color Vision—Ishihara Test

Name: _____   Date: _____

Evaluated by: _____   Score: _____

Performance Objective

Outcome:	Assess color vision.
Conditions:	Given an Ishihara book of color plates and a cotton swab.
Standards:	Time: 10 minutes. Student completed procedure in _____ minutes.
	Accuracy: Satisfactory score on the Performance Evaluation Checklist.

Performance Evaluation Checklist

Trial 1	Trial 2	Point Value	Performance Standards
		•	Sanitized hands.
		•	Assembled equipment.
		•	Conducted the test in a quiet room illuminated by natural daylight.
		▷	Stated why natural daylight should be used.
		•	Greeted the patient and introduced yourself.
		•	Identified the patient.
		•	Explained the procedure using the practice plate.
		▷	Stated the purpose of the practice plate.
		•	Held the first plate 30 inches from the patient at a right angle to the patient's line of vision.
		•	Instructed patient to keep both eyes open.
		•	Told patient that he or she would have 3 seconds to identify each plate.
		•	Asked the patient to identify the number on the plate.
		•	Asked the patient to trace plates that have a winding line with a cotton swab.
		▷	Stated why a cotton swab should be used to make the tracing.
		•	Documented the results after identification of each plate.
		•	Continued until the patient viewed all plates.
		•	Documented the results correctly.
		★	The results were identical to the evaluator's results.
		•	Returned the Ishihara book to its proper place, storing it in a closed position.
		▷	Explained why the book should be stored in a closed position.

Trial 1	Trial 2	Point Value	Performance Standards
		■	Demonstrated critical thinking skills.
		★	Completed the procedure within 10 minutes.
			Totals

CHART		
Plate No.	Normal Person	Results
1	12	
2	8	
3	5	
4	29	
5	74	
6	7	
7	45	
8	2	
9	X	
10	16	
11	Traceable	
Date:		
Evaluated by:		

Evaluation of Student Performance

EVALUATION CRITERIA			COMMENTS
Symbol	**Category**	**Point Value**	
★	Critical Step	16 points	
•	Essential Step	6 points	
■	Affective Competency	6 points	
▷	Theory Question	2 points	

Score calculation: 100 points

− _____ points missed

_____ Score

Satisfactory score: 85 or above

CAAHEP Competencies Achieved

Psychomotor (Skills)
☑ I. 8. Instruct and prepare a patient for a procedure or a treatment.

Affective (Behavior)
☑ A. 1. Demonstrate critical thinking skills.

ABHES Competencies Achieved

☑ 4. a. Follow documentation guidelines.
☑ 8. e. Perform specialty procedures, including but not limited to pediatric care, minor surgery, cardiac, respiratory, OB-GYN, neurological, and gastroenterology.

Notes

Procedure 6-3: Performing an Eye Irrigation

Name: _____ Date: _____

Evaluated by: _____ Score: _____

Performance Objective

Outcome:	Perform an eye irrigation.
Conditions:	Given the following: disposable gloves, irrigating solution, solution container, disposable rubber bulb syringe, basin, moisture-resistant towel, and sterile gauze pads.
Standards:	Time: 5 minutes. Student completed procedure in _____ minutes.
	Accuracy: Satisfactory score on the Performance Evaluation Checklist.

Performance Evaluation Checklist

Trial 1	Trial 2	Point Value	Performance Standards
		•	Sanitized hands.
		•	Assembled equipment.
		•	Checked the solution label with the provider's instructions.
		•	Checked expiration date of the solution.
		▷	Stated the reason for checking the expiration date.
		•	Warmed the irrigating solution to body temperature.
		▷	Explained why the solution should be at body temperature.
		•	Checked the label a second time and poured the solution into a basin.
		•	Checked the label a third time before returning the container to storage.
		•	Greeted the patient and introduced yourself.
		•	Identified the patient and explained the procedure.
		•	Asked patient to remove glasses or contact lenses.
		•	Positioned patient in a sitting or lying position.
		•	Placed a moisture-resistant towel on the patient's shoulder.
		•	Positioned a basin tightly against the patient's cheek under the affected eye.
		•	Asked the patient to tilt head in the direction of the affected eye and hold the basin in place.
		▷	Explained why the patient's head is turned in the direction of the affected eye.
		•	Applied gloves.
		•	Cleansed the eyelids from inner to outer canthus.
		▷	Stated why eyelids are cleansed.
		•	Filled irrigating syringe.
		•	Instructed patient to keep both eyes open and to look at a focal point.

Trial 1	Trial 2	Point Value	Performance Standards
		▷	Stated the reason for looking at a focal point.
		•	Separated eyelids.
		•	Held tip of syringe 1 inch above the eye at the inner canthus.
		•	Allowed solution to flow over the eye at a moderate rate from the inner canthus to the outer canthus and directed solution to the lower conjunctiva.
		▷	Explained why the syringe should be directed toward the lower conjunctiva.
		'	Did not allow syringe to touch the eye.
		•	Refilled the syringe and continued irrigating until the desired results were obtained or all the solution was used.
		•	Dried the eyelids with a gauze pad from inner to outer canthus.
		•	Removed gloves and sanitized hands.
		•	Documented the procedure correctly.
		•	Returned equipment.
		■	Demonstrated critical thinking skills.
		■	Reassured patients.
		■	Demonstrated empathy for patients' concerns.
		★	Completed the procedure within 5 minutes.
			Totals

CHART

Date	

Evaluation of Student Performance

EVALUATION CRITERIA			COMMENTS
Symbol	**Category**	**Point Value**	
★	Critical Step	16 points	
•	Essential Step	6 points	
■	Affective Competency	6 points	
▷	Theory Question	2 points	

Score calculation: 100 points

     –   points missed

         ___Score

Satisfactory score: 85 or above

CAAHEP Competencies Achieved

Psychomotor (Skills)
- ☑ I. 8. Instruct and prepare a patient for a procedure or a treatment.
- ☑ II. 1. Calculate proper dosages of medication for administration.
- ☑ X.3. Document patient care accurately in the medical record.

Affective (Behavior)
- ☑ A. 1. Demonstrate critical thinking skills.
- ☑ A. 2. Reassure patients.
- ☑ A. 3. Demonstrate empathy for patients' concerns.

ABHES Competencies Achieved

- ☑ 2. c. Identify diagnostic and treatment modalities as they relate to each body system.
- ☑ 4. a. Follow documentation guidelines.
- ☑ 8. e. Perform specialty procedures, but not limited to pediatric care, minor surgery, cardiac, respiratory, OB-GYN, neurological, and gastroenterology.

Notes

Procedure 6-4: Performing an Eye Instillation

Name: _____   Date: _____

Evaluated by: _____   Score: _____

Performance Objective

Outcome:	Perform an eye instillation.
Conditions:	Given the following: disposable gloves, ophthalmic medication, tissues, and gauze pads.
Standards:	Time: 5 minutes. Student completed procedure in _____ minutes.
	Accuracy: Satisfactory score on the Performance Evaluation Checklist.

Performance Evaluation Checklist

Trial 1	Trial 2	Point Value	Performance Standards
		•	Sanitized hands.
		•	Assembled equipment.
		•	Checked the drug label when removing it from storage.
		▷	Stated what word must appear on the medication label.
		•	Checked drug label and dosage against the provider's instructions.
		•	Checked the expiration date of the medication.
		•	Greeted the patient and introduced yourself.
		•	Identified the patient and explained the procedure.
		•	Positioned patient in a sitting or supine position.
		•	Applied gloves.
		•	Prepared the medication.
		•	Checked the drug label and removed the cap.
		•	Asked patient to look up and exposed the lower conjunctival sac.
		▷	Explained the reason for asking patient to look up.
		•	Drew the skin of the cheek downward and exposed the conjunctival sac.
		•	Inserted the medication correctly.
		▷	Explained how to instill eye drops and eye ointment.
		•	Instructed the patient to close his or her eyes gently and move the eyeballs.
		▷	Stated the reason for closing the eyes and moving the eyeballs.
		•	Told the patient that the instillation may temporarily blur vision.
		•	Dried the eyelids with a gauze pad from inner to outer canthus.

Trial 1	Trial 2	Point Value	Performance Standards
		•	Removed gloves and sanitized hands.
		•	Documented the procedure correctly.
		•	Returned equipment.
		■	Demonstrated critical thinking skills.
		■	Reassured patients.
		■	Demonstrated empathy for patients' concerns.
		★	Completed the procedure within 5 minutes.
			Totals

CHART	
Date	

Evaluation of Student Performance

EVALUATION CRITERIA			COMMENTS
Symbol	**Category**	**Point Value**	
★	Critical Step	16 points	
•	Essential Step	6 points	
■	Affective Competency	6 points	
▷	Theory Question	2 points	

Score calculation: 100 points

      −   points missed

      ___Score

Satisfactory score: 85 or above

CAAHEP Competencies Achieved

Psychomotor (Skills)
- ☑ I. 8. Instruct and prepare a patient for a procedure or a treatment.
- ☑ II. 1. Calculate proper dosages of medication for administration.
- ☑ X.3. Document patient care accurately in the medical record.

Affective (Behavior)
- ☑ A. 1. Demonstrate critical thinking skills.
- ☑ A. 2. Reassure patients.
- ☑ A. 3. Demonstrate empathy for patients' concerns.

ABHES Competencies Achieved

- ☑ 2. c. Identify diagnostic and treatment modalities as they relate to each body system.
- ☑ 4. a. Follow documentation guidelines.
- ☑ 8. e. Perform specialty procedures, including including but not limited to pediatric care, minor surgery, cardiac, respiratory, OB-GYN, neurological, and gastroenterology.

Notes

Procedure 6-5: Performing an Ear Irrigation

Name: _____   Date: _____

Evaluated by: _____   Score: _____

Performance Objective

Outcome:	Perform an ear irrigation.
Conditions:	Given the following: disposable gloves, irrigating solution, solution basin, bath thermometer, ear irrigating syringe or Elephant Ear Wash System, ear basin, moisture-resistant towel, gauze pads, and ear wick.
Standards:	Time: 10 minutes. Student completed procedure in _____ minutes. Accuracy: Satisfactory score on the Performance Evaluation Checklist.

Performance Evaluation Checklist

Trial 1	Trial 2	Point Value	Performance Standards
		•	Sanitized hands.
		•	Assembled equipment.
		•	Checked the label of the irrigating solution with the provider's instructions.
		•	Checked expiration date of the solution.
		•	Warmed the irrigating solution to body temperature.
		•	Used a bath thermometer to make sure the temperature of the water did not exceed body temperature.
		▷	Stated the reason for warming the irrigating solution.
		•	Checked the label a second time and poured the solution: a. Irrigating syringe: Poured the solution into the basin and replaced the cap without contaminating it. Covered the basin to keep it warm. b. Elephant system: Removed the top of the spray bottle and poured the solution into the bottle and replaced the top of the spray bottle.
		•	Checked the label a third time before returning the container to storage.
		•	Greeted the patient and introduced yourself.
		•	Identified the patient and explained the procedure.
		•	Positioned the patient in a sitting position.
		•	Placed a towel on the patient's shoulder under the ear to be irrigated.
		•	Positioned a basin under the affected ear and asked the patient to hold it in place.
		•	Asked the patient to tilt his or her head toward the affected ear.
		▷	Explained why the head should be tilted toward the affected ear.
		•	Applied gloves.
		•	Cleansed the outer ear.

Trial 1	Trial 2	Point Value	Performance Standards
		▷	Explained why the outer ear should be cleansed.

		•	Filled the irrigating syringe:
			  a. Irrigating syringe: Filled the syringe with the irrigating solution and expelled air from the syringe.
			  b. Elephant system: Twisted a disposable tip onto the nozzle of the tube, making sure to screw it firmly into place.

		▷	Explained why air should be expelled from the irrigating syringe.
		•	Properly straightened the ear canal.
		▷	Stated why the canal must be straightened.
		•	Inserted the tip of the irrigating device into the ear.
		•	Did not insert the tip of the irrigating device too deeply.
		•	Made sure that the tip of the syringe did not obstruct the canal opening.
		▷	Stated why the canal should not be obstructed.

		•	Performed the irrigation:
			  a. Irrigating syringe: Injected the irrigating solution toward the roof of the ear canal by slowly depressing the plunger of the syringe.
			  b. Elephant system: Sprayed the irrigating solution toward the roof of the ear canal by depressing the trigger handle and made sure to keep the tubing straight.

		▷	Stated why solution should be injected toward the roof of the canal.
		•	Continued irrigating until the desired results were obtained or all the solution was used.
		•	Observed the returning solution to note the material present and the amount.
		•	Dried outside of the ear with a gauze pad.
		•	Informed the patient that the ear will feel sensitive for a short time.
		•	Instructed the patient to lie on the affected side on the treatment table.
		▷	Explained why the patient should lie on the affected side.
		•	Inserted a cotton wick loosely in the ear canal for 15 minutes.
		▷	Stated the purpose of the cotton wick.
		•	Removed gloves and sanitized hands.
		•	Documented the procedure correctly.
		•	Returned equipment.
		■	Demonstrated critical thinking skills.
		■	Reassured patients.
		■	Demonstrated empathy for patients' concerns.
		★	Completed the procedure within 10 minutes.
			Totals

CHART	
Date	

Evaluation of Student Performance

EVALUATION CRITERIA			COMMENTS
Symbol	**Category**	**Point Value**	
★	Critical Step	16 points	
•	Essential Step	6 points	
■	Affective Competency	6 points	
▷	Theory Question	2 points	

Score calculation: 100 points

$-$ _____ points missed

_____ Score

Satisfactory score: 85 or above

CAAHEP Competencies Achieved

Psychomotor (Skills)
- ☑ I. 8. Instruct and prepare a patient for a procedure or a treatment.
- ☑ II. 1. Calculate proper dosages of medication for administration.
- ☑ X.3. Document patient care accurately in the medical record.

Affective (Behavior)
- ☑ A. 1. Demonstrate critical thinking skills.
- ☑ Reassured patients.
- ☑ A. 3. Demonstrate empathy for patients' concerns.

ABHES Competencies Achieved

- ☑ 2. c. Identify diagnostic and treatment modalities as they relate to each body system.
- ☑ 4. a. Follow documentation guidelines.
- ☑ 8. e. Perform specialty procedures, including but not limited to pediatric care, minor surgery, cardiac, respiratory, OB-GYN, neurological, and gastroenterology.

Notes

Chapter **6** **Eye and Ear Assessment and Procedures**

Procedure 6-6: Performing an Ear Instillation

Name: _____   Date: _____

Evaluated by: _____   Score: _____

Performance Objective

Outcome:	Perform an ear instillation.
Conditions:	Given the following: disposable gloves, otic drops, and gauze pad.
Standards:	Time: 5 minutes. Student completed procedure in _____ minutes.
	Accuracy: Satisfactory score on the Performance Evaluation Checklist.

Performance Evaluation Checklist

Trial 1	Trial 2	Point Value	Performance Standards
		•	Sanitized hands.
		•	Assembled equipment.
		•	Checked the drug label when removing the medication from storage.
		▷	Stated what word must appear on the medication label.
		•	Checked the drug label and dosage against the provider's instructions.
		•	Checked the expiration date of the medication.
		▷	Explained what might occur if the medication is outdated.
		•	Greeted the patient and introduced yourself.
		•	Identified the patient and explained the procedure.
		•	Positioned patient in a sitting position.
		•	Warmed the eardrops with your hands.
		•	Applied gloves.
		•	Mixed medication if required, by shaking the container.
		•	Checked the drug label and removed the cap.
		•	Asked the patient to tilt the head in the direction of the unaffected ear.
		•	Properly straightened the ear canal.
		▷	Stated the reason for straightening the canal.
		•	Placed tip of dropper at the opening of the ear canal and inserted the proper amount of medication.
		•	Did not touch the tip of the dropper to the ear.
		•	Instructed the patient to lie on the unaffected side for 2 to 3 minutes.
		▷	Explained why the patient should lie on the unaffected side.

Trial 1	Trial 2	Point Value	Performance Standards
		•	Placed a moistened cotton wick loosely in the ear canal for 15 minutes.
		▷	Stated the reason for moistening the wick.
		•	Removed gloves and sanitized hands.
		•	Documented the procedure correctly.
		•	Returned equipment.
		■	Incorporated critical thinking skills when performing patient care.
		■	Showed awareness of a patient's concerns related to the procedure being performed.
		■	Explained to a patient the rationale for performance of a procedure.
		★	Completed the procedure within 5 minutes.
			Totals

CHART	
Date	

Evaluation of Student Performance

EVALUATION CRITERIA			COMMENTS
Symbol	**Category**	**Point Value**	
★	Critical Step	16 points	
•	Essential Step	6 points	
■	Affective Competency	6 points	
▷	Theory Question	2 points	

Score calculation: 100 points

    −   points missed

        Score

Satisfactory score: 85 or above

Psychomotor (Skills)
☑ I. 8. Instruct and prepare a patient for a procedure or a treatment.
☑ II. 1. Calculate proper dosages of medication for administration.
☑ X.3. Document patient care accurately in the medical record.

Affective (Behavior)
☑ I. 2. Incorporate critical thinking skills when performing patient care.
☑ I. 3. Show awareness of a patient's concerns related to the procedure being performed.
☑ V. 4. Explain to a patient the rationale for performance of a procedure.

ABHES Competencies Achieved

☑ 2. c. Identify diagnostic and treatment modalities as they relate to each body system.
☑ 4. a. Follow documentation guidelines.
☑ 8. e. Perform specialty procedures, but not limited to minor surgery, cardiac, respiratory, OB-GYN, neurological, and gastroenterology.

7 Physical Agents to Promote Tissue Healing

CHAPTER ASSIGNMENTS

√ After Completing	Date Due	Study Guide Pages	STUDY GUIDE ASSIGNMENTS (CTA = Critical Thinking Activity)	Possible Points	Points You Earned
		261	📋 Pretest	10	
		262	🔑 Term Key Term Assessment	16	
		262-266	📑 Evaluation of Learning questions	34	
		266	CTA A: Dear Gabby	10	
		266-267	CTA B: Cast Care	20	
		269	CTA C: Crutch Guidelines	8	
		270	CTA D: Accessibility for Physical Disabilities	7	
		271	CTA E: Crossword Puzzle	26	
		272-274	CTA F: Bone and Joint Conditions	40	
			Evolve: Quiz Show (Record points earned)		
			Evolve: Apply Your Knowledge questions	10	
			Evolve: Video Evaluation	63	
		261	📋 Posttest	10	
			ADDITIONAL ASSIGNMENTS		
			Total points		

√ When Assigned by Your Instructor	Study Guide Page(s)	Practices Required	LABORATORY ASSIGNMENTS (Procedure Number and Name)	Score*
	275-276	3	**Practice for Competency** 7-1: Applying a Heating Pad	
	277-278		**Evaluation of Competency** 7-1: Applying a Heating Pad	*
	275-276	3	**Practice for Competency** 7-2: Applying a Hot Soak	
	279-281		**Evaluation of Competency** 7-2: Applying a Hot Soak	*
	275-276	3	**Practice for Competency** 7-3: Applying a Hot Compress	
	283-285		**Evaluation of Competency** 7-3: Applying a Hot Compress	*
	275-276	3	**Practice for Competency** 7-4: Applying an Ice Bag	
	287-288		**Evaluation of Competency** 7-4: Applying an Ice Bag	*
	275-276	3	**Practice for Competency** 7-5: Applying a Cold Compress	
	289-290		**Evaluation of Competency** 7-5: Applying a Cold Compress	*
	275-276	3	**Practice for Competency** 7-6: Applying a Chemical Pack	
	291-292		**Evaluation of Competency** 7-6: Applying a Chemical Pack	*
	275-276	3	**Practice for Competency** 7-A: Applying a Gel Pack	
	293-294		**Evaluation of Competency** 7-A: Applying a Gel Pack	*
	275-276	3	**Practice for Competency** 7-7: Measuring for Axillary Crutches	
	295-296		**Evaluation of Competency** 7-7: Measuring for Axillary Crutches	*
	275-276	3 × for each gait	**Practice for Competency** 7-8: Instructing a Patient in Crutch Gaits	
	297-299		**Evaluation of Competency** 7-8: Instructing a Patient in Crutch Gaits	*

Chapter **7 Physical Agents to Promote Tissue Healing**

√ When Assigned by Your Instructor	Study Guide Page(s)	Practices Required	LABORATORY ASSIGNMENTS (Procedure Number and Name)	Score*
	275-276	Cane: 3 Walker: 3	**Practice for Competency** 7-9 and 7-10: Instructing a Patient in the Use of a Cane and Walker	
	301-302		**Evaluation of Competency** 7-9 and 7-10: Instructing a Patient in the Use of a Cane and Walker	*
			ADDITIONAL ASSIGNMENTS	

Name: _____ Date: _____

True or False

_____ 1. A hot compress is an example of moist heat.

_____ 2. Erythema is redness of the skin caused by dilation of superficial blood vessels.

_____ 3. The local application of cold may be used to relieve muscle spasms.

_____ 4. Chemical cold packs should be stored in the refrigerator.

_____ 5. An orthodontist is a physician who specializes in the diagnosis and treatment of disorders of the musculo-skeletal system.

_____ 6. The most frequent reason for applying a cast is to aid in the nonsurgical correction of a deformity.

_____ 7. Numbness of the fingers or toes may indicate that a cast is too tight.

_____ 8. A coat hanger can be used to scratch under a cast, if itching occurs.

_____ 9. Ambulation refers to the inability to walk.

_____ 10. A patient using crutches should be instructed to support his or her weight on the axilla.

POSTTEST

True or False

_____ 1. The recommended time for the application of heat is 15 to 30 minutes.

_____ 2. The local application of heat results in constriction of blood vessels in the area to which it is applied.

_____ 3. The most frequent cause of low back pain is poor posture.

_____ 4. An ice bag should be filled with large pieces of ice.

_____ 5. If axillary crutches have been fitted properly, the elbow will be flexed at an angle of 30 degrees.

_____ 6. A wet cast can cause a pressure area to occur.

_____ 7. The purpose of cast padding is to prevent pressure areas.

_____ 8. It usually takes 10 to 12 weeks for a fracture to heal.

_____ 9. Incorrectly fitted crutches may cause crutch palsy.

_____ 10. A cane should be held on the strong side of the body.

Directions: Match each key term with its definition.

_____ 1. Ambulation

_____ 2. Brace

_____ 3. Cast

_____ 4. Compress

_____ 5. Edema

_____ 6. Erythema

_____ 7. Exudate

_____ 8. Long arm cast

_____ 9. Maceration

_____ 10. Orthopedist

_____ 11. Short leg cast

_____ 12. Soak

_____ 13. Splint

_____ 14. Sprain

_____ 15. Strain

_____ 16. Suppuration

A. A discharge produced by the body's tissues
B. An overstretching of a muscle caused by trauma
C. A soft, moist, absorbent cloth that is folded in several layers and applied to a part of the body in the local application of heat or cold
D. Walking or moving from one place to another
E. The direct immersion of a body part in water or a medicated solution
F. The retention of fluid in the tissues, resulting in swelling
G. An orthopedic device used to support and hold a part of the body in the correct position to allow for functioning of the body part while healing takes place
H. A cast that extends from the axilla to the fingers of the hand, usually with a bend in the elbow.
I. Reddening of the skin caused by dilation of superficial blood vessels in the skin
J. Trauma to a joint that causes injury to the ligaments
K. The process of pus formation
L. A physician who specializes in the diagnosis and treatment of disorders of the musculoskeletal system
M. The softening and breaking down of the skin as a result of prolonged exposure to moisture
N. A cast that begins just below the knee and extends to the toes
O. An orthopedic device used to support and immobilize a part of the body
P. A stiff cylindrical casing that is used to immobilize a body part until healing occurs.

EVALUATION OF LEARNING

Directions: Fill in each blank with the correct answer.

1. State whether the following is an example of dry heat, moist heat, dry cold, or moist cold.

   a. Hot compress

   _____

   b. Ice bag

   _____

   c. Heating pad

   _____

   d. Chemical hot pack

   _____

   e. Cold compress

   _____

2. List three factors that must be taken into consideration when applying heat or cold.

   _____

   _____

3. How does the local application of heat to an affected area for a short period of time influence the following?

   a. The diameter of the blood vessels in the affected area

   _____

   b. The blood supply to the affected area

   _____

   c. Tissue metabolism in the affected area

   _____

4. What happens to the diameter of blood vessels if heat is applied for a prolonged period (more than 1 hour)?

   _____

   _____

5. List three reasons for applying heat locally.

   _____

   _____

   _____

6. How does the local application of cold for a short period of time to an affected area influence the following?

   a. The diameter of the blood vessels in the affected area

   _____

   _____

   b. The blood supply to the affected area

   _____

   _____

   c. Tissue metabolism in the affected area

   _____

   _____

7. List two reasons for applying cold locally.

   _____

   _____

8. What are three reasons for applying a cast?

   _____

   _____

9. What causes a pressure area?

   _____

   _____

263

10. What are the symptoms of a pressure area?

_____

11. What are the complications of a pressure ulcer?

_____

_____

12. What is the purpose of covering the body part with a stockinette before applying a cast?

_____

_____

13. What is the purpose of applying cast padding during cast application?

_____

_____

14. Why should each of the following precautions be taken when applying a synthetic cast?

    a. Removing synthetic casting particles using an alcohol swab

    _____

    b. Checking the circulation, sensation, and movement of the extremity

    _____

15. How soon can a synthetic cast bear weight following application?

_____

16. What can be done to prevent or decrease swelling following application of a cast?

_____

_____

_____

17. Why is it important to prevent foreign particles from being trapped under a cast?

_____

_____

18. Why is it important not to insert anything under a cast to relieve itching?

_____

_____

19. Why is it important to dry a synthetic cast as soon as possible after it gets wet?

_____

20. If a cast becomes wet, how should it be dried?

_____

_____

21. What symptoms may indicate that a cast is too tight and an infection is developing?

_____

_____

22. How is a cast removed?

_____

_____

23. What will the affected extremity look like after a cast has been removed?

_____

24. List two examples of conditions for which a splint may be applied.

_____

_____

25. List one example of a condition for which a brace may be applied.

_____

26. What factors does the provider take into consideration when prescribing an ambulatory assistive device?

_____

_____

27. Describe one advantage of the forearm crutch.

_____

28. What may occur if axillary crutches are not fitted properly?

_____

_____

29. List eight guidelines that must be followed during crutch use to ensure safety.

_____

_____

_____

_____

_____

_____

_____

_____

30. List one use for each of the following crutch gaits:

a. Four-point gait _____

b. Three-point gait _____

c. Swing gaits _____

31. List and describe the three types of canes.

_____

_____

32. List two reasons for prescribing a cane.

_____

_____

33. List two reasons for prescribing a walker.

_____

_____

34. What are two disadvantages of using a walker?

_____

_____

CRITICAL THINKING ACTIVITIES

A. Dear Gabby

Gabby was called out of town unexpectedly and wants you to fill in for her. In the space provided, respond to the following letter.

Dear Gabby:

I am 15 years old and in the 10th grade. I need your help. I have a backpack; my dad weighed it and said it was 40 pounds. I only weigh 105 pounds. My back and neck hurt from lugging it around. I have to walk almost one-half mile to the bus stop. I do not have time to use my locker between classes because it is down a flight of stairs and at the end of the hall. Once, when I started using my locker, my science teacher got upset with me because I was late getting to class. Gabby, what should I do?

Signed,
Pain in the Neck

_____

_____

_____

_____

_____

_____

_____

_____

B. Cast Care

1. You are employed by a pediatric orthopedic surgeon. She is concerned because many of her school-aged patients do not follow proper guidelines for the care of their fiberglass casts, even with their parents' constant reminders. She asks you to develop a creative and colorful instruction sheet in the shape of a cast that presents cast care instructions at a level that can be understood by this age group (8 to 12 years old). Use the illustration of the cast on the next page to design your instruction sheet.

2. After developing your instruction sheet, get into a group of three or four students and share your sheets. Have the group decide whether the instructions on each sheet are appropriate for a school-aged child and whether the sheet would be visually appealing to this age group.

Instruction Sheet for Cast Care

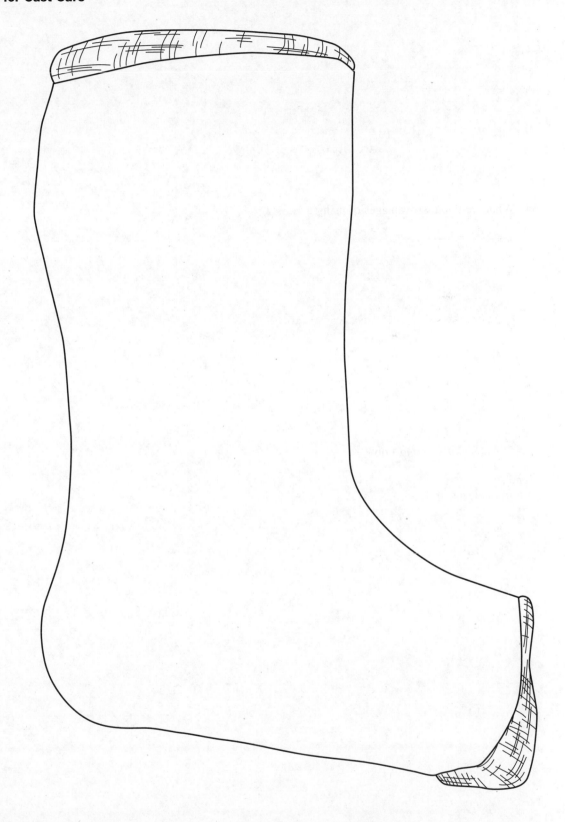

C. Crutch Guidelines

Each of the following patients is wearing a long leg cast because of a broken tibia and is using wooden axillary crutches to ambulate. Evaluate the crutch technique being practiced by each patient. Write **C** if the technique is correct and **I** if the technique is incorrect. If the technique is correct, explain why it should be performed this way. If incorrect, indicate what may happen from performing the technique in this manner.

1. Andy Morris wears Nike sports shoes when ambulating with his crutches.

_____

_____

2. Susan Yang does not stand up straight when using her crutches.

_____

_____

3. Miguel Saldivia puts his weight on the axilla when getting around on his crutches.

_____

_____

4. Lindy Campbell has a lot of decorative throw rugs in her house, and she does not want to remove them.

_____

_____

5. LeBron Jamar likes to move quickly on his crutches, so he advances them forward about 20 inches with each step when using the swing-through gait.

_____

_____

6. Hanna Romes has tingling in her hands but thinks it is just part of what happens when one uses crutches.

_____

_____

7. Tamra Hetrick pads both the shoulder rests and the handgrips of her crutches.

_____

_____

8. Erica Anderson's crutch tips get wet, but she does not take the time to dry them before going into a shopping mall.

_____

_____

D. Accessibility for Physical Disabilities

Next to each of the following facilities, list the features you have observed that facilitate accessibility of individuals with a physical disability.

1. Schools

   _____

   _____

2. Grocery stores

   _____

   _____

3. Shopping malls

   _____

   _____

4. Movie theaters

   _____

   _____

5. Restaurants

   _____

   _____

6. Doctors' offices

   _____

   _____

7. Community parks

   _____

   _____

E. Crossword Puzzle: Physical Agents to Promote Tissue Healing

Directions: Complete the crossword puzzle using the clues presented below.

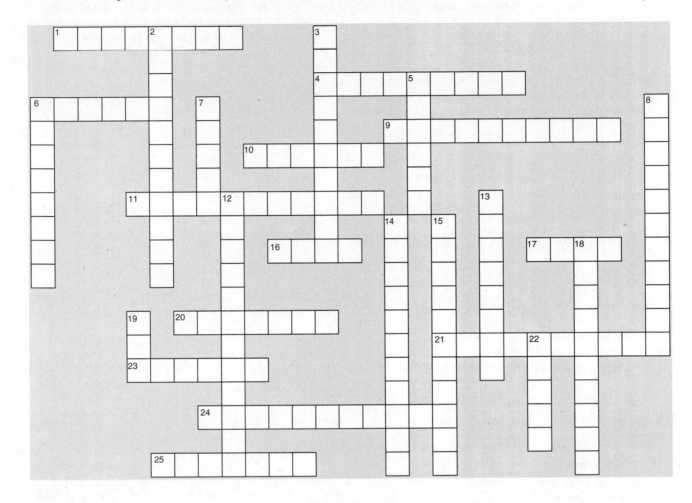

Across
- **1** Transfers weight from legs to arms
- **4** Cold blood vessels do this
- **6** Removable immobilizer
- **9** Popular synthetic cast
- **10** Warm blood vessels do this
- **11** Prevents pressure areas
- **16** Examples: standard, tripod, or quad
- **17** Takes 4 to 6 weeks for fracture to do this
- **20** Discharge
- **21** Purpose of a cast
- **23** Needed after knee replacement
- **24** Bone doctor
- **25** Cutting a cast in half

Down
- **2** "Too long" crutches may cause this
- **3** Soft and broken down skin
- **5** Maximum minutes for heat application
- **6** Elevate cast to prevent this
- **7** Do not bend here to lift!
- **8** Prevents LBP
- **12** Cast is rubbing against the skin
- **13** Red skin
- **14** Pus formation
- **15** Located between skin and cast padding
- **18** Walking
- **19** Blow-dry a cast on this heat setting
- **22** Holds body part in correct position

F. Bone and Joint Conditions

1. It is National Bone and Joint Week. The mayor has asked you and your classmates to develop informative, creative, and colorful brochures for the community about bone and joint conditions. Choose a condition below and design a brochure using the blank Frequently Asked Questions (FAQs) brochure provided on the following page. Each student in the class should select a different topic. On a separate sheet of paper, write 5 true or false questions relating to the information in your brochure.

2. Present your brochure to the class. After all the brochures have been presented, students should ask their questions to the class to see how well they understand bone and joint conditions. (*Note:* You can take notes during the presentations and refer to them when answering the questions.)

   1. Bursitis

   2. Congenital hip dysplasia

   3. Epicondylitis

   4. Fibromyalgia

   5. Gout

   6. Hammer toe

   7. Herniated disk

   8. Juvenile rheumatoid arthritis

   9. Knee replacement surgery

   10. Kyphosis

   11. Osteoarthritis

   12. Osteomyelitis

   13. Osteoporosis

   14. Paget's disease

   15. Rheumatoid arthritis

   16. Scoliosis

   17. Sprain

   18. Strain

   19. Tendinitis

FAQ ON:

Q:

A:

Q:

A:

Q:

A:

Q:

A:

Illustration

Chapter **7 Physical Agents to Promote Tissue Healing**

Local Application of Heat and Cold

Procedures 7-1, 7-2, 7-3, and 7A: Application of Heat

Apply the following heat treatments, and document the procedure in the chart provided: heating pad, hot soak, hot compress, chemical hot pack, gel hot pack.

Procedures 7-4, 7-5, 7-6 and 7-A: Application of Cold

Apply the following cold treatments, and document the results in the chart provided: ice bag, cold compress, chemical cold pack, and gel cold pack.

Ambulatory Aids

Procedure 7-7: Axillary Crutch Measurement

Measure an individual for axillary crutches, and document the procedure in the chart provided.

Procedure 7-8: Crutch Gaits

Instruct an individual in mastering the following crutch gaits: four-point, two-point, three-point, swing-to, and swing-through. Document the procedure in the chart provided.

Procedure 7-9: Cane

Instruct an individual in the use of a cane, and document the procedure in the chart provided.

Procedure 7-10: Walker

Instruct an individual in the use of a walker, and document the procedure in the chart provided.

CHART	
Date	

CHART	
Date	

Procedure 7-1: Applying a Heating Pad

Name: _____   Date: _____

Evaluated by: _____   Score: _____

Performance Objective

Outcome:	Apply a heating pad.
Conditions:	Given a heating pad with a protective covering.
Standards:	Time: 5 minutes. Student completed procedure in _____ minutes.
	Accuracy: Satisfactory score on the Performance Evaluation Checklist.

Performance Evaluation Checklist

Trial 1	Trial 2	Point Value	Performance Standards
		•	Sanitized hands.
		•	Assembled the equipment.
		•	Greeted the patient and introduced yourself.
		•	Identified the patient and explained the procedure.
		•	Placed the heating pad in a protective covering.
		•	Connected the plug to an electrical outlet and set the selector switch to the proper setting.
		•	Placed the heating pad on patient's affected body area and asked how the temperature felt.
		•	Instructed the patient not to lie on the pad or turn the temperature setting higher.
		▷	Stated why the patient should be instructed not to lie on the heating pad.
		▷	Explained why the patient may want to increase the temperature.
		•	Checked the patient's skin periodically.
		•	Administered treatment for the proper length of time as designated by the provider.
		•	Sanitized hands.
		•	Documented the procedure correctly.
		•	Properly cared for and returned the equipment to its storage place.
		■	Demonstrated critical thinking skills.
		■	Reassured patients.
		★	Completed the procedure within 5 minutes.
			Totals

Evaluation of Student Performance

EVALUATION CRITERIA			COMMENTS
Symbol	**Category**	**Point Value**	
★	Critical Step	16 points	
•	Essential Step	6 points	
■	Affective Competency	6 points	
★	Theory Question	2 points	

Score calculation: 100 points

− _____ points missed

_____ Score

Satisfactory score: 85 or above

CAAHEP Competencies Achieved

Psychomotor (Skills)
☑ I. 8. Instruct and prepare a patient for a procedure or a treatment.
☑ X. 3. Document patient care accurately in the patient record.

Affective (Behavior)
☑ A. 1. Incorporate Demonstrate critical thinking skills.
☑ A. 2. Reassure patients.

ABHES Competencies Achieved

☑ 2. c. Identify diagnostic and treatment modalities as they relate to each body system.
☑ 7. g. Display professionalism through written and verbal communications.
☑ 8. e. Perform specialty procedures including but not limited to pediatric care, minor surgery, cardiac, respiratory, OB-GYN, neurological and gastroenterology.

Procedure 7-2: Applying a Hot Soak

Name: _____ Date: _____

Evaluated by: _____ Score: _____

Performance Objective

Outcome:	Apply a hot soak.
Conditions:	Given the following: soaking solution, bath thermometer, basin, and bath towels.
Standards:	Time: 10 minutes. Student completed procedure in _____ minutes.
	Accuracy: Satisfactory score on the Performance Evaluation Checklist.

Performance Evaluation Checklist

Trial 1	Trial 2	Point Value	Performance Standards
		•	Sanitized hands.
		•	Assembled the equipment.
		•	Checked the label on the solution container.
		•	Warmed the soaking solution.
		•	Greeted the patient and introduced yourself.
		•	Identified the patient and explained the procedure.
		•	Filled a basin one-half to two-thirds full with the warmed soaking solution.
		•	Checked the temperature of the solution with a bath thermometer.
		▷	Stated the safe temperature range that should be used for an adult patient (105–110° F).
		•	Assisted the patient into a comfortable position and padded the side of the basin with a towel.
		•	Slowly and gradually immersed the affected body part into the solution and asked the patient how the temperature felt.
		•	Kept the solution at a constant temperature by removing cooler solution and adding hot solution.
		•	Placed a hand between the patient and the solution when adding more solution.
		•	Stirred the solution with your hand while pouring it.
		•	Checked the patient's skin periodically.
		•	Applied the hot soak for the proper length of time as designated by the provider.
		•	Completely dried the affected part.
		•	Sanitized hands.
		•	Documented the procedure correctly.
		•	Properly cared for and returned the equipment to its storage place.

Trial 1	Trial 2	Point Value	Performance Standards
		■	Demonstrated critical thinking skills.
		■	Reassured patients.
		★	Completed the procedure within 10 minutes.
			Totals

CHART	
Date	

Evaluation of Student Performance

EVALUATION CRITERIA			COMMENTS
Symbol	**Category**	**Point Value**	
★	Critical Step	16 points	
•	Essential Step	6 points	
■	Affective Competency	6 points	
▷	Theory Question	2 points	

Score calculation: 100 points

    − ____ points missed

    ___Score

Satisfactory score: 85 or above

CAAHEP Competencies Achieved

Psychomotor (Skills)
☑   I. 8. Instruct and prepare a patient for a procedure or a treatment.
☑   X. 3. Document patient care accurately in the medical record.

Affective (Behavior)
☑   A. 1. Demonstrate critical thinking skills.
☑   A. 2. Reassure patients.

ABHES Competencies Achieved

☑   2. c. Identify diagnostic and treatment modalities as they relate to each body system.
☑   7. g. Display professionalism through written and verbal communications.
☑   8. e. Perform specialty procedures including but not limited to pediatric care, minor surgery, cardiac, respiratory, OB-GYN, neurological, and gastroenterology.

Notes

Chapter **7 Physical Agents to Promote Tissue Healing**

EVALUATION OF COMPETENCY

Procedure 7-3: Applying a Hot Compress

Name: _____ Date: _____

Evaluated by: _____ Score: _____

Performance Objective

Outcome:	Apply a hot compress.
Conditions:	Given the following: solution for the compresses, bath thermometer, basin, washcloths, and a towel.
Standards:	Time: 10 minutes. Student completed procedure in _____ minutes.
	Accuracy: Satisfactory score on the Performance Evaluation Checklist.

Performance Evaluation Checklist

Trial 1	Trial 2	Point Value	Performance Standards
		•	Sanitized hands.
		•	Assembled the equipment.
		•	Checked the label on the solution container.
		•	Warmed the soaking solution.
		•	Greeted the patient and introduced yourself.
		•	Identified the patient and explained the procedure.
		•	Filled the basin half full with the warmed solution.
		•	Checked the temperature of the solution with a bath thermometer.
		▷	Stated the safe temperature range that should be used for an adult patient (105° F to 110° F).
		•	Completely immersed the compress in the solution.
		•	Squeezed excess solution from the compress.
		•	Applied the compress to the affected body part and asked the patient how the temperature felt.
		•	Placed additional compresses in the solution.
		•	Repeated the application every 2 to 3 minutes for the duration of time specified by the provider.
		•	Checked the patient's skin periodically.
		•	Checked the temperature of the solution periodically, removed cooler fluid, and added hot fluid if needed.
		•	Administered the treatment for the proper length of time as designated by a provider.
		•	Thoroughly dried the affected part.
		•	Sanitized hands.

Chapter **7** Physical Agents to Promote Tissue Healing

Trial 1	Trial 2	Point Value	Performance Standards
		•	Documented the procedure correctly.
		•	Properly cared for and returned the equipment to its storage place.
		■	Demonstrated critical thinking skills.
		■	Reassured patients.
		★	Completed the procedure within 10 minutes.
			Totals

CHART

Date	

Evaluation of Student Performance

EVALUATION CRITERIA			COMMENTS
Symbol	**Category**	**Point Value**	
★	Critical Step	16 points	
•	Essential Step	6 points	
■	Affective Competency	6 points	
▷	Theory Question	2 points	

Score calculation: 100 points

−   points missed

_____ Score

Satisfactory score: 85 or above

CAAHEP Competencies Achieved

Psychomotor (Skills)
☑ I. 8. Instruct and prepare a patient for a procedure or a treatment.
☑ X. 3. Document patient care accurately in the medical record.

Affective (Behavior)
☑ A. 1. Demonstrate critical thinking skills.
☑ A. 2. Reassured patients.

ABHES Competencies Achieved

☑ 2. c. Identify diagnostic and treatment modalities as they relate to each body system.
☑ 7. g. Display professionalism through written and verbal communications.
☑ 8. e. Perform specialty procedures including but not limited to pediatric care, minor surgery, cardiac, respiratory, OB-GYN, neurological, and gastroenterology.

Notes

Procedure 7-4: Applying an Ice Bag

Name: _____   Date: _____

Evaluated by: _____   Score: _____

Performance Objective

Outcome:	Apply an ice bag.
Conditions:	Given the following: ice bag and protective covering, and small pieces of ice.
Standards:	Time: 10 minutes. Student completed procedure in _____ minutes.
	Accuracy: Satisfactory score on the Performance Evaluation Checklist.

Performance Evaluation Checklist

Trial 1	Trial 2	Point Value	Performance Standards
		•	Sanitized hands.
		•	Assembled the equipment.
		•	Greeted the patient and introduced yourself.
		•	Identified the patient and explained the procedure.
		•	Checked the ice bag for leakage.
		•	Filled the bag one-half to two-thirds full with small pieces of ice.
		▷	Explained why small pieces of ice are used.
		•	Expelled air from the bag.
		▷	Explained the reason for expelling air from bag.
		•	Placed the bag in a protective covering.
		▷	Stated the purpose of placing the bag in a protective covering.
		•	Placed the bag on the affected body area and asked the patient how the temperature felt.
		•	Checked the patient's skin periodically.
		▷	Listed skin changes that would warrant removal of the bag.
		•	Refilled the bag with ice and changed the protective covering when needed.
		•	Administered the treatment for the proper length of time as designated by the provider.
		•	Sanitized hands.
		•	Documented the procedure correctly.
		•	Properly cared for and returned the equipment to its storage place.
		■	Demonstrated critical thinking skills.

Trial 1	Trial 2	Point Value	Performance Standards
		■	Demonstrated critical thinking skills.
		★	Completed the procedure within 10 minutes.
			Totals

CHART

Date	

Evaluation of Student Performance

EVALUATION CRITERIA			COMMENTS
Symbol	**Category**	**Point Value**	
★	Critical Step	16 points	
•	Essential Step	6 points	
■	Affective Competency	6 points	
▷	Theory Question	2 points	

Score calculation: 100 points

    −   points missed

      ___Score

Satisfactory score: 85 or above

CAAHEP Competencies Achieved

Psychomotor (Skills)
- ☑ I. 8. Instruct and prepare a patient for a procedure or a treatment.
- ☑ X. 3. Document patient care accurately in the medical record.

Affective (Behavior)
- ☑ A. 1. Demonstrate critical thinking skills.
- ☑ A. 2. Reassure patients.

ABHES Competencies Achieved

- ☑ 2. c. Identify diagnostic and treatment modalities as they relate to each body system.
- ☑ 7. g. Display professionalism through written and verbal communications.
- ☑ 8. e. Perform specialty procedures including but not limited to pediatric care, minor surgery, cardiac, respiratory, OB-GYN, neurological, and gastroenterology.

Procedure 7-5: Applying a Cold Compress

Name: _____   Date: _____

Evaluated by: _____   Score: _____

Performance Objective

Outcome:	Apply a cold compress.
Conditions:	Given the following: ice cubes, a basin, and washcloths.
Standards:	Time: 10 minutes. Student completed procedure in _____ minutes.
	Accuracy: Satisfactory score on the Performance Evaluation Checklist.

Performance Evaluation Checklist

Trial 1	Trial 2	Point Value	Performance Standards
		•	Sanitized hands.
		•	Assembled the equipment.
		•	Checked the label on the solution.
		•	Greeted the patient and introduced yourself.
		•	Identified the patient and explained the procedure.
		•	Placed large ice cubes in the basin and added the solution until the basin is half full.
		▷	Explained why larger pieces of ice are used.
		•	Completely immersed the compress in the solution.
		•	Squeezed excess solution from the compress.
		•	Applied the compress to the affected body part and asked the patient how the temperature felt.
		•	Placed additional compresses in the solution.
		•	Repeated the application every 2 to 3 minutes for the duration of time specified by the provider.
		•	Checked the patient's skin periodically.
		•	Added ice if needed to keep the solution cold.
		•	Administered the treatment for the proper length of time as designated by the provider.
		•	Thoroughly dried the affected part.
		•	Sanitized hands.
		•	Documented the procedure correctly.
		•	Properly cared for and returned the equipment to its storage place.
		■	Demonstrated critical thinking skills.

Trial 1	Trial 2	Point Value	Performance Standards
		■	Reassured patients.
		★	Completed the procedure within 10 minutes.
			Totals

CHART	
Date	

Evaluation of Student Performance

EVALUATION CRITERIA			COMMENTS
Symbol	**Category**	**Point Value**	
★	Critical Step	16 points	
•	Essential Step	6 points	
■	Affective Competency	6 points	
▷	Theory Question	2 points	

Score calculation: 100 points

− _____ points missed

_____ Score

Satisfactory score: 85 or above

CAAHEP Competencies Achieved

Psychomotor (Skills)
☑ I. 8. Instruct and prepare a patient for a procedure or a treatment.
☑ X. 3. Document patient care accurately in the medical record.

Affective (Behavior)
☑ A. 1. Demonstrate critical thinking skills.
☑ A. 2. Reassured patients.

ABHES Competencies Achieved

☑ 2. c. Identify diagnostic and treatment modalities as they relate to each body system.
☑ 7. g. Display professionalism through written and verbal communications.
☑ 8. e. Perform specialty procedures including but not limited to pediatric care, minor surgery, cardiac, respiratory, OB-GYN, neurological, and gastroenterology.

Procedure 7-6: Applying a Chemical Pack

Name: _____ Date: _____

Evaluated by: _____ Score: _____

Performance Objective

Outcome:	Apply a chemical cold and hot pack.
Conditions:	Given a chemical cold and hot pack.
Standards:	Time: 5 minutes. Student completed procedure in _____ minutes.
	Accuracy: Satisfactory score on the Performance Evaluation Checklist.

Performance Evaluation Checklist

Trial 1	Trial 2	Point Value	Performance Standards
		•	Sanitized hands.
		•	Assembled the equipment.
		•	Greeted the patient and introduced yourself.
		•	Identified the patient and explained the procedure.
		•	Shook the crystals to the bottom of bag.
		•	Squeezed the bag firmly to break the inner water bag.
		•	Shook the bag vigorously to mix the contents.
		•	Covered the bag with a protective covering.
		•	Applied the bag to the affected area.
		•	Checked the patient's skin periodically.
		•	Administered the treatment for the proper length of time.
		•	Discarded the bag in an appropriate receptacle.
		•	Sanitized hands.
		•	Documented the procedure correctly.
		■	Demonstrated critical thinking skills.
		■	Reassured patients.
		★	Completed the procedure within 5 minutes.
			Totals

Evaluation of Student Performance

EVALUATION CRITERIA			COMMENTS
Symbol	**Category**	**Point Value**	
★	Critical Step	16 points	
•	Essential Step	6 points	
■	Affective Competency	6 points	
▷	Theory Question	2 points	

Score calculation: 100 points
       −   points missed
         ___Score
Satisfactory score: 85 or above

CAAHEP Competencies Achieved

Psychomotor (Skills)
☑ I. 8. Instruct and prepare a patient for a procedure or a treatment.
☑ X. 3. Document patient care accurately in the medical record.

Affective (Behavior)
☑ A. 1. Demonstrate critical thinking skills.
☑ A. 2. Reassure patients.

ABHES Competencies Achieved

☑ 2. c. Identify diagnostic and treatment modalities as they relate to each body system.
☑ 7. g. Display professionalism through written and verbal communications.
☑ 8. e. Perform specialty procedures including but not limited to pediatric care, minor surgery, cardiac, respiratory, OB-GYN, neurological, and gastroenterology.

Procedure 7-A: Applying a Gel Pack

Name: _____   Date: _____

Evaluated by: _____   Score: _____

Performance Objective

Outcome:	Apply a gel pack.
Conditions:	Given a gel pack and a protective covering.
Standards:	Time: 10 minutes. Student completed procedure in _____ minutes.
	Accuracy: Satisfactory score on the Performance Evaluation Checklist.

Performance Evaluation Checklist

Trial 1	Trial 2	Point Value	Performance Standards
		•	Sanitized hands.
		•	Assembled the equipment.
		•	Greeted the patient and introduced yourself.
		•	Identified the patient and explained the procedure.
		•	Checked the gel pack for rupture or leakage.
		•	Stated what should be done if the gel pack is damaged.
			Preparing a gel hot pack for application:
		•	Evenly distributed the gel in the pack.
		•	Laid the pack flat in a microwave.
		•	Microwaved the pack on high power for the length of time specified in the instructions accompanying the pack.
		•	Removed the gel pack from the microwave from the microwave using heat resistant gloves.
		•	Kneaded the gel pack using heat resistant gloves.
		▷	Stated the reason for kneading the pack.
		•	If the pack is too hot, allowed it to cool before application.
		•	If the pack is not hot enough, returned it to the microwave and heated it in 10 second intervals until the desired temperature is reached.
		•	Did not overheat the gel pack.
		▷	Explained what might happen if the pack is overheated.
			Preparing a gel cold pack for application:
		•	Removed the gel pack from the freezer.
		▷	Stated how long a gel pack must be placed in the freezer prior to application.

Trial 1	Trial 2	Point Value	Performance Standards
			Applying the gel pack:
		•	Wrapped the gel pack in a protective covering.
		•	Applied the gel pack to the affected area.
		•	Checked the patient's skin periodically.
		•	Administered the treatment for the proper length of time.
		•	Documented the procedure correctly.
		•	Returned the gel pack to its proper storage location.
		■	Demonstrated critical thinking skills.
		■	Reassured patients.
		★	Completed the procedure within 10 minutes.
			Totals

Evaluation of Student Performance

EVALUATION CRITERIA			COMMENTS
Symbol	**Category**	**Point Value**	
★	Critical Step	16 points	
•	Essential Step	6 points	
■	Affective Competency	6 points	
▷	Theory Question	2 points	

Score calculation: 100 points

      −   points missed

        ___Score

Satisfactory score: 85 or above

CAAHEP Competencies Achieved

Psychomotor (Skills)
☑ I. 8. Instruct and prepare a patient for a procedure or a treatment.
☑ X. 3. Document patient care accurately in the medical record.

Affective (Behavior)
☑ A. 1. Demonstrate critical thinking skills.
☑ A. 2. Reassure patients.

ABHES Competencies Achieved

☑ 2. c. Identify diagnostic and treatment modalities as they relate to each body system.
☑ 7. g. Display professionalism through written and verbal communications.
☑ 8. e. Perform specialty procedures including but not limited to pediatric care, minor surgery, cardiac, respiratory, OB-GYN, neurological, and gastroenterology.

Procedure 7-7: Measuring for Axillary Crutches

Name: _____   Date: _____

Evaluated by: _____   Score: _____

Performance Objective

Outcome:	Measure an individual for axillary crutches.
Conditions:	Given the following: axillary crutches and a tape measure.
Standards:	Time: 10 minutes. Student completed procedure in _____ minutes.
	Accuracy: Satisfactory score on the Performance Evaluation Checklist.

Performance Evaluation Checklist

Trial 1	Trial 2	Point Value	Performance Standards
		•	Greeted the patient and introduced yourself.
		•	Identified the patient and explained the procedure.
		•	Discussed the importance of properly fitted crutches with the patient.
		•	Asked the patient to stand erect.
		•	Positioned the crutches with the tips at a distance of 2 inches in front of, and 4 to 6 inches to the side of, each foot.
		•	Adjusted crutch length so that the shoulder rests were approximately 1½ to 2 inches below the axilla.
		•	Asked the patient to support his or her weight by the handgrips.
		•	Adjusted the handgrips so that the patient's elbow was flexed approximately 30 degrees.
		•	Checked the fit of the crutches by placing two fingers between the top of the crutch and the patient's axilla.
		•	Documented the procedure correctly.
		■	Demonstrated critical thinking skills.
		■	Reassured patients.
		★	Completed the procedure within 10 minutes.
			Totals

CHART	
Date	

Evaluation of Student Performance

EVALUATION CRITERIA			COMMENTS
Symbol	**Category**	**Point Value**	
★	Critical Step	16 points	
•	Essential Step	6 points	
■	Affective Competency	6 points	
▷	Theory Question	2 points	

Score calculation: 100 points

      −   points missed

      ___Score

Satisfactory score: 85 or above

CAAHEP Competencies Achieved

Psychomotor (Skills)
☑ I. 8. Instruct and prepare a patient for a procedure or a treatment.

Affective (Behavior)
☑ A. 1. Demonstrate critical thinking skills.
☑ A. 2. Reassure patients.

ABHES Competencies Achieved

☑ 7. g. Display professionalism through written and verbal communications.
☑ 8. j. Accommodate patients with special needs (psychological or physical limitations).

Procedure 7-8: Instructing a Patient in Crutch Gaits

Name: _____ Date: _____

Evaluated by: _____ Score: _____

Performance Objective

Outcome:	Instruct an individual in the following crutch gaits: four-point, two-point, three-point, swing-to, and swing-through.
Conditions:	Given axillary crutches.
Standards:	Time: 15 minutes. Student completed procedure in _____ minutes.
	Accuracy: Satisfactory score on the Performance Evaluation Checklist.

Performance Evaluation Checklist

Trial 1	Trial 2	Point Value	Performance Standards
			Tripod Position
			Instructed the patient:
		•	Stand erect and face straight ahead.
		•	Place the tips of crutches 4 to 6 inches in front of, and 4 to 6 inches to side of, each foot.
		▷	Stated one use of the tripod position.
			Four-Point Gait
			Instructed the patient:
		•	Begin in the tripod position.
		•	Move the right crutch forward.
		•	Move the left foot forward to the level of the left crutch.
		•	Move the left crutch forward.
		•	Move the right foot forward to the level of the right crutch.
		•	Repeat the above sequence.
		▷	Stated one use of the four-point gait.
			Two-Point Gait
			Instructed the patient:
		•	Begin in the tripod position.
		•	Move the left crutch and the right foot forward at the same time.
		•	Move the right crutch and the left foot forward at the same time.
		•	Repeat the above sequence.
		▷	Stated one use of the two-point gait.

297

Trial 1	Trial 2	Point Value	Performance Standards
			Three-Point Gait
			Instructed the patient:
		•	Begin in the tripod position.
		•	Move both crutches and the affected leg forward.
		•	Move the unaffected leg forward while balancing weight on both crutches.
		•	Repeat the above sequence.
		▷	Stated two uses of the three-point gait.
			Swing-To Gait
			Instructed the patient:
		•	Begin in the tripod position.
		•	Move both crutches forward together.
		•	Lift and swing body to the crutches.
		•	Repeat the above sequence.
		▷	Stated one use of the swing-to gait.
			Swing-Through Gait
			Instructed the patient:
		•	Begin in the tripod position.
		•	Move both crutches forward together.
		•	Lift and swing the body past the crutches.
		•	Repeat the above sequence.
		▷	Stated one use of the swing-through gait.
		■	Demonstrated empathy for patients' concerns.
		★	Completed the procedure within 15 minutes.
			Totals
CHART			
Date			

Evaluation of Student Performance

EVALUATION CRITERIA			COMMENTS
Symbol	**Category**	**Point Value**	
★	Critical Step	16 points	
•	Essential Step	6 points	
■	Affective Competency	6 points	
▷	Theory Question	2 points	

Score calculation: 100 points

−   points missed

_____

_____Score

Satisfactory score: 85 or above

CAAHEP Competencies Achieved

Psychomotor (Skills)
☑   I. 8. Instruct and prepare a patient for a procedure or a treatment.
☑   V. 3. Coach patients regarding: a. office policies b. medical encounters.

Affective (Behavior)
☑   A. 3. Demonstrate empathy for patients' concerns.

ABHES Competencies Achieved

☑   7. g. Display professionalism through written and verbal communications.
☑   8. j. Accommodate patients with special needs (psychological or physical limitations).

Notes

Procedures 7-9 and 7-10: Instructing a Patient in Use of a Cane and Walker

Name: _____   Date: _____

Evaluated by: _____   Score: _____

Performance Objective

Outcome:	Instruct an individual in the use of a cane and walker.
Conditions:	Given the following: a cane and a walker.
Standards:	Time: 10 minutes. Student completed procedure in _____ minutes.
	Accuracy: Satisfactory score on the Performance Evaluation Checklist.

Performance Evaluation Checklist

Trial 1	Trial 2	Point Value	Performance Standards
			Cane
			Instructed the patient:
		•	Hold the cane on the strong side of body.
		•	Place the tip of the cane 4 to 6 inches to the side of foot.
		•	Move the cane forward approximately 12 inches.
		•	Move the affected leg forward to the level of the cane.
		•	Move the strong leg forward and ahead of the cane and weak leg.
		•	Repeat the above sequence.
		▷	Stated one condition for which a cane is used.
			Walker
			Instructed the patient:
		•	Pick up the walker and move it forward approximately 6 inches.
		•	Move the right foot and then the left foot up to the walker.
		•	Repeat the above sequence.
		▷	Stated one condition for which a walker is used.
		■	Demonstrated empathy for patients' concerns.
		★	Completed the procedure within 10 minutes.
			Totals

CHART	
Date	

Evaluation of Student Performance

EVALUATION CRITERIA			COMMENTS
Symbol	**Category**	**Point Value**	
★	Critical Step	16 points	
•	Essential Step	6 points	
■	Affective Competency	6 points	
▷	Theory Question	2 points	

Score calculation: 100 points

$-$ _____ points missed

_____ Score

Satisfactory score: 85 or above

CAAHEP Competencies Achieved

Psychomotor (Skills)
- ☑ I. 8. Instruct and prepare a patient for a procedure or a treatment.
- ☑ V. 3. Coach patients regarding: a. office policies b. medical encounters.

Affective (Behavior)
- ☑ A. 3. Demonstrate empathy for patients' concerns.

ABHES Competencies Achieved

- ☑ 7. g. Display professionalism through written and verbal communications.
- ☑ 8. j. Accommodate patients with special needs (psychological or physical limitations).

8 The Gynecologic Examination and Prenatal Care

CHAPTER ASSIGNMENTS

√ After Completing	Date Due	Study Guide Pages	STUDY GUIDE ASSIGNMENTS (CTA = Critical Thinking Activity)	Possible Points	Points You Earned
		307	⬚ Pretest	10	
			🔑Term Key Term Assessment		
		308-309	A. Definitions	52	
		310	B. Word Parts	22	
			(Add 1 point for each key term)		
		311-319	⬚ Evaluation of Learning questions	79	
		320	CTA A: Breast Cancer (5 points per question)	15	
			Evolve: What's on Your Tray? (Record points ea rned)		
		321-325	CTA B: Methods of Contraception (3 points per each method)	42	
		326	CTA C: Signs and Symptoms of Pregnancy	16	
		327	CTA D: Calculation of the Expected Date of Delivery	5	
		327	CTA E: Documenting Gravidity and Parity	4	
		327-328	CTA F: Nutrition During Pregnancy	8	
		329	CTA G: Minor Discomforts of Pregnancy	10	
		330	CTA H: Health Promotion During Pregnancy	7	
		331	CTA I: Breastfeeding	8	
		331	CTA J: Prenatal Ultrasound	5	
		332	CTA K: Crossword Puzzle	30	

√ After Completing	Date Due	Study Guide Pages	STUDY GUIDE ASSIGNMENTS (CTA = Critical Thinking Activity)	Possible Points	Points You Earned
			Evolve: Road to Recovery Game OB/GYN Terminology (Record points earned)		
			Evolve: Apply Your Knowledge questions	15	
			Evolve: Video Evaluation	48	
		307	Posttest	10	
			ADDITIONAL ASSIGNMENTS		
			Total points		

√ When Assigned By Your Instructor	Study Guide Pages	Practices Required	LABORATORY ASSIGNMENTS (Procedure Number and Name)	Score*
	333	5	**Practice for Competency** 8-1: Breast Self-Examination Instructions	
	341-344		**Evaluation of Competency** 8-1: Breast Self-Examination Instructions	*
	333	5	**Practice for Competency** 8-A: Patient-Collected Vaginal Specimen Instructions	
	345-347		**Evaluation of Competency** 8-A: Patient-Collected Vaginal Specimen Instructions	*
	333-334	5	**Practice for Competency** 8-2: Assisting with a Gynecologic Examination	
	349-353		**Evaluation of Competency** 8-2: Assisting with a Gynecologic Examination	*
	335-340	5	**Practice for Competency** 8-3: Assisting with a Return Prenatal Examination	
	355-358		**Evaluation of Competency** 8-3: Assisting with a Return Prenatal Examination	*
			ADDITIONAL ASSIGNMENTS	

Notes

Name: _____ Date: _____

True or False

_____ 1. A complete gynecologic examination consists of a breast examination and a pelvic examination.

_____ 2. The American Cancer Society states that a breast self-examination is an option for women starting in their 20s.

_____ 3. The purpose of the Pap test is for the early detection of cervical cancer.

_____ 4. The patient should be instructed to douche before having a Pap test.

_____ 5. Bacterial vaginosis is the most common cause of abnormal discharge in women of childbearing age.

_____ 6. Another name for vulvovaginal candidiasis is a yeast infection.

_____ 7. Prenatal refers to the care of the pregnant woman before delivery of the infant.

_____ 8. During each return prenatal visit, the mother's urine is tested for glucose and protein.

_____ 9. The normal range for the fetal pulse rate is between 120 and 160 beats per minute.

_____ 10. Amniocentesis can be used to diagnose certain genetically transmitted conditions.

? POSTTEST

True or False

_____ 1. The patient position for a breast examination is the lithotomy position.

_____ 2. Most breast lumps are discovered by the provider.

_____ 3. Trichomoniasis is caused by a virus.

_____ 4. Chlamydia often occurs in association with syphilis.

_____ 5. In the absence of complications, the first prenatal visit should be scheduled after a woman misses her first period.

_____ 6. True labor pains are referred to as Braxton Hicks contractions.

_____ 7. The purpose of measuring fundal height is to determine the degree of cervical dilation and effacement.

_____ 8. The fetal heart tones can first be detected between 4 and 6 weeks of gestation using a Doppler fetal pulse detector.

_____ 9. Obstetric ultrasound scanning is used to assess fetal lung maturity.

_____ 10. The perineum is the period of time in which the body systems are returning to their prepregnant state.

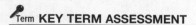 **KEY TERM ASSESSMENT**

A. Definitions
Gynecologic Examination
Directions: Match each key term with its definition.

_____ 1. Amenorrhea

_____ 2. Cervix

_____ 3. Colposcopy

_____ 4. Cytology

_____ 5. Dysmenorrhea

_____ 6. Dyspareunia

_____ 7. Dysplasia

_____ 8. Ectocervix

_____ 9. Endocervix

_____ 10. External os

_____ 11. Gynecology

_____ 12. Menopause

_____ 13. Menorrhagia

_____ 14. Metrorrhagia

_____ 15. Perimenopause

_____ 16. Perineum

_____ 17. Risk factor

_____ 18. Vulva

A. The opening of the cervical canal of the uterus into the vagina
B. The inner part of the cervix that forms a narrow canal that connects the vagina to the uterus.
C. The permanent cessation of menstruation.
D. The external region between the vaginal orifice and the anus in a female and between the scrotum and the anus in a male
E. The outermost layer of the cervix.
F. The absence or cessation of the menstrual period
G. The region of the female external genital organs
H. The science that deals with the study of cells, including their origin, structure, function, and pathology
I. The branch of medicine that deals with the health maintenance and diseases of the female reproductive system.
J. Anything that increases an individual's chance of developing a disease
K. The growth of abnormal cells
L. Before the onset of menopause, the phase during which a woman with regular periods changes to irregular cycles and increased periods of amenorrhea
M. Pain in the vagina or pelvis experienced by a woman during sexual intercourse
N. Examination of the cervix using a lighted instrument with a magnifying lens
O. Bleeding between menstrual periods
P. Excessive bleeding during a menstrual period
Q. The lower narrow end of the uterus that opens into the vagina
R. Pain associated with the menstrual period

Prenatal Care

Directions: Match each key term with its definition.

_____ 1. Abortion

_____ 2. Braxton Hicks contractions

_____ 3. Dilation (of the cervix)

_____ 4. EDD

_____ 5. Effacement

_____ 6. Embryo

_____ 7. Engagement

_____ 8. Fetal heart rate

_____ 9. Fetal heart tones

_____ 10. Fetus

_____ 11. Fundus

_____ 12. Gestation

_____ 13. Gestational age

_____ 14. Gravidity

_____ 15. Infant

_____ 16. Lochia

_____ 17. Multigravida

_____ 18. Multipara

_____ 19. Nullipara

_____ 20. Obstetrics

_____ 21. Parity

_____ 22. Position

_____ 23. Postpartum

_____ 24. Preeclampsia

_____ 25. Prenatal

_____ 26. Presentation

_____ 27. Preterm birth

_____ 28. Primigravida

_____ 29. Primipara

_____ 30. Puerperium

_____ 31. Quickening

_____ 32. Term birth

_____ 33. Toxemia

_____ 34. Trimester

A. A woman who has completed two or more pregnancies to the age of viability, regardless of whether they ended in live infants or stillbirths

B. The entrance of the fetal head or the presenting part into the pelvic inlet

C. Before birth

D. Three months, or one third, of the gestational period of pregnancy

E. The condition of having borne offspring regardless of the outcome

F. The period, usually 4 to 6 weeks, after delivery, in which the uterus and the body systems are returning to normal

G. The termination of the pregnancy before the fetus reached the age of viability (20 weeks)

H. The dome-shaped upper portion of the uterus between the fallopian tubes

I. The number of times per minute the fetal heart beats

J. The first movements of the fetus in utero as felt by the mother

K. The child in utero, from the third month after conception to birth

L. A woman who has been pregnant more than once

M. Projected birth date of the infant

N. A woman who has carried a pregnancy to fetal viability for the first time, regardless of whether the infant was stillborn or alive at birth

O. The stretching of the external os from an opening a few millimeters wide to an opening large enough to allow the passage of an infant (approximately 10 cm)

P. The period of intrauterine development from conception to birth

Q. A discharge from the uterus after delivery consisting of blood, tissue, white blood cells, and some bacteria

R. The thinning and shortening of the cervical canal from its normal length of 1 to 2 cm to a structure with paper-thin edges in which there is no canal at all

S. The total number of pregnancies a woman has had regardless of duration, including a current pregnancy

T. A woman who has not carried a pregnancy to the point of viability (20 weeks of gestation)

U. The branch of medicine concerned with the care of the woman during pregnancy, childbirth, and the postpartal period

V. A woman who is pregnant for the first time

W. Occurring after childbirth

X. Intermittent and irregular painless uterine contractions that occur throughout pregnancy

Y. The relation of the presenting part of the fetus to the maternal pelvis

Z. The sounds of the heartbeat of the fetus heard through the mother's abdominal wall

AA. A child from birth to 12 months of age

BB. The child in utero from the time of conception through the first 8 weeks of development.

CC. The age of the fetus between conception and birth

DD. A major complication of pregnancy characterized by increasing hypertension, albuminuria, and edema

EE. Indication of the part of the fetus that is closest to the cervix and will be delivered first

FF. Delivery occurring between 20 and 37 weeks, regardless of whether the child was born alive or stillborn

GG. Delivery occurring after 37 weeks, regardless of whether the child was born alive or stillborn

HH. A condition occurring in pregnant women that includes preeclampsia and eclampsia

B. Word Parts

Directions: Indicate the meaning of each word part in the space provided. List as many medical terms as possible that incorporate the word part in the space provided.

Word Part	Meaning of Word Part	Medical Terms That Incorporate Word Part
1. a-		
2. men/o		
3. -orrhea		
4. colp/o		
5. -scopy		
6. cyt/o		
7. -ology		
8. dys-		
9. -plasia		
10. ecto-		
11. endo-		
12. gynec/o		
13. multi-		
14. par/o		
15. nulli-		
16. peri-		
17. post-		
18. pre-		
19. nat/o		
20. -al		
21. prim/i		
22. tri-		

Gynecologic Examination

Directions: Fill in each blank with the correct answer.

1. What is the purpose of the gynecologic examination?

_____

_____

2. What is the purpose of performing a breast examination?

_____

_____

3. What should a woman do if a lump or other change is discovered during a breast self-examination?

_____

4. What is the purpose of the pelvic examination?

_____

_____

5. What are the components of the pelvic examination?

_____

_____

6. What position is generally used for the pelvic examination?

_____

7. How can the medical assistant help the patient to relax during the pelvic examination?

_____

8. What is the function of a vaginal speculum?

_____

_____

9. What is the purpose of performing a visual examination of the vagina and the cervix?

_____

_____

10. What are three examples of vaginal infections that cause a discharge?

_____

_____

11. What is the purpose of cervical cancer screening?

_____

12. What causes most cervical cancers?

_____

13. What factors place a woman at higher risk for the development of cervical cancer?

_____

_____

14. What are the cervical cancer screening guidelines for the following age groups?

    a. Ages 21 to 29: _____

    b. Ages 30 to 65: _____

_____

    c. Women over 65 years of age who have had regular cervical cancer screening during the past 10 years:

_____

15. What is the primary purpose of the Pap test?

_____

_____

16. What is the purpose of the HPV test?

_____

_____

17. Why is an HPV test not necessary under the age of 30 years?

_____

_____

18. Why should the medical assistant instruct the patient not to douche or insert vaginal medications for 2 days before coming to the medical office to have a Pap test?

_____

_____

_____

19. What are the three types of specimens that may be obtained for a Pap test? Where is each collected?

_____

20. What are the advantages of using the liquid-based Pap test method?

_____

_____

21. Why must a Pap slide be stained before it is evaluated?

_____

_____

22. How does an automated cytology computer-imaging device assist in the evaluation of a Pap slide?

_____

_____

23. List three conditions that the maturation index can help to evaluate.

_____

_____

24. Describe each of the following categories included on a cytology report:

    a. Specimen adequacy: _____

       • Satisfactory for Evaluation: _____

       • Unsatisfactory for Evaluation: _____

    b. General categorization: _____

       • Negative for Intraepithelial Lesions or Malignancy: _____

         _____

       • Epithelial Cell Abnormality: _____

25. What is the cause of most abnormal Pap test results?

_____

26. Describe the following procedures that may be performed following an abnormal Pap test result.

    a. Colposcopy:

       _____

       _____

    b. Cervical biopsy:

       _____

       _____

    c. LEEP:

       _____

       _____

    d. Cervical cryotherapy:

       _____

       _____

    e. Laser treatment:

       _____

       _____

f. Conization:

_____

_____

27. What is the purpose of performing the bimanual pelvic examination?

_____

_____

28. What is the purpose of the rectal–vaginal examination?

_____

_____

29. What is the difference between a vaginal infection and a sexually transmitted infection?

_____

_____

30. List the symptoms of each of the following gynecologic infections:

a. Bacterial vaginosis in the female:

_____

_____

b. Vulvovaginal candidiasis in the female:

_____

_____

c. Trichomoniasis in the female:

_____

_____

d. Chlamydia

Female:

_____

_____

Male:

_____

_____

e. Gonorrhea

Female:

_____

_____

Male:

_____

_____

314

f. Genital herpes:

      _____

      _____

g. Low-risk HPV infection:

      _____

31. What activities increase the risk of developing bacterial vaginosis?

      _____

      _____

32. What gynecologic infections can be diagnosed through a DNA-probe test?

      _____

      _____

33. List the conditions that might precipitate the development of vulvovaginal candidiasis.

      _____

      _____

34. Describe the laboratory procedure that can be used to identify *Candida albicans* in the medical office.

      _____

      _____

35. Describe the microscopic appearance of *Trichomonas vaginalis.*

      _____

36. Describe the laboratory procedure that can be used to identify *Trichomonas vaginalis* in the medical office.

      _____

      _____

37. What are the CDC screening recommendations for chlamydia?

      _____

      _____

38. What is the recommended test method for chlamydia and gonorrhea?

      _____

39. How can a vaginal specimen be obtained to test for chlamydia if a woman does not need a pelvic examination?

      _____

40. What are the symptoms of PID? What complications can occur from PID?

      _____

      _____

315

41. What conditions may result from infection with the following?

   a. Herpes simplex virus 1: _____

   b. Herpes simplex virus 2: _____

42. What may occur from being infected with persistent high-risk HPVs?

   _____

   _____

43. What is the purpose of the HPV vaccine?

   _____

Prenatal Care

Directions: Fill in each blank with the correct answer.

1. What is the purpose of prenatal care?

   _____

   _____

2. List the three categories of medical office visits for provision of prenatal and postnatal care to the pregnant woman.

   _____

   _____

3. List the four components of the first prenatal visit.

   _____

   _____

4. What is the purpose of the prenatal record?

   _____

   _____

5. List two types of information included in the past medical history (of the prenatal record).

   _____

   _____

6. What is the purpose of the obstetric history?

   _____

7. List three types of information included in the present pregnancy history.

   _____

   _____

8. What are the warning signs of a spontaneous abortion?

   _____

   _____

9. What are the warning signs of preeclampsia?

_____

_____

10. What is the purpose of the interval prenatal history?

_____

11. Explain the importance of performing a physical examination on the prenatal patient.

_____

_____

12. What is the importance of making sure a pregnant woman does not have gonorrhea before delivery of the infant?

_____

_____

13. Why is a pregnant woman tested for group B streptococcus (GBS)? When is the woman tested for GBS?

_____

_____

14. What is the purpose of performing hemoglobin and hematocrit tests on a prenatal patient?

_____

15. What is the importance of assessing the Rh factor and ABO blood type of a pregnant woman?

_____

16. What is the purpose of performing a glucose challenge test on a pregnant woman?

_____

17. List two tests that can be used to screen for the presence of syphilis.

_____

18. What is the purpose of performing a rubella titer test on a pregnant woman?

_____

19. Why is RH immune globulin (RhoGAM) administered to an Rh-negative pregnant woman?

_____

20. Why does the CDC recommend that pregnant women have a blood test to screen for exposure to the hepatitis B virus?

_____

_____

21. What is the CDC recommendation for HIV testing on pregnant women?

_____

_____

317

22. What is the purpose of the return prenatal visit? List the usual schedule for return prenatal visits.

_____

_____

_____

23. What tests are performed on the patient's urine specimen at each return visit and why is each performed?

_____

_____

24. List two purposes of measuring the fundal height.

_____

_____

25. What is the normal range for the fetal heart rate?

_____

26. What is the purpose of performing a vaginal examination as the patient nears term?

_____

_____

27. What is the purpose for performing each of the following special tests and procedures?

a. Carrier screening _____

_____

b. First trimester prenatal screening test _____

_____

c. Non-invasive prenatal test _____

_____

d. Multiple marker test _____

_____

e. Obstetric ultrasound scan _____

_____

f. Amniocentesis _____

_____

g. Fetal heart rate monitoring _____

_____

28. What conditions might warrant performing a carrier screening test?

_____

_____

29. What type of patient preparation is required for a transabdominal ultrasound scan?

_____

30. What conditions might warrant performing an amniocentesis?

_____

_____

31. What is the difference between the following fetal heart rate monitoring tests: nonstress test and contraction stress test?

_____

_____

_____

32. What occurs during the puerperium?

_____

_____

33. Describe the changes in the lochia when they should normally occur during the puerperium.

a. Lochia rubra _____

_____

b. Lochia serosa _____

_____

c. Lochia alba _____

34. When should the patient contact the medical office during the puerperium with respects to the characteristics of the lochia?

_____

_____

_____

35. When does menstruation typically occur following delivery?

a. Nonnursing mother _____

b. Nursing mother _____

36. List the procedures generally included in the 6-week postpartum examination.

_____

_____

_____

CRITICAL THINKING ACTIVITIES

A. Breast Cancer

Select three of the following questions that interest you the most. Using the following Internet sites, answer these questions in the space provided.

National Cancer Institute: www.cancer.gov
American Cancer Society: www.cancer.org
Cancer Treatment Center: www.cancercenter.com

1. Can a male develop breast cancer? Elaborate on your answer.
2. How does tamoxifen work in treating breast cancer?
3. What are the pros and cons of being tested for the breast cancer gene?
4. What methods are used to reconstruct the breast after a mastectomy?
5. What new diagnostic methods are being explored to detect breast cancer?
6. What complementary and alternative therapies are being used in the treatment of breast cancer?

Question # _____

_____

_____

_____

_____

_____

Question # _____

_____

_____

_____

_____

Question # _____

_____

_____

_____

_____

B. Methods of Contraception

Gynecologic patients often ask the medical assistant questions regarding methods of contraception. The medical assistant should have knowledge of the various types of contraceptives, how they work to prevent pregnancy, and the advantages and disadvantages of each. A list of common contraceptive methods is provided. List the information requested for each in the spaces provided. Internet sites on the topic of contraception can be used to complete this activity.

Contraceptive Method	Mode of Action	Advantages	Disadvantages
Oral contraceptives			
Contraceptive injections			
Contraceptive patch			

Contraceptive Method	Mode of Action	Advantages	Disadvantages
Birth control implant			
Male condom			
Female condom			

Contraceptive Method	Mode of Action	Advantages	Disadvantages
Spermicide			
Diaphragm			
Cervical cap			

Chapter **8** **The Gynecologic Examination and Prenatal Care**

Contraceptive Method	Mode of Action	Advantages	Disadvantages
Vaginal sponge			
Vaginal ring			
Intrauterine device (IUD)			

Contraceptive Method	Mode of Action	Advantages	Disadvantages
Fertility awareness-based method			
Surgical sterilization			
Emergency contraception			

C. Signs and Symptoms of Pregnancy

Listed here are the common signs and symptoms of pregnancy. Describe each of them and, if possible, explain what causes the sign or symptom to occur. Pregnancy internet sites can be used to obtain information to complete this activity.

1. Amenorrhea

   _____

   _____

2. Fatigue

   _____

   _____

3. Urinary frequency _____

   _____

4. Quickening

   _____

   _____

5. Goodell's sign _____

   _____

6. Hegar's sign

   _____

   _____

7. Braxton Hicks contractions

   _____

   _____

8. Skin changes: striae gravidarum, chloasma, linea nigra

   _____

   _____

   _____

D. Calculation of the Expected Date of Delivery

Calculate the expected date of delivery (EDD) for the following patients using a (cardboard) gestation calculator or an online gestation calculator and document the results below.

1. February 10, 2023 _____

2. April 28, 2023 _____

3. July 20, 2023 _____

4. October 2, 2023 _____

5. December 22, 2023 _____

E. Documenting Gravidity and Parity

The following patients are at your medical office for their first prenatal visit. In the space provided, document the following information in terms of gravidity and parity.

1. Auset Salah is pregnant for the third time. Her first pregnancy resulted in the birth of a baby boy, now alive and well. She lost her second pregnancy at 16 weeks' gestation.

   G: _____   T: _____   P: _____   A: _____   L: _____

2. Amanda Schuster is pregnant for the third time. Her first pregnancy resulted in the birth of twin girls, now alive and well. Her second pregnancy resulted in the birth of a baby girl, now alive and well.

   G: _____   T: _____   P: _____   A: _____   L: _____

3. Florencia Ramos is pregnant for the fourth time. She lost her first pregnancy at 2 months' gestation. Her second pregnancy was carried to term but resulted in the birth of a stillborn. Her third pregnancy resulted in the birth of a baby girl, now alive and well.

   G: _____   T: _____   P: _____   A: _____   L: _____

4. Rose Samson is pregnant for the fifth time. She carried her first pregnancy to 24 weeks and delivered a stillborn baby. Her second pregnancy resulted in the birth of a baby girl, now alive and well. She lost her third pregnancy at 12 weeks' gestation. Her fourth pregnancy resulted in the birth of a baby boy, now alive and well.

   G: _____   T: _____   P: _____   A: _____   L: _____

F. Nutrition During Pregnancy

1. Zamira Silva is in your medical office for her first prenatal visit. This is her first pregnancy, and she is concerned about adequate nutrition during her pregnancy. Explain why the following nutrients are of particular importance during pregnancy and provide good food sources of each. Pregnancy internet sites can be used to obtain information to complete this activity.

2. In a classroom situation, select a partner. In a role-playing situation, one student takes the role of the medical assistant, and the other plays the role of the patient. Explain to the patient the importance of these nutrients, and list good food sources of each.

327

Nutrient	Importance During Pregnancy	Food Sources
Iron		
Calcium		
Protein		
Folic acid		

G. Minor Discomforts of Pregnancy

1. Listed here are the minor discomforts that a prenatal patient may experience during pregnancy. Indicate measures the patient can take to help prevent or relieve each discomfort. Pregnancy internet sites listed can be used to obtain information to complete this activity.

2. In a classroom situation, select a partner. In a role-playing situation, one student takes the role of the medical assistant, and the other plays the role of the patient. The patient should indicate that she has a problem with each of these discomforts, and the medical assistant should respond by describing measures the patient can take to help prevent or relieve each problem.

a. Nausea (morning sickness)

_____

_____

b. Heartburn

_____

_____

c. Fatigue

_____

_____

d. Constipation

_____

_____

e. Backache

_____

_____

f. Breathing difficulties

_____

_____

g. Varicose veins

_____

_____

h. Hemorrhoids

_____

_____

i. Leg cramps

_____

_____

j. Swelling of the lower legs and feet

_____

_____

H. Health Promotion During Pregnancy

1. Identify the guidelines a prenatal patient should follow with respect to each of the areas listed below. Pregnancy internet sites can be used to obtain information to complete this activity.

2. In a classroom situation, select a partner. In a role-playing situation, one student takes the role of the medical assistant, and the other plays the role of the prenatal patient. The patient should ask for guidance regarding each of these areas, and the medical assistant should respond with appropriate information.

a. Nutrition

_____

_____

b. Exercise

_____

_____

c. Travel

_____

_____

d. Smoking

_____

_____

e. Alcohol

_____

_____

f. Medication

_____

_____

I. Breast feeding

1. Lucy Clark asks you for information regarding the advantages and disadvantages of breastfeeding and bottle–feeding. Pregnancy and childbirth internet sites can be used to obtain information to complete this activity.

2. In a classroom situation, select a partner. In a role-playing situation, one student takes the role of the medical -assistant, and the other plays the role of the patient. The patient should ask for information regarding the advantages and disadvantages of both methods, and the medical assistant should respond with appropriate information.

Breastfeeding	
Advantages	*Disadvantages*

Bottle-Feeding	
Advantages	*Disadvantages*

J. Prenatal Ultrasound

View obstetric ultrasound scans at the following Internet site:

www.ob-ultrasound.net/frames.htm

The following scans can be viewed at this site

1. Gestational sac

2. Fetus at various gestational ages

3. Fetal measurements

4. Fetal organs

5. Three-dimensional (3D) and four-dimensional (4D) images of the fetus

K. Crossword Puzzle: Gynecology and Obstetrics

Directions: Complete the crossword puzzle using the clues presented below.

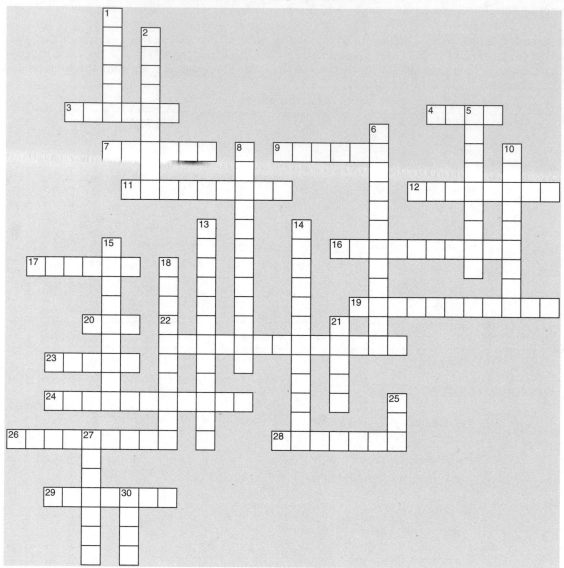

Across
3 STI preventer
4 Definite minor Pap changes
7 Malignant or benign?
9 Breast exam position
11 Growth of abnormal cells
12 Holds walls of vagina apart
16 Examination of the cervix
17 Early sign of pregnancy
19 Extreme cold to destroy cervical cells
20 Cervical cancer risk factor
22 Phase before menopause
23 Slightly abnormal Pap cells
24 Serious STI complication
26 Breast radiograph
28 Used to diagnose gonorrhea
29 Med for GDM

Down
1 What most breast lumps are
2 Pelvic exam position
5 Cause of most abnormal Pap tests
6 Genital HPV symptom
8 Removal of the uterus
10 Most frequently reported STI
13 Pregnant more than once
14 Menstrual pain
15 Menstrual cycle ceases
18 Uterus is returning to normal
21 Birth size of macrosomia baby
25 Screening test for GDM
27 Risk factor for GDM
30 Warning sign of breast cancer

PRACTICE FOR COMPETENCY

Procedure 8-1: Breast Self-Examination. Instruct an individual in the procedure for performing a breast self-examination and document the procedure in the chart provided.

Procedure 8-A: Patient-Collected Vaginal Specimen. Instruct a patient in the procedure for obtaining a patient-collected vaginal specimen and document the procedure in the chart provided.

Procedure 8-2: Gynecologic Examination

1. Complete the cytology request form provided using a female classmate as the patient.

2. Practice the procedure for assisting with a gynecologic examination. Document the vital signs and height and weight in the chart provided.

CHART	
Date	

333

Chapter **8** The Gynecologic Examination and Prenatal Care

GYN CYTOLOGY REQUISITION

THOMAS WOODSIDE, MD
501 MAIN ST
ST. LOUIS, MO 63146
(314) 883–0093

PATIENT INFO

Patient's Name (Last)	(First)	(MI)	Date of Birth MO | DAY | YR	Collection Time : AM PM	Collection Date MO | DAY | YR	Patient's ID #

Patient's Address	Phone
City	State	ZIP

RESP. PARTY

Name of Responsible Party (if different from patient)
Address of Responsible Party	APT #
City	State	ZIP

INSURANCE

Patient's Relationship to Responsible Party: ☐ 1. Self ☐ 2. Spouse ☐ 3. Child ☐ 4. Other

Insurance Company Name	Plan	Carrier Code
Subscriber/Member #	Location	Group #
Insurance Address		Physician's Provider #
	State	ZIP
Employer's Name or Number	Insured SSN	

Diagnosis/Signs/Symptoms in ICD-9 Format (Highest Specificity)

REQUIRED

ICD-9 codes are the internationally accepted method of describing the clinical picture of the patient. All diagnoses should be provided by the ordering physician or his or her authorized designee. The following is a partial list of common diagnoses in ICD-9 format. Most third party payers require an ICD-9 code to indicate the medical necessity of the test(s) and/or profile(s) ordered. For a complete list of all ICD-9 codes, please refer to a current ICD-9 manual.

V76.2	Routine Cervical Pap Smear	616.0	Cervicitis	626.8	Abnormal Bleeding
V15.89	High Risk Cervical Screening	616.10	Vaginitis	627.1	Postmenopausal Bleeding
V22.2	Pregnancy	617.0	Endometriosis, Uterus	627.3	Atrophic Vaginitis
079.4	Human Papillomavirus	622.1	Dysplasia, Cervix	795.0	Abnormal Cervical Pap Smear
180.0	Malignant Neoplasm, Cervix	623.0	Dysplasia, Vagina		

COLLECTION METHOD

Liquid-Based Prep

192055 ☐ Thin Prep Pap Test

192039 ☐ Thin Prep Pap Test w/reflex to HPV Hybrid Capture when ASC-US or SIL

192047 ☐ Thin Prep Pap Test w/reflex to high-risk only HPV Hybrid Capture when ASC-US

Pap Smear

009100 ☐ 1 Slide   009191 ☐ 2 Slides

Pap Smear and Maturation Index

009209 ☐ 1 Slide   190074 ☐ 2 Slides

SOURCE OF SPECIMEN

☐ Cervical
☐ Endocervical
☐ Vaginal

Date LMP

___ / ___ / ___
Mo   Day   Year

COLLECTION TECHNIQUE

☐ Spatula
☐ Brush
☐ Broom
☐ Other
_____

PATIENT HISTORY

☐ Pregnant
☐ Lactating
☐ Oral Contraceptives
☐ Postmenopausal
☐ Hormone Replacement Therapy

☐ PMP Bleeding
☐ Postpartum
☐ IUD
☐ Postcoital Bleeding
☐ DES Exposure
☐ Previous Abnormal Pap Test

☐ Other _____

PREVIOUS TREATMENT   Date/Results

☐ None
☐ Colposcopy and Bx   _____
☐ Cryosurgery   _____
☐ LEEP   _____
☐ Laser Vaporization   _____
☐ Conization   _____
☐ Hysterectomy   _____
☐ Radiation   _____
☐ Chemotherapy   _____

Procedure 8-3: Return Prenatal Examination

1. Complete the prenatal health history form provided using a female classmate as the patient.

2. Prepare the patient and assist with a return prenatal examination. Document the results of procedures you performed on the chart provided.

CHART	
Date	

335

CHART	
Date	

Chapter **8** **The Gynecologic Examination and Prenatal Care**

PRENATAL HEALTH HISTORY

PATIENT INFORMATION

Date: _____ EDD: _____

Name: _____
         LAST   FIRST   MIDDLE

Address: _____

_____
    CITY   STATE   ZIP

Referred By: _____

Phone (home): _____

Phone (work): _____

Emergency Contact: _____

Phone: _____

Date of Birth: ___/___/___ Age: ____ Marital Status: _____

Occupation: _____

Education: ☐ High School ☐ College ☐ Post-graduate

PAST MEDICAL HISTORY

	○ Neg + Pos	DETAIL POSITIVE REMARKS INCLUDE DATE AND TREATMENT		○ Neg + Pos	DETAIL POSITIVE REMARKS INCLUDE DATE AND TREATMENT
1. DIABETES			16. D (Rh) SENSITIZED		
2. HYPERTENSION			17. PULMONARY (TB, ASTHMA)		
3. HEART DISEASE			18. RHEUMATIC FEVER		
4. AUTOIMMUNE DISORDER			19. BLEEDING TENDENCY		
5. KIDNEY DISEASE/UTI			20. GYN SURGERY		
6. NEUROLOGIC/EPILEPSY					
7. PSYCHIATRIC			21. OPERATIONS/HOSPITALIZATIONS (YEAR AND REASON)		
8. HEPATITIS/LIVER DISEASE					
9. VARICOSITIES/PHLEBITIS					
10. THYROID DYSFUNCTION			22. ANESTHETIC COMPLICATIONS		
11. TRAUMA/DOMESTIC VIOLENCE			23. HISTORY OF ABNORMAL PAP		
12. BLOOD TRANSFUSION			24. UTERINE ANOMALY/DES		

	AMT/DAY PREPREG.	AMT/DAY PREG.	# YEARS USE			
				25. INFERTILITY		
13. TOBACCO				26. SEXUALLY TRANSMITTED DISEASE		
14. ALCOHOL						
15. STREET DRUGS				27. OTHER		

IMMUNIZATIONS:

Mark an X next to those you have had.

☐ Influenza   ☐ Chickenpox

☐ Hepatitis B   ☐ Pneumococcal

☐ Hib   ☐ Tuberculin Test

☐ Polio   ☐ Tetanus Booster

☐ MMR

ALLERGIES:

List all allergies (foods, drugs, environment). ☐ None

_____

_____

_____

_____

_____

_____

MENSTRUAL HISTORY

Menarche: Age of Onset _____

Frequency: Q _____ Days

Duration: _____ Days

Amount of Flow: ☐ Small ☐ Moderate ☐ Large

GYN Disorders (List): _____

_____

_____

On contraceptive at conception? ☐ Yes ☐ No

OBSTETRIC HISTORY

G _____ T _____ P _____ A _____ L _____
(Total Pregnancies)   (Term)   (Preterm)   (Abortions)   (Living Children)

PREVIOUS PREGNANCIES:

DATE MONTH/ YEAR	WEEKS GEST.	LENGTH OF LABOR	BIRTH WEIGHT	SEX M/F	TYPE DELIVERY	ANES.	MATERNAL COMPLICATIONS	INFANT COMPLICATIONS

PRESENT PREGNANCY HISTORY

NAUSEA			ABDOMINAL PAIN		
VOMITING			URINARY COMPLAINTS		
FATIGUE			VAGINAL BLEEDING		
BREAST CHANGES			VAGINAL DISCHARGE		
INDIGESTION			PRURITUS		
CONSTIPATION			ACCIDENTS		
PERSISTENT HEADACHES			SURGERY		
DIZZINESS			X-RAYS		
VISUAL DISTURBANCE			RUBELLA EXPOSURE		
EDEMA (SPECIFY AREA)			OTHER VIRAL INFECTIONS		

LMP _____ / _____ / _____   Amount of Flow: ☐ Small   ☐ Moderate   ☐ Large
        Mo   Day   Year

CURRENT MEDICATIONS: (Include prescription, OTC, herbal, and vitamins). ☐ None

Medication _____ **Frequency** _____

_____

_____

INITIAL PHYSICAL EXAMINATION

DATE ____ / ____ / ____

1. HEENT	☐ NORMAL	☐ ABNORMAL	12. VULVA	☐ NORMAL	☐ CONDYLOMA	☐ LESIONS
2. FUNDI	☐ NORMAL	☐ ABNORMAL	13. VAGINA	☐ NORMAL	☐ INFLAMMATION	☐ DISCHARGE
3. TEETH	☐ NORMAL	☐ ABNORMAL	14. CERVIX	☐ NORMAL	☐ INFLAMMATION	☐ LESIONS
4. THYROID	☐ NORMAL	☐ ABNORMAL	15. UTERUS SIZE _____ WEEKS			☐ FIBROIDS
5. BREASTS	☐ NORMAL	☐ ABNORMAL	16. ADNEXA	☐ NORMAL	☐ MASS	
6. LUNGS	☐ NORMAL	☐ ABNORMAL	17. RECTUM	☐ NORMAL	☐ ABNORMAL	
7. HEART	☐ NORMAL	☐ ABNORMAL	18. DIAGONAL CONJUGATE	☐ REACHED	☐ NO	_____ CM
8. ABDOMEN	☐ NORMAL	☐ ABNORMAL	19. SPINES	☐ AVERAGE	☐ PROMINENT	☐ BLUNT
9. EXTREMITIES	☐ NORMAL	☐ ABNORMAL	20. SACRUM	☐ CONCAVE	☐ STRAIGHT	☐ ANTERIOR
10. SKIN	☐ NORMAL	☐ ABNORMAL	21. SUBPUBIC ARCH	☐ NORMAL	☐ WIDE	☐ NARROW
11. LYMPH NODES	☐ NORMAL	☐ ABNORMAL	22. GYNECOID PELVIC TYPE	☐ YES	☐ NO	

COMMENTS (Number and explain abnormals): _____

_____

_____

_____ **EXAM BY** _____

PATIENT'S NAME _____

	INTERVAL PRENATAL HISTORY																	

Date 20__	Weeks Gestation	Height of Fundus (cm)	Weight	B/P	Urine Glucose	Urine Protein	FHT	Vaginal Examination	Presentation	Edema	Discharge	Bleeding	Contractions	Fetal Activity	NST	Next Appt.	Initials

PLANS/EDUCATION (COUNSELED ✓)

☐ ANESTHESIA PLANS _____
☐ TOXOPLASMOSIS PRECAUTIONS (CATS/RAW MEAT) _____
☐ CHILDBIRTH CLASSES _____
☐ PHYSICAL/SEXUAL ACTIVITY _____
☐ LABOR SIGNS _____
☐ NUTRITION COUNSELING _____
☐ BREAST OR BOTTLE FEEDING _____
☐ NEWBORN CAR SEAT _____
☐ POSTPARTUM BIRTH CONTROL _____
☐ ENVIRONMENTAL/WORK HAZARDS _____

☐ TUBAL STERILIZATION _____
☐ VBAC COUNSELING _____
☐ CIRCUMCISION _____
☐ TRAVEL _____
☐ LIFESTYLE, TOBACCO, ALCOHOL _____

REQUESTS _____
_____

TUBAL STERILIZATION   DATE   INITIALS
CONSENT SIGNED   ___/___/___   _____

339

LABORATORY		PATIENT'S NAME _____			
INITIAL LABS	DATE	RESULTS		REVIEWED	COMMENTS
BLOOD TYPE	/ /	A B AB O			
Rh FACTOR	/ /	☐ Pos ☐ Neg			
Rh ANTIBODY SCREEN	/ /	☐ Pos ☐ Neg			
HCT/HGB	/ /	_____% _____ g/dL			
RUBELLA ANTIBODY TITER	/ /	Immune Nonimmune			
VDRL	/ /	☐ NR ☐ R			
HBsAg (HEPATITIS B)	/ /	☐ Pos ☐ Neg			
HIV	/ /	☐ Pos ☐ Neg ☐ Declined			
URINE CULTURE/SCREEN	/ /				
PAP TEST	/ /	☐ Normal ☐ Abnormal			
CHLAMYDIA (DNA PROBE)	/ /	☐ Pos ☐ Neg			
GONORRHEA (DNA PROBE)	/ /	☐ Pos ☐ Neg			
7–20 WEEK LABS (WHEN INDICATED/ELECTED)	DATE	RESULTS		REVIEWED	COMMENTS
ULTRASOUND #1 (7–13 WEEKS)	/ /	EDD:			
ULTRASOUND #2 (18–20 WEEKS)	/ /	EFW:			
Multiple marker test (15–20 WEEKS)	/ /				
CVS	/ /				
AMNIOCENTESIS	/ /				
24–28 WEEK LABS (WHEN INDICATED)	DATE	RESULTS		REVIEWED	COMMENTS
HCT/HGB	/ /	_____ % _____ g/dL			
GCT (24–28 WKS)	/ /	1 Hour _____			
GTT (IF SCREEN ABNORMAL)	/ /	_____ FBS _____ 1 Hour _____ 2 Hour _____ 3 Hour			
D (Rh) ANTIBODY SCREEN	/ /				
D IMMUNE GLOBULIN (RhIG) GIVEN (28 WKS)	/ /	SIGNATURE			
32–36 WEEK LABS	DATE	RESULTS		REVIEWED	COMMENTS
HCT/HGB (32 WKS)	/ /	_____ % _____ g/dL			
ULTRASOUND #3 (34 WKS)	/ /	EFW:			
GROUP B STREP (35–37 WKS)	/ /	☐ Pos ☐ Neg			
ADDITIONAL LAB TESTS	DATE	RESULTS		REVIEWED	COMMENTS
	/ /				
	/ /				
	/ /				
	/ /				
	/ /				

Procedure 8-1: Breast Self-Examination Instructions

Name: _____   Date: _____

Evaluated by: _____   Score: _____

Performance Objective

Outcome:	Instruct a patient in the procedure for performing a breast self-examination.
Conditions:	Small pillow.
Standards:	Time: 10 minutes. Student completed procedure in _____ minutes.
	Accuracy: Satisfactory score on the performance evaluation checklist.

Performance Evaluation Checklist

Trial 1	Trial 2	Point Value	Performance Standards
		•	Greeted the patient and introduced yourself.
		•	Identified patient and explained that you will be instructing the patient in a BSE.
		•	Explained the purpose of the exam, when to perform it, and the three methods of examination.
		▷	Explained why three methods are used to examine the breasts.
			Instructed the patient:
			1. Before a mirror
		•	Remove clothing from the waist up and stand in front of a large mirror.
		•	Place arms at sides.
		•	Inspect the breasts for a change in size or shape; swelling, puckering, or dimpling; change in skin texture; nipple retraction; change in nipple size or position compared with other breast.
		▷	Described what may cause puckering or dimpling of the skin.
		•	Slowly raise arms over head and repeat the same inspection.
		▷	Stated what should normally occur when the arms are moved at the same time.
		•	Rest palms on hips, press down firmly to flex the chest muscles, and repeat the breast inspection.
		▷	Stated the purpose of flexing the chest muscles.
		•	Gently squeeze each nipple and look for a discharge.
			2. Lying down
		•	Place a small pillow (or folded towel) under right shoulder.
		•	Place the right hand behind the head.
		▷	Stated the purpose of the pillow and the hand placement.

Trial 1	Trial 2	Point Value	Performance Standards
		•	Use the finger pads of the middle three fingers of the left hand to perform the examination.
		▷	Explained why the finger pads should be used.
		•	Use small rotating motions and continuous firm pressure with the finger pads.
		•	Use one of the following patterns to move around the breast: circular, vertical strip, or wedge.
		▷	Stated why a pattern is used.
			Circular pattern:
		•	Visualize the breast as a clock face.
		•	Start at outside edge of breast.
		•	Proceed clockwise around the outer rim of the breast until you return to the starting point.
		•	Move in 1 inch, and repeat the circle.
		•	Continue around the breast in smaller circles until the nipple is reached.
			Vertical strip:
		•	Mentally divide the breast into strips.
		•	Start at the underarm.
		•	Slowly move fingers down until they are below the breast.
		•	Move fingers 1 inch toward middle and move back up.
		•	Repeat until entire breast has been examined.
			Wedge:
		•	Mentally divide the breasts into wedges.
		•	Start at outer edge of the breast.
		•	Move fingers toward the nipple and back to edge of breast.
		•	Repeat until the entire breast has been examined.
			Used the following techniques during the examination:
			Used the finger pads and the pattern selected to examine the right breast.
		•	Press firmly enough to feel the different breast tissues.
		•	Palpate for lumps, hard knots, and thickening.
		▷	Explained how normal breast tissue feels.
		•	Examine the entire chest area from the collarbone to the base of a properly fitted bra and from the breastbone to the underarm.
		•	Pay special attention to the area between the breast and underarm including the under-arm itself.
		▷	Explained why the underarm should be examined.

Trial 1	Trial 2	Point Value	Performance Standards
		•	Continue the examination until every part of the right breast has been examined, including the nipple.
		•	Repeat the procedure on the left breast, with a small pillow or rolled towel under the left shoulder, the left hand behind the head, and using the right hand to palpate.
			3. In the shower
		•	Gently lather each breast.
		▷	Explained why the breasts should be examined in the shower.
		•	Place right hand behind the head.
		•	Use the finger pads of the middle three fingers of the left hand.
		•	Use small, rotating motions and continuous, firm pressure to examine the right breast.
		•	Use your preferred pattern to palpate the breast and underarm for lumps, hard knots, and thickening.
		•	Repeat the procedure on the left breast by placing the left arm behind the head and using the pads of the right fingers.
		•	Instructed the patient to report any lumps or changes to the provider immediately.
		•	Documented the procedure correctly.
		■	Reassured patients.
		■	Demonstrated tactfulness.
		*	Completed the procedure within 10 minutes.
			Totals

CHART	
Date	

Evaluation of Student Performance

EVALUATION CRITERIA			COMMENTS
Symbol	**Category**	**Point Value**	
★	Critical Step	16 points	
•	Essential Step	6 points	
■	Affective Competency	6 points	
▷	Theory Question	2 points	

Score calculation: 100 points

− points missed

___Score

Satisfactory score: 85 or above

CAAHEP Competencies Achieved

Psychomotor (Skills)

☑ V. 3. Coach patients regarding: a. office policies b. medical encounters.
☑ X. 3. Document patient care accurately in the medical record.

Affective (Behavior)

☑ A. 2 Reassure patients.
☑ A. 7. Demonstrate tactfulness.

ABHES Competencies Achieved

☑ 4. a. Follow documentation guidelines.
☑ 7. g. Display professionalism through written and verbal communications.
☑ 8. h. Teach self-examination, disease management and health promotion.

Procedure 8-A: Patient-Collected Vaginal Specimen Instructions

Name: _____ Date: _____

Evaluated by: _____ Score: _____

Performance Objective

Outcome:	Instruct a patient in the procedure for obtaining a patient-collected vaginal specimen.
Conditions:	Given the following: Disposable gloves, specimen collection kit, laboratory requisition form, and a biohazard specimen transport bag.
Standards:	Time: 10 minutes. Student completed procedure in _____ minutes.
	Accuracy: Satisfactory score on the performance evaluation checklist.

Performance Evaluation Checklist

Trial 1	Trial 2	Point Value	Performance Standards
		•	Sanitized hands
		•	Assembled equipment. Checked the expiration date on the specimen collection kit.
		•	Completed a laboratory requisition and labeled the transport tube.
		▷	Stated what information should be included on the transport tube label.
		•	Greeted the patient and introduced yourself.
		•	Identified patient and explained that you will be instructing the patient how to collect a vaginal specimen.
		•	Escorted the patient to the rest room and placed the transport tube on a flat surface.
		•	Partially opened the swab package and placed it on a flat surface within easy reach of the patient.
			Instructed the patient:
		•	Wash hands thoroughly and dry them.
		•	Do not cleanse or wipe the genital area.
		•	Remove all clothing from the waist down.
		•	Comfortably position yourself by either sitting on the toilet or standing with the legs spread apart.
		•	Remove the swab from the package making sure not to touch the tip, drop it, or lay it down.
		▷	Stated what the patient should do if the swab becomes contaminated.
		•	Hold the swab in your dominant hand and place your thumb and forefinger in the middle of the shaft covering the black score line.
		•	Expose the vaginal opening by spreading apart the folds of skin around the vaginal opening with your nondominant hand.
		•	Insert the tip of the swab into your vagina about 2 inches past the opening of the vagina (approximately the length of your little finger).

345

Trial 1	Trial 2	Point Value	Performance Standards
		•	Gently rotate the swab for 10 to 30 seconds making sure the swab touches the walls of the vagina.
		•	Withdraw the swab without touching the skin outside the vagina.
		•	While still holding the swab in your dominant hand, unscrew the cap from the transport tube.
		•	Lower the swab into the tube until the visible black score line on the swab shaft is lined up with the rim of the tube.
		•	Break the swab shaft at the score line by leaning the shaft against the tube rim being careful not to spill the liquid in the tube.
		•	Dispose of the broken-off end of the shaft in a biohazard waste container.
		•	Tightly screw the cap onto the transport tube.
		•	Thoroughly wash hands and return the transport tube to the medical assistant.
			Performed the following:
		•	Applied gloves and placed the transport tube in a biohazard specimen transport bag. Insert the laboratory requisition in the outside pocket.
		•	Removed gloves and sanitized the hands.
		•	Placed the specimen in the proper place for pickup by the laboratory.
		•	Documented the procedure correctly.
		■	Reassured patients.
		■	Demonstrated empathy for patients' concerns.
		★	Completed the procedure within 10 minutes.
			Totals

CHART	
Date	

Evaluation of Student Performance

EVALUATION CRITERIA			COMMENTS
Symbol	**Category**	**Point Value**	
★	Critical Step	16 points	
•	Essential Step	6 points	
■	Affective Competency	6 points	
▷	Theory Question	2 points	

Score calculation: 100 points

    −   points missed

       ___Score

Satisfactory score: 85 or above

CAAHEP Competencies Achieved

Psychomotor (Skills)

☑   I. 8. Instruct and prepare a patient for a procedure or treatment.

Affective (Behavior)

☑   A. 2. Reassure patients.
☑   A. 3. Demonstrate empathy for patients' concerns.

ABHES Competencies Achieved

☑   5. h. Display effective interpersonal skills with patients and health care team members.
☑   7. g. Display professionalism through written and verbal communications.

Notes

Procedure 8-2: Assisting with a Gynecologic Examination

Name: _____   Date: _____

Evaluated by: _____   Score: _____

Performance Objective

Outcome:	Assist with a gynecologic examination.
Conditions:	Given the following: disposable gloves, examining gown and drape, disposable vaginal speculum, collection vial, cytospatula and cytobrush or cytobroom, lubricant, gauze pads, fecal occult blood test, tissues, cytology request form, biohazard specimen transport bag.
	Using an examining table
Standards:	Time: 15 minutes. Student completed procedure in _____ minutes.
	Accuracy: Satisfactory score on the Performance Evaluation Checklist.

Performance Evaluation Checklist

Trial 1	Trial 2	Point Value	Performance Standards
		•	Sanitized hands.
		•	Assembled equipment.
		•	Completed as much of the cytology request form as possible.
		•	Checked expiration date and labeled the collection vial.
		•	Greeted the patient and introduced yourself.
		•	Escorted the patient to the examining room.
		•	Identified the patient.
		•	Asked patient if she has any problems or concerns and documented the information.
		•	Completed the rest of the cytology request by asking necessary questions.
		•	Measured vital signs and height and weight and documented the results correctly.
			Prepared patient for the examination:
		•	Asked patient if she needs to empty the bladder or instructed the patient in the collection of a urine specimen.
		▷	Explained why the bladder should be empty for the examination.
		•	Instructed the patient to undress and put on the examining gown with opening in front and to have a seat on the examining table.
		•	Left the room to provide patient privacy.
		•	Made medical record available for review by the provider (if using a PPR).
		•	Knocked lightly on the door and checked to make sure the patient is ready.
		•	Informed the provider that the patient was ready.

349

Trial 1	Trial 2	Point Value	Performance Standards
			Assisted the provider:
		•	Positioned and draped patient in a supine position for the breast examination.
		•	Positioned and draped patient in the lithotomy position for the pelvic examination.
		•	Prepared the vaginal speculum with lubricant and handed it to the provider.
		•	Prepared the light for the provider.
		•	Handed vaginal speculum to the provider.
		•	Reassured patient and helped the patient relax **during the examination.**
		▷	Explained why patient should be relaxed during the examination.
			Assisted with Pap specimen collection:
		•	Applied gloves.
			ThinPrep Cytospatula and Cytobrush Method
		•	Removed cap and held the vial to receive the cytospatula from the provider.
		•	Rinsed the cytospatula in the preservative by vigorously swirling it 10 times.
		▷	Explained why the cytospatula should be swirled vigorously.
		•	Discarded the cytospatula in a biohazard waste container.
		•	Held the vial to receive the cytobrush from the provider.
		•	Rinsed the cytobrush in the preservative by vigorously rotating it 10 times while pushing it against the vial wall.
		•	Swirl the cytobrush in the solution to further release cellular material and discarded it in a biohazard waste container.
		•	Securely tightened the cap on the vial.
			ThinPrep Cytobroom Method
		•	Removed cap and held the vial to receive the cytobroom from the provider.
		•	Rinsed the cytobroom in the preservative by pushing it vigorously into the bottom of the vial 10 times.
		•	Swirl the cytobroom vigorously to further release cellular material.
		•	Discarded the cytobroom in a biohazard waste container.
		•	Securely tightened the cap on the vial.
			SurePath spatula and brush method
		•	Removed cap and held the vial to receive each collection device from the provider.
		•	Broke off or disconnected tip of each collection device.
		•	Discarded each handle in a regular waste container.
		•	Securely tightened the cap on the vial.

Trial 1	Trial 2	Point Value	Performance Standards
			Assisted with the remainder of the examination:
		•	Removed light source.
		•	Discarded vaginal speculum in a biohazard waste container.
		•	Provided the provider with lubricant for the bimanual and rectal-vaginal examinations.
		•	Assisted as required with the collection of the fecal occult blood specimen.
		•	Assisted the patient into a sitting position and allowed her to rest.
		▷	Explained why the patient should be allowed to rest.
		•	Offered the patient tissues to remove lubricant from the perineum.
		•	Assisted patient from the examining table.
		•	Instructed the patient to get dressed.
		•	Informed patient of the method used by the medical office to relay test results.
		•	Tested the fecal occult blood specimen and documented the results.
		•	Prepared Pap specimen for transport to the laboratory.
		•	Placed specimen in a biohazard specimen bag and sealed the bag.
		•	Inserted the cytology requisition into the outside pocket of bag.
		•	Placed bag in appropriate location for pickup by the laboratory.
		•	Documented the transport of the Pap specimen to an outside laboratory.
		•	Cleaned the examining room.
		■	Reassured patients.
		■	Demonstrated empathy for patients' concerns.
		■	Demonstrated active listening.
		★	Completed the procedure within 15 minutes.
			Totals

CHART	
Date	

Evaluation of Student Performance

EVALUATION CRITERIA			COMMENTS
Symbol	**Category**	**Point Value**	
★	Critical Step	16 points	
•	Essential Step	6 points	
■	Affective Competency	6 points	
▷	Theory Question	2 points	

Score calculation: 100 points

− _____ points missed

_____ Score

Satisfactory score: 85 or above

CAAHEP Competencies Achieved

Psychomotor (Skills)

☑ I. 3. Perform patient screening following established protocols.
☑ I. 8. Instruct and prepare a patient for a procedure or a treatment.
☑ I. 9. Assist provider with a patient exam.
☑ II. 2. Record laboratory test results in the patient's record.
☑ V. 1. Respond to nonverbal communication.
☑ X. 2. Apply HIPAA rules in regard to: a. privacy b. release of information.
☑ X. 3. Document patient care accurately in the medical record.

Affective (Behavior)

☑ Reassure patients.
☑ A. 3. Demonstrate empathy for patients' concerns.
☑ A. 4. Demonstrate active listening.

ABHES Competencies Achieved

☑ 4. a. Follow documentation guidelines.
☑ 8. b. Obtain and document chief complaint, patient history, and vital signs.
☑ 8. d. Assist provider with specialty examination including pediatric care, cardiac, respiratory, OB-GYN, neurological, and gastroenterology procedures.
☑ 8. e. Perform specialty procedures including but not limited to pediatric care, minor surgery, cardiac, respiratory, OB-GYN, neurological, and gastroenterology.
☑ 8. h. Teach self-examination, disease management and health promotion.

GYN CYTOLOGY REQUISITION

THOMAS WOODSIDE, MD
501 MAIN ST
ST. LOUIS, MO 63146
(314) 883–0093

PATIENT INFO

Patient's Name (Last)	(First)	(MI)	Date of Birth MO DAY YR	Collection Time : AM PM	Collection Date MO DAY YR	Patient's ID #

Patient's Address   Phone

City   State   ZIP

RESP. PARTY

Name of Responsible Party (if different from patient)

Address of Responsible Party   APT #

City   State   ZIP

INSURANCE

Patient's Relationship to Responsible Party   ☐ 1. Self   ☐ 2. Spouse   ☐ 3. Child   ☐ 4. Other

Insurance Company Name	Plan	Carrier Code
Subscriber/Member #	Location	Group #
Insurance Address		Physician's Provider #
City	State	ZIP
Employer's Name or Number	Insured SSN	

Diagnosis/Signs/Symptoms in ICD-9 Format (Highest Specificity)

REQUIRED

ICD-9 codes are the internationally accepted method of describing the clinical picture of the patient. All diagnoses should be provided by the ordering physician or his or her authorized designee. The following is a partial list of common diagnoses in ICD-9 format. Most third party payers require an ICD-9 code to indicate the medical necessity of the test(s) and/or profile(s) ordered. For a complete list of all ICD-9 codes, please refer to a current ICD-9 manual.

V76.2	Routine Cervical Pap Smear	616.0	Cervicitis	626.8	Abnormal Bleeding
V15.89	High Risk Cervical Screening	616.10	Vaginitis	627.1	Postmenopausal Bleeding
V22.2	Pregnancy	617.0	Endometriosis, Uterus	627.3	Atrophic Vaginitis
079.4	Human Papillomavirus	622.1	Dysplasia, Cervix	795.0	Abnormal Cervical Pap Smear
180.0	Malignant Neoplasm, Cervix	623.0	Dysplasia, Vagina		

COLLECTION METHOD	SOURCE OF SPECIMEN	COLLECTION TECHNIQUE

Liquid-Based Prep

192055 ☐ Thin Prep Pap Test

192039 ☐ Thin Prep Pap Test w/reflex to HPV Hybrid Capture when ASC-US or SIL

192047 ☐ Thin Prep Pap Test w/reflex to high-risk only HPV Hybrid Capture when ASC-US

Pap Smear
009100 ☐ 1 Slide   009191 ☐ 2 Slides

Pap Smear and Maturation Index
009209 ☐ 1 Slide   190074 ☐ 2 Slides

☐ Cervical
☐ Endocervical
☐ Vaginal

Date LMP
___/___/___
Mo   Day   Year

☐ Spatula
☐ Brush
☐ Broom
☐ Other _____

PATIENT HISTORY	PREVIOUS TREATMENT	Date/Results

☐ Pregnant
☐ Lactating
☐ Oral Contraceptives
☐ Postmenopausal
☐ Hormone Replacement Therapy

☐ PMP Bleeding
☐ Postpartum
☐ IUD
☐ Postcoital Bleeding
☐ DES Exposure
☐ Previous Abnormal Pap Test

☐ Other _____

☐ None
☐ Colposcopy and Bx _____
☐ Cryosurgery _____
☐ LEEP _____
☐ Laser Vaporization _____
☐ Conization _____
☐ Hysterectomy _____
☐ Radiation _____
☐ Chemotherapy _____

353

Notes

Procedure 8-3: Assisting with a Return Prenatal Examination

Name: _____   Date: _____

Evaluated by: _____   Score: _____

Performance Objective

Outcome:	Prepare the patient and assist with a return prenatal examination.
Conditions:	Using an examining table. Given the following: urine specimen container, centimeter tape measure, Doppler fetal pulse detector, ultrasound coupling agent, paper towel, disposable vaginal speculum, disposable gloves, lubricant, gauze pads, and an examining gown and drape.
Standards:	Time: 15 minutes. Student completed procedure in _____ minutes. Accuracy: Satisfactory score on the Performance Evaluation Checklist.

Performance Evaluation Checklist

Trial 1	Trial 2	Point Value	Performance Standards
		•	Sanitized hands.
		•	Set up the tray for the prenatal examination.
		•	Greeted the patient and introduced yourself.
		•	Identified the patient and explained the procedure.
		•	Provided a specimen container and asked the patient to obtain a urine specimen.
		•	Escorted the patient to the examining room and asked her to be seated.
		•	Asked the patient if she has experienced any problems since her last visit and documented information in the prenatal record.
		•	Measured the patient's blood pressure and documented the results correctly.
		•	Weighed the patient and documented the results correctly.
		▷	Stated the importance of weighing the patient.
		•	Instructed and prepared the patient for the examination and told her to take a seat on the examining table.
		•	Left the room to provide the patient with privacy.
		•	Tested the urine specimen for glucose and protein, and documented the results correctly.
		▷	Explained why the urine specimen is tested for glucose and protein.
		•	Made the medical record available for review by the provider (PPR).
		•	Knocked lightly on the door and checked to make sure the patient is ready to be seen by the provider.
		•	Informed the provider that patient is ready.
		▷	Stated how the provider can be informed that the patient is ready.

Trial 1	Trial 2	Point Value	Performance Standards
		•	Assisted the patient into a supine position and properly draped her.
		•	Provided support and reassurance to the patient.
			Assisted the provider during the examination:
		•	Handed the provider the tape measure for determination of fundal height.
		•	Applied coupling gel to the patient's abdomen and handed the provider the Doppler device.
			Removed gel from patient's abdomen
		•	Cleaned the probe head of the Doppler device and placed it back in its holder.
		•	Assisted the patient into the lithotomy position if a vaginal specimen is to be obtained or if vaginal examination is to be performed.
			After completion of the examination:
		•	Assisted the patient into a sitting position and allowed her to rest.
		▷	Explained why the patient should be allowed to rest.
		•	Assisted the patient from examining table and instructed her to get dressed.
		•	Left the room to provide patient privacy.
		•	Provided prenatal patient teaching and explanation of the provider's instructions as required.
		•	Escorted the patient to the reception area.
		•	Cleaned the examining room in preparation for the next patient.
		•	Prepared any specimens collected for transport to an outside laboratory.
		■	Reassured patients.
		■	Demonstrated empathy for patients' concerns.
		■	Demonstrated active listening.
		★	Completed the procedure within 15 minutes.
			Totals

CHART

Date	

Evaluation of Student Performance

EVALUATION CRITERIA			COMMENTS
Symbol	**Category**	**Point Value**	
★	Critical Step	16 points	
•	Essential Step	6 points	
■	Affective Competency	6 points	
▷	Theory Question	2 points	

Score calculation: 100 points

        –   points missed

           ___Score

Satisfactory score: 85 or above

CAAHEP Competencies Achieved

Psychomotor (Skills)

☑ I. 3. Perform patient screening following established protocols.
☑ I. 8. Instruct and prepare a patient for a procedure or a treatment.
☑ I. 9. Assist provider with a patient exam.
☑ II. 2. Record laboratory test results in the patients' record.
☑ V. 3. Coach patients regarding a. office policies b. medical encounters.
☑ V. 3. Coach patients regarding: a. office policies b. medical encounters.
☑ X. 2. Apply HIPAA rules in regard to: a. privacy b. release of information.
☑ X. 3. Document patient care accurately in the medical record.

Affective (Behavior)

☑ V. 2. Reassured patients.
☑ A. 3. Demonstrate empathy for patients' concerns.
☑ A. 4. Demonstrate active listening.

ABHES Competencies Achieved

☑ 4. a. Follow documentation guidelines.
☑ 7. g. Display professionalism through written and verbal communications.
☑ 8. b. Obtain and document chief complaint, patient history, and vital signs.
☑ 8. d. Assist provider with specialty examination including pediatric care, cardiac, respiratory, OB-GYN, neurological, and gastroenterology procedures.
☑ 8. e. Perform specialty procedures including but not limited to pediatric care, minor surgery, cardiac, respiratory, OB-GYN, neurological, and gastroenterology.
☑ 8. h. Teach self-examination, disease management and health promotion.

PATIENT'S NAME _____

INTERVAL PRENATAL HISTORY																	
Date 20___	Weeks Gestation	Height of Fundus (cm)	Weight	B/P	Urine Glucose	Urine Protein	FHT	Vaginal Examination	Presentation	Edema	Discharge	Bleeding	Contractions	Fetal Activity	NST	Next Appt.	Initials

9 The Pediatric Examination

CHAPTER ASSIGNMENTS

√ After Completing	Date Due	Study Guide Pages	STUDY GUIDE ASSIGNMENTS (CTA = Critical Thinking Activity)	Possible Points	Points You Earned
		363	Pretest	10	
		364	Term Key Term Assessment	12	
		364-368	Evaluation of Learning questions	40	
		368	CTA A: Pediatric Weight	7	
			Evolve: Pounds and Ounces (Record points earned)		
		369	CTA B: Pediatric Length	8	
			Evolve: Inch by Inch (Record points earned)		
		369-370	CTA C: Growth Charts	18	
		371	CTA D: Motor and Social Development (5 points per each category)	65	
		372	CTA E: Intramuscular Injection	15	
		372-373	CTA F: Vaccine Information Statement	11	
		373	CTA G: Locating and Interpreting a Vaccine Information Statement	20	
		373-374	CTA H: Immunization Administration Record	40	
		375	CTA I: Crossword Puzzle	28	
			Evolve: Apply Your Knowledge questions (Record points earned)	10	
			Evolve: Video Evaluation	31	
		363	Posttest	10	

√ After Completing	Date Due	Study Guide Pages	STUDY GUIDE ASSIGNMENTS (CTA = Critical Thinking Activity)	Possible Points	Points You Earned
			ADDITIONAL ASSIGNMENTS		
			Total points		

√ When Assigned By Your Instructor	Study Guide Pages	Practices Required	LABORATORY ASSIGNMENTS (Procedure Number and Name)	Score*
	377	3	**Practice for Competency** 9-A: Carrying an Infant	
	381-382		**Evaluation of Competency** 9-A: Carrying an Infant	*
	378	5	**Practice for Competency** 9-1: Measuring the Weight and Length of an Infant	
	383-385		**Evaluation of Competency** 9-1: Measuring the Weight and Length of an Infant	*
	378	5	**Practice for Competency** 9-2: Measuring Head and Chest Circumference of an Infant	
	387-388		**Evaluation of Competency** 9-2: Measuring Head and Chest Circumference of an Infant	*
	378	5	**Practice for Competency** 9-3: Calculating Growth Percentiles	
	389-390		**Evaluation of Competency** 9-3: Calculating Growth Percentiles	*
	379-380	5	**Practice for Competency** 9-4: Applying a Pediatric Urine Collector	
	391-393		**Evaluation of Competency** 9-4: Applying a Pediatric Urine Collector	*
	379-380	5	**Practice for Competency** 9-5: Newborn Screening Test	
			Evaluation of Competency 9-5: Newborn Screening Test	*
			ADDITIONAL ASSIGNMENTS	

Notes

Name: _____ Date: _____

True or False

_____ 1. A pediatrician is a medical doctor who specializes in the diagnosis and treatment of disease in children.

_____ 2. The first well-child visit is usually scheduled 4 weeks after birth of the infant.

_____ 3. Length is measured with the child standing with his or her back to the measuring device.

_____ 4. Blood pressure should be taken for a child starting at 8 years of age.

_____ 5. It is best not to tell a child that an immunization will hurt.

_____ 6. The vastus lateralis muscle site is recommended for administering an injection to an infant.

_____ 7. An MMR injection includes the following immunizations: measles, meningitis, and rubella.

_____ 8. A Vaccine Information Statement (VIS) explains the benefits and risks of a vaccine in lay terminology.

_____ 9. The hepatitis B vaccine can be given to a newborn.

_____ 10. The blood specimen for a newborn screening test is obtained from the infant's earlobe.

📄 **POSTTEST**

True or False

_____ 1. A well-child visit is also referred to as a health maintenance visit.

_____ 2. A reason for weighing a child is to determine proper medication dosage.

_____ 3. Growth charts can be used to identify children with growth abnormalities.

_____ 4. Measuring pediatric blood pressure helps to identify children at risk for type 1 diabetes.

_____ 5. Using a blood pressure cuff that is too large for the child can result in a falsely low reading.

_____ 6. The length of the needle used for a pediatric IM injection depends on the amount of medication being administered.

_____ 7. The resistance of the body to pathogenic microorganisms or their toxins is known as inflammation.

_____ 8. The recommended route of administration for an MMR vaccine is subcutaneous.

_____ 9. Before administering a pediatric immunization, the National Childhood Vaccine Injury Act (NCVIA) requires that the parent sign a consent form.

_____ 10. If phenylketonuria (PKU) is left untreated, it can lead to malnutrition.

Directions: Match each key term with its definition.

_____ 1. Immunity

_____ 2. Immunization

_____ 3. Infant

_____ 4. Length

_____ 5. Pediatrician

_____ 6. Pediatrics

_____ 7. Preschool child

_____ 8. School-age child

_____ 9. Toddler

_____ 10. Toxoid

_____ 11. Vaccine

_____ 12. Vertex

A. A physician who specializes in the care and development of children and the diagnosis and treatment of children's diseases

B. A child between 1 and 3 years old

C. The top of the head

D. The resistance of the body to the effects of a harmful agent such as a pathogenic microorganism or its toxins

E. The branch of medicine that deals with the care and development of children and the diagnosis and treatment of children's diseases

F. A suspension of attenuated or killed microorganisms administered to an individual to prevent an infectious disease

G. The process of becoming immune or of rendering an individual immune through the use of a vaccine or toxoid

H. The measurement from the vertex of the head to the heel of the foot in a supine position

I. A toxin that has been treated by heat or chemicals to destroy its harmful properties administered to an individual to prevent an infectious disease

J. A child from birth to 12 months old

K. A child from 3 to 6 years old

L. A child from 6 to 12 years old

EVALUATION OF LEARNING

Directions: Fill in each blank with the correct answer.

1. What is the purpose of the well-child visit?

_____

2. What are the components of the well-child visit?

_____

_____

3. What topics are commonly included in anticipatory guidance?

_____

_____

4. What is the usual schedule for well-child visits?

_____

_____

5. What is the purpose of the sick-child visit?

_____

_____

6. What procedures are often performed by the medical assistant during pediatric office visits?

_____

_____

7. Why is it important for the medical assistant to develop a rapport with the pediatric patient?

_____

_____

8. List the two positions that can be used to safely carry an infant.

_____

9. Why is it important to measure the growth (weight and height or length) of the child during each office visit?

_____

10. What is the difference between height and length?

_____

_____

11. What is the purpose of measuring head circumference?

_____

12. What is the primary use of growth charts?

_____

_____

13. What is the primary cause of childhood obesity?

_____

14. What problems are associated with childhood obesity?

_____

_____

15. List five guidelines for preventing childhood obesity.

_____

_____

_____

16. According to the American Academy of Pediatrics, at what age and how often should blood pressure be measured in children?

_____

365

17. What is the importance of measuring blood pressure in children?

_____

18. What can cause high blood pressure in children?

_____

19. What criteria must be followed to determine the correct cuff size for a child?

_____

_____

20. What occurs if the blood pressure cuff is too small or too large?

_____

_____

21. Why is it important for a child to be relaxed before taking his or her blood pressure?

_____

22. What three factors must be taken into consideration when determining if a child has hypertension?

_____

23. List three reasons for collecting a urine specimen from a child.

_____

_____

24. Why should the child's genitalia be cleansed before applying a pediatric urine collector?

_____

25. What gauge and length (range) of needle are recommended for administering the following injections to a child?

Intramuscular: _____

Subcutaneous: _____

26. Why is the dorsogluteal site not recommended for use as an intramuscular injection site in infants and young children?

_____

_____

_____

27. Why is the vastus lateralis muscle recommended as a good site for giving an intramuscular injection to an infant or young child? How is this site located?

_____

_____

_____

28. When might the length of the needle used to administer an intramuscular injection to a child need to be decreased or increased?

    a. Decreased needle length: _____

    b. Increased needle length: _____

29. At what age can the deltoid site be used to administer an IM injection to a child? Explain the reason for this.

    _____

    _____

30. Why should a child be held and comforted following an injection?

    _____

31. What is the recommended subcutaneous injection site for each of the following?

    a. An infant younger than 12 months of age: _____

    b. A child that is 12 months of age or older: _____

32. What is the difference between a vaccine and a toxoid?

    _____

    _____

    _____

33. What immunizations are included in the following?

    a. DTaP: _____

    b. MMR: _____

34. According to the American Academy of Pediatrics, at what ages should the following immunizations be administered to a child?

    a. Hepatitis B: _____

    b. DTaP: _____

    c. IPV: _____

    d. MMR: _____

    e. Influenza: _____

35. What information must be provided to parents as required by the NCVIA?

    _____

    _____

36. What information is included in a VIS?

    _____

    _____

    _____

367

37. According to the NCVIA, what information must be documented in the patient's medical record after a pediatric immunization has been administered?

_____

_____

_____

38. The newborn screening test screens for which metabolic diseases?

_____

_____

39. What are the symptoms of PKU, if left untreated?

_____

40. Why can the PKU screening test be performed earlier on infants on formula compared with breast-fed babies?

_____

_____

CRITICAL THINKING ACTIVITIES

A. Pediatric Weight

Locate the following weight values on a pediatric balance scale. Place a check mark next to each one after it has been correctly located.

1. 7 lb, 9 oz _____

2. 8 lb, 5 oz _____

3. 12 lb, 10 oz _____

4. 15 lb, 11 oz _____

5. 19 lb, 7 oz _____

6. 23 lb, 6 oz _____

7. 25 lb, 3 oz _____

B. Pediatric Length

Locate the following length values on a pediatric balance scale. Place a check mark next to each after it has been correctly located.

1. 20½ inches _____

2. 22½ inches _____

3. 9 inches _____

4. 25¾ inches _____

5. 28½ inches _____

6. 31 inches _____

7. 33¼ inches _____

8. 36½ inches _____

C. Growth Charts

Matthew Williams, age 2 years (9 months), has had health maintenance visits at the intervals listed below. His length and weight measurements were taken during each visit and are documented here. Plot these on the growth chart on the following page. Calculate the percentile for each and document it in the space provided. (Note: Matthew William's birth weight was 7 lb, 8 oz and his length was 20 inches.)

Well-Child Visits				
Age	Weight	Percentile	Length	Percentile
1 month	9 lb, 10 oz		22 in	
2 months	12 lb, 4 oz		23½ in	
4 months	16 lb, 5 oz		25¼ in	
6 months	18 lb, 8 oz		27 in	
9 months	22 lb, 4 oz		29¼ in	
12 months	24 lb, 4 oz		30½ in	
15 months	26 lb, 8 oz		31½ in	
18 months	27 lb		32½ in	
24 months	28 lb		35¾ in	

Chapter **9** The Pediatric Examination

Birth to 36 months: Boys
Length-for-age and Weight-for-age percentiles

NAME _____

RECORD# _____

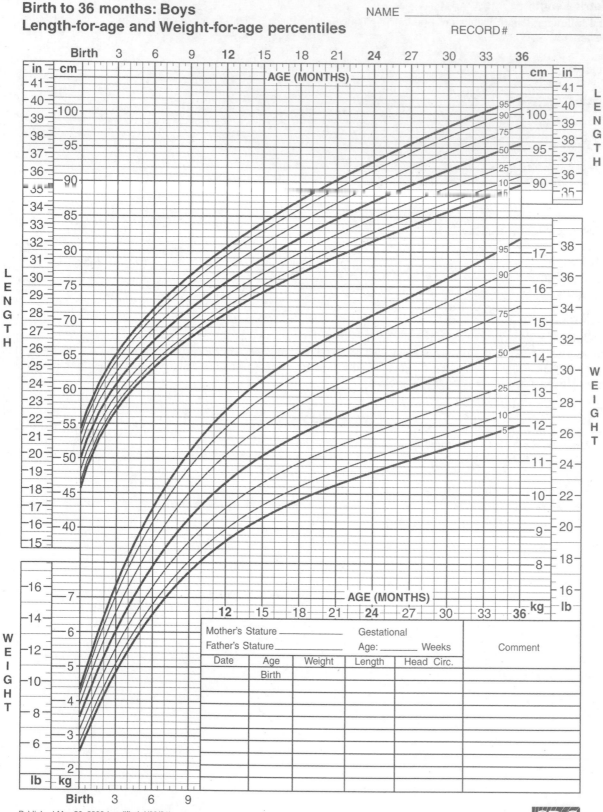

Published May 30, 2000 (modified 4/20/01).
SOURCE: Developed by the National Center for Health Statistics in collaboration with
the National Center for Chronic Disease Prevention and Health Promotion (2000).
http://www.cdc.gov/growthcharts

CDC
SAFER · HEALTHIER · PEOPLE™

Chapter **9 The Pediatric Examination**

D. Motor and Social Development

Using a reference source, describe the motor and social development of the age groups listed here. The first one is done for you.

Age	Motor and Social Development
Birth to 3 months	Raises head but not stable, can turn head from side to side, activities are limited to reflexes, cries when hungry, responsive social smile, coos, eyes can focus on an object and follow a moving object 180 degrees.
4 to 6 months	
7 to 9 months	
10 to 12 months	

E. Intramuscular Injection

How would you prepare the following children for an intramuscular injection of penicillin to reduce apprehension and fear? Techniques for Interaction with Children (Table 9.2) in your textbook can be used as a reference for this activity.

a. Katie Waugh, age 5

_____

_____

_____

b. Patrick Williams, age 8

_____

_____

_____

c. Julie Anderson, age 15

_____

_____

_____

F. Vaccine Information Statement

Refer to the Diphtheria, Tetanus, and Pertussis Vaccine Information Statement (VIS) in your textbook (Fig. 9.12), and answer the following questions:

1. How does an individual contract diphtheria, pertussis, and tetanus?

_____

_____

2. What are the symptoms of the following diseases?

a. Diphtheria _____

_____

b. Tetanus _____

_____

c. Pertussis _____

_____

3. What is the immunization schedule for DTaP?

_____

_____

4. What information should be relayed to the health care provider regarding the patient getting the vaccine with respect to allergies?

_____

_____

5. What should be done in the following situations?

a. The patient has a minor illness such as a cold: _____

b. The patient has a moderate or severe illness: _____

372

6. What mild reactions may occur from a DTaP vaccine?

_____

_____

7. What serious reactions may occur from a DTaP vaccine?

_____

_____

8. What are the symptoms of a severe allergic reaction to a DTaP vaccine?

_____

_____

9. What should be done if a severe allergic reaction occurs from the vaccine after the patient leaves the office?

_____

10. What is the National Vaccine Injury Compensation Program?

_____

_____

G. Locating and Interpreting a Vaccine Information Statement

Obtain a VIS for a vaccine that you would like to know more about (other than the DTaP vaccine already included in your textbook). List the information that would be important for a parent to know before this immunization is administered to his or her child. The following Internet site can be used to obtain a VIS:

www.immunize.org/vis

Name of Immunization: _____

Publication Date: _____
Information to Relay to a Parent:

_____

_____

_____

_____

_____

_____

_____

_____

_____

_____

H. Immunization Administration Record

Complete the following immunization record form for an infant at his or her 2-month, 4-month, and 6-month visits using Figure 9-10 (immunization schedule) in the textbook to determine which immunizations are administered during these well-child visits. The website (www.immunize.org/catg.d/p2022.pdf) provides an example of a completed immunization administration form to assist you in completing this form.

IMMUNIZATION ADMINISTRATION RECORD

Name _____
      (first)   (MI)   (last)

DOB _____

Physician _____

Address _____

_____

SITE ABBREVIATIONS:

RVL: Right vastus lateralis

LVL: Left vastus lateralis

RD: Right deltoid

LD: Left deltoid

PO: By mouth

IN: Intranasal

Vaccine	Type of Vaccine[1]	Date Given (mo/day/yr)	+Dose	Site	Vaccine Information Statement				Signature and Title of Vaccinator
					Lot #	Mfr.	Date on VIS	Date Given	
Hepatitis B[2] (e.g., HepB, Hib-HepB, DTaP-HepB-IPV) Give IM.									
Diphtheria, Tetanus, Pertussis[2] (e.g., DTaP, DTaP-Hib, DTaP-HepB-IPV, DT, DTaP-HiB-IPV, Tdap, DTaP-IPV, Td) Give IM.									
Haemophilus influenzae **type b**[2] (e.g., Hib, Hib-HepB, DTaP-HiB-IPV, DTaP-Hib) Give IM.									
Polio[2] (e.g., IPV, DTaP-HepB-IPV, DTaP-HiB-IPV, DTaP-IPV) Give IPV SC or IM. Give all others IM.									
Pneumococcal (e.g., PCV, conjugate; PPV, polysaccharide) Give PCV IM. Give PPV SC or IM.									
Rotovirus (RV1, RV5 Give orally (po).									
Measles, Mumps, Rubella (e.g., MMR, MMRV) Give SC.									
Varicella (e.g., Var, MMRV) Give SC.									
Hepatitis A (HepA) Give IM									
Meningococcal (e.g., MCV4, MPSV4) Give MCV4 IM and MPSV4 SC.									
Human papillomavirus (e.g., HPV) Give IM									
Influenza (e.g., TIV, inactivated; LAIV, live attenuated) Give TIV IM. Give LAIV IN.									
Other									

1. Record the generic abbreviation for the type of vaccine given (e.g., DTaP-Hib, PCV), *not* the trade name.
2. For combination vaccines, fill in a row for each separate antigen in the combination.

374

I. Crossword Puzzle: The Pediatric Examination

Directions: Complete the crossword puzzle using the clues provided.

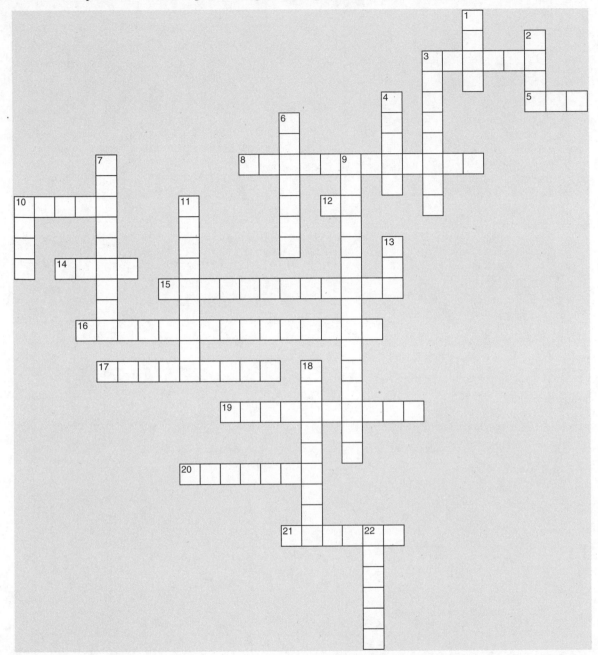

Across
- **3** Birth to 12 months
- **5** No phenylalanine enzyme disease
- **8** Baby doctor
- **10** Common immunization side effect
- **12** Begin at 3 years
- **14** PKU puncture site
- **15** MMR administration route
- **16** Injection site for infants
- **17** First breast milk
- **19** Can give at birth vaccine
- **20** German measles
- **21** Hold-me position

Down
- **1** Right size for child's BP?
- **2** 3-in-1 vaccine
- **3** Resistance to microorganisms
- **4** Child's vaccine act
- **6** From 1 to 3 years
- **7** Not caused by chickens
- **9** Childhood obesity can cause this
- **10** Don't use as a reward
- **11** Whooping cough
- **13** Immunization explainer
- **18** Do not weigh infant in this
- **22** Vertex to heel

Notes

Procedure 9-A: Carrying an Infant

Practice the procedure for carrying an infant, using a pediatric training mannequin in the following positions: cradle and upright.

Carrying Position	Number Of Practices

Procedure 9-1: Weight and Length.

Weight and Length. Measure the weight and length of an infant using a pediatric training mannequin. Document the results in the chart provided.

Procedure 9-2: Head and Chest Circumference. Measure the head and chest circumference of an infant using a pediatric training mannequin. Document the results in the chart provided.

Procedure 9-3: Growth Charts. Calculate growth percentiles on a growth chart using the values presented below. Assume these values were taken from the same (female) child over the course of her first year of life. You can use the *Girls: Birth to 36 months* growth chart accompanying Procedure 9-3 in your textbook to plot the growth values and calculate the percentiles. You can also print out a growth chart using your computer by going to the following website: http://www.cdc.gov/growthcharts www.cdc.gov/growthcharts.

Age	Weight	Length
2 months	9 pounds	21 inches
4 months	11 pounds, 8 ounces	23½ inches
6 months	14 pounds, 8 ounces	25¼ inches
9 months	18 pounds, 8 ounces	27¼ inches
12 months	21 pounds, 6 ounces	28¾ inches

CHART	
Date	

378

Procedure 9-4: Pediatric Urine Collector. Practice the procedure for applying a pediatric urine collector, using a pediatric training mannequin. Document the procedure in the chart provided.

Procedure 9-5: Newborn Screening Test

1. Complete the information section of the Newborn Screening Test Card provided for you.

2. Practice the procedure for specimen collection for the newborn screening test using a pediatric training mannequin. Document the procedure in the chart provided.

CHART	
Date	

Newborn Screening Test

USE BALL-
POINT PEN-
PRESS HARD

ALL
INFORMATION
MUST BE
PRINTED

Birth date: ___/___/___

Baby's name:
(last, first)

Hospital provider number:

Hospital of birth
or transfer:

Mom's name:
(last, first, initial)

Mom's address:

Mom's city: Ohio   Zip:

Mom's race:

Mom's age:

Mom's phone: (___)___-___   Mom's SSN: ___-___-___

Mom's ID: Mom's county:

Specimen date ___/___/___   Baby's ID:

Time ___:___   Time ___:___ (Use 24-hour time only)

Baby's physician:
(last name first)

Physician address:

Physician   City: Ohio   Zip

Physician phone: (___)___-___   Physician
                                 provider number:

Time ___:___ (Use 24-hour time only)

1. SPECIMEN: [ ] FIRST [ ] SECOND
   [ ] other _____

2. BIRTH NUMBER/ SEX:
   [ ] SINGLE   [ ] MULTIPLE A, B, C, etc.
   [ ] FEMALE   [ ] MALE

3. BIRTH WEIGHT: [ ][ ][ ][ ] GRAMS

4. PREMATURE: [ ] YES [ ] NO

5. ANTIBIOTICS: [ ] YES [ ] NO

6. TRANSFUSION: [ ] YES [ ] NO

7. FEEDING: [ ] YES [ ] NO
   [ ] Type 1. Breast 2. Milk-base
   NO. 3. Soy 4. TPN 5. IV-only

8. SUBMITTER:
   [ ] HOSPITAL/BIRTH CENTER
   [ ] HEALTH DEPARTMENT
   [ ] PHYSICIAN
   [ ] HOME HEALTH CARE AGENCY
   [ ] CLINICAL LAB
   [ ] OTHER

[ ] SPECIMEN REJECTED _____

EVALUATION OF COMPETENCY

Procedure 9-A: Carrying an Infant

Name: _____   Date: _____

Evaluated by: _____   Score: _____

Performance Objective

Outcome:	Carry an infant in the following positions: cradle and upright.
Conditions:	Given a pediatric training mannequin.
Standards:	Time: 5 minutes. Student completed procedure in _____ minutes.
	Accuracy: Satisfactory score on the performance evaluation checklist.

Performance Evaluation Checklist

Trial 1	Trial 2	Point Value	Performance Standards
			Cradle position:
		•	Slid the left hand and arm under infant's back.
		•	Grasped infant's upper arm from behind.
		•	Encircled infant's upper arm with the thumb and fingers.
		•	Supported infant's head, shoulders, and back on your arm.
		•	Slipped the right arm up and under the infant's buttocks.
		•	Cradled infant in your arms with the infant's body resting against your chest.
			Upright position:
		•	Slipped the right hand under infant's head and shoulders.
		•	Spread the fingers apart to support infant's head and neck.
		•	Slipped the left forearm under infant's buttocks.
		•	Allowed infant to rest against your chest.
		■	Reassured patients.
		★	Completed the procedure within 5 minutes.
			Totals

CHART	
Date	

Evaluation of Student Performance

<table>
<tr><th colspan="3">EVALUATION CRITERIA</th><th>COMMENTS</th></tr>
<tr><th>Symbol</th><th>Category</th><th>Point Value</th><th></th></tr>
<tr><td>★</td><td>Critical Step</td><td>16 points</td><td></td></tr>
<tr><td>•</td><td>Essential Step</td><td>6 points</td><td></td></tr>
<tr><td>■</td><td>Affective Competency</td><td>6 points</td><td></td></tr>
<tr><td>▷</td><td>Theory Question</td><td>2 points</td><td></td></tr>
<tr><td colspan="3">Score calculation: 100 points
      −   points missed
        ___Score
Satisfactory score: 85 or above</td><td></td></tr>
</table>

CAAHEP Competencies Achieved

Psychomotor (Skills)

☑ I. 8. Instruct and prepare a patient for a procedure or a treatment.

Affective (Behavior)

☑ A. 2. Reassure patients.

ABHES Competencies Achieved

☑ 9. c. Assist provider with general/physical examination.

Procedure 9-1: Measuring the Weight and Length of an Infant

Name: _____ Date: _____

Evaluated by: _____ Score: _____

Performance Objective

Outcome:	Measure the weight and length of an infant.
Conditions:	Using a pediatric training mannequin and a pediatric balance scale (table model). Given a paper protector.
Standards:	Time: 5 minutes Student completed procedure in _____ minutes. Accuracy: Satisfactory score on the performance evaluation checklist.

Performance Evaluation Checklist

Trial 1	Trial 2	Point Value	Performance Standards
			Weight:
		•	Sanitized hands.
		•	Greeted the infant's parent and introduced yourself.
		•	Identified the infant.
		•	Explained the procedure to the child's parent.
		•	Based on the medical office policy asked parent to: Remove infant's clothing and put on a dry diaper. Remove infant's clothing including the diaper.
		▷	Stated why the infant should not be weighed with a wet diaper.
		•	Unlocked pediatric scale and placed a clean paper protector on it.
		▷	Stated the purpose of the paper protector.
		•	Checked the balance scale for accuracy.
		▷	Stated the purpose for balancing the scale.
		•	Gently placed infant on his or her back on the scale.
		•	Placed one hand slightly above infant.
		•	Balanced the scale.
		•	Read results while infant was lying still.
		•	Jotted down value or made a mental note of it.
		*	The result was identical to the evaluator's result.
		•	Returned balance to its resting position and locked the scale.
			Length:
		•	Placed the vertex of infant's head against the headboard at the zero mark.
		•	Asked parent to hold infant's head in position.

383

Trial 1	Trial 2	Point Value	Performance Standards
		•	Straightened infant's knees and placed soles of infant's feet firmly against the upright footboard.
		•	Read infant's length in inches from the measure.
		•	Jotted down value or made a mental note of it.
		*	The result was identical to the evaluator's results.
		•	Removed infant from the scale and handed him or her to the parent.
		•	Returned headboard and footboard to their resting positions.
		•	Sanitized hands.
		•	Documented the results correctly.
		■	Demonstrated critical thinking skills.
		■	Demonstrated empathy for patients' concerns.
		★	Completed the procedure within 5 minutes.
			Totals
CHART			
Date			

Evaluation of Student Performance

EVALUATION CRITERIA			COMMENTS
Symbol	**Category**	**Point Value**	
★	Critical Step	16 points	
•	Essential Step	6 points	
■	Affective Competency	6 points	
▷	Theory Question	2 points	

Score calculation: 100 points

− _____ points missed

_____ Score

Satisfactory score: 85 or above

CAAHEP Competencies Achieved

Psychomotor (Skills)

- ☑ I. 1. f. Measure and record weight (adult and infant).
- ☑ I. 1. g. Accurately measure and record length (infant)
- ☑ II. 3. Document on a growth chart.

Affective (Behavior)

- ☑ A. 1. Demonstrate critical thinking skills.
- ☑ A. 3. Demonstrated empathy for patients' concerns.

ABHES Competencies Achieved

- ☑ 4. a. Follow documentation guidelines.
- ☑ 5. d. Discuss developmental stages of life.
- ☑ 9. c. Assist provider with general/physical examination.

Notes

Procedure 9-2: Measuring Head and Chest Circumference of an Infant

Name: _____ Date: _____

Evaluated by: _____ Score: _____

Performance Objective

Outcome:	Measure the head and chest circumference of an infant.
Conditions:	Given a flexible, nonstretch tape measure (in centimeters).
Standards:	Time: 5 minutes Student completed procedure in _____ minutes.
	Accuracy: Satisfactory score on the performance evaluation checklist.

Performance Evaluation Checklist

Trial 1	Trial 2	Point Value	Performance Standards
			Measurement of head circumference:
		•	Sanitized hands.
		•	Assembled equipment.
		•	Positioned the infant.
		▷	Stated what positions can be used to measure head circumference.
		•	Positioned the tape measure around the infant's head.
		•	The tape measure was placed slightly above the eyebrows and pinna of the ears, and around the occipital prominence at the back of the skull.
		•	Read the results in centimeters (or inches).
		•	Jotted down value or made a mental note of it.
		★	The result was identical to the evaluator's result.
		•	Sanitized hands.
		•	Documented the results correctly.
			Measurement of chest circumference:
		•	Positioned the infant on his or her back on the examining table.
		•	Encircled the measuring device around the infant's chest at the nipple line.
		•	Ensured that the measuring device was snug but not too tight.
		•	Read the results in centimeters (or inches).
		•	Jotted down this value or made a mental note of it.
		★	The reading was identical to the evaluator's reading.
		•	Documented the results correctly.
		■	Demonstrated critical thinking skills.

Trial 1	Trial 2	Point Value	Performance Standards
		★	Completed the procedure within 5 minutes.
			Totals

CHART

Date	

Evaluation of Student Performance

EVALUATION CRITERIA			COMMENTS
Symbol	**Category**	**Point Value**	
★	Critical Step	16 points	
•	Essential Step	6 points	
■	Affective Competency	6 points	
■	Theory Question	2 points	

Score calculation: 100 points

− _____ points missed

_____ Score

Satisfactory score: 85 or above

CAAHEP Competencies Achieved

Psychomotor (Skills)

☑ I. 1. h. Accurately measure and record head circumference (infant).

Affective (Behavior)

☑ A. 1. Demonstrate critical thinking skills.

ABHES Competencies Achieved

☑ 4. a. Follow documentation guidelines.
☑ 9. c. Assist provider with general/physical examination.

EVALUATION OF COMPETENCY

Procedure 9-3: Calculating Growth Percentiles

Name: _____   Date: _____

Evaluated by: _____   Score: _____

Performance Objective

Outcome:	Plot a pediatric growth value on a growth chart.
Conditions:	Given a pediatric growth chart.
Standards:	Time: 5 minutes Student completed procedure in _____ minutes.
	Accuracy: Satisfactory score on the performance evaluation checklist.

Performance Evaluation Checklist

Trial 1	Trial 2	Point Value	Performance Standards
		•	Selected the proper growth chart.
		•	Located the child's age in the horizontal column at the bottom of the chart.
		•	Located the growth value in the vertical column under the appropriate category.
		•	Drew a (imaginary) vertical line from the child's age mark and an imaginary horizontal line from the growth mark.
		•	Found the site at which the two lines intersected on the graph.
		•	Placed a dot on this site.
		•	Determined the percentile by following the curved percentile line upward.
		•	Read the value located on the right side of the chart.
		•	Estimated the results if the value did not fall exactly on a percentile line.
		•	Documented the results correctly.
		★	The value was within ±2 percentage points of the evaluator's determination.
		■	Demonstrated critical thinking skills.
		★	Completed the procedure within 5 minutes.
			Totals

CHART	
Date	

Evaluation of Student Performance

EVALUATION CRITERIA			COMMENTS
Symbol	**Category**	**Point Value**	
★	Critical Step	16 points	
•	Essential Step	6 points	
■	Affective Competency	6 points	
▷	Theory Question	2 points	

Score calculation: 100 points

− _____ points missed

_____ Score

Satisfactory score: 85 or above

CAAHEP Competencies Achieved

Psychomotor (Skills)

☑ II. 3. Document on a growth chart.

Affective (Behavior)

☑ A. 1. Demonstrate critical thinking skills.

ABHES Competencies Achieved

☑ 4. a. Follow documentation guidelines.
☑ 5. d. Discuss developmental stages of life.

Procedure 9-4: Applying a Pediatric Urine Collector

Name: _____   Date: _____

Evaluated by: _____   Score: _____

Performance Objective

Outcome:	Apply a pediatric urine collector.
Conditions:	Using a pediatric training mannequin.
	Given the following: disposable gloves, personal antiseptic wipes, pediatric urine collector bag, urine specimen container and label, and a waste container.
Standards:	Time: 10 minutes Student completed procedure in _____ minutes.
	Accuracy: Satisfactory score on the performance evaluation checklist.

Performance Evaluation Checklist

Trial 1	Trial 2	Point Value	Performance Standards
		•	Sanitized hands.
		•	Assembled equipment.
		•	Greeted the child's parent and introduced yourself.
		•	Identified the child and explained the procedure to the parent.
		•	Applied gloves.
		•	Positioned child on his or her back with legs spread apart.
			Cleanse the area and apply the bag:
			Females
		•	Cleansed each side of the meatus with a separate wipe using a front-to-back motion.
		•	Cleansed directly down the middle with a third wipe.
		•	Discarded each wipe after cleansing.
		▷	Stated the reason for cleansing the urinary meatus.
		•	Allowed the area to dry completely.
		▷	Explained why the area should be allowed to dry.
		•	Removed paper backing from urine collector bag.
		•	Placed the bottom of the adhesive ring on the perineum and work upward.
		•	Firmly pressed the adhesive surface firmly to the skin surrounding the external genitalia.
		•	Made sure there was no puckering.
		•	Opening of the bag was placed directly over the urinary meatus.
		•	Excess length of the bag was positioned toward the feet.

391

Trial 1	Trial 2	Point Value	Performance Standards
			Males
		•	Retracted the foreskin of the penis if the child is not circumcised.
		•	Cleansed each side of the urethral orifice with a separate wipe.
		•	Cleansed directly over the urethral orifice.
		•	Cleansed the scrotum.
		•	Discarded each wipe after cleansing.
		•	Allowed the area to dry completely.
		•	Removed the paper backing from urine collector bag.
		•	Positioned the bag so that child's penis and scrotum are projected through the opening of the bag.
		•	Firmly pressed the adhesive surface firmly to the skin.
		•	Excess length of the bag was positioned toward the feet.
			Completed the procedure:
		•	Loosely diapered child.
		•	Checked bag every 15 minutes until urine specimen was obtained.
		•	Gently removed collector bag from top to bottom.
		•	Cleansed genital area with a personal antiseptic wipe and rediapered child.
		•	Transferred urine specimen into specimen container and tightly applied the lid.
		•	Applied label to the container.
		•	Disposed of collector bag in a regular waste container.
		•	Tested the specimen or prepared it for transfer to an outside laboratory.
		▷	Explained why the urine specimen should not be allowed to stand at room temperature.
		•	Removed gloves and sanitized hands.
		•	Documented the procedure correctly.
		■	Demonstrated critical thinking skills.
		★	Completed the procedure within 5 minutes.
			Totals

CHART

Date	

Evaluation of Student Performance

EVALUATION CRITERIA			COMMENTS
Symbol	**Category**	**Point Value**	
★	Critical Step	16 points	
•	Essential Step	6 points	
■	Affective Competency	6 points	
▷	Theory Question	2 points	

Score calculation: 100 points

        −   points missed

              ___Score

Satisfactory score: 85 or above

CAAHEP Competencies Achieved

Psychomotor (Skills)

☑   I. 11. c. Collect specimens and perform CLIA waived urinalysis.

Affective (Behavior)

☑   A. 1. Demonstrate critical thinking skills.

ABHES Competencies Achieved

☑   4. a. Follow documentation guidelines.
☑   10. d. Collect, label and process specimens.

Notes

EVALUATION OF COMPETENCY

Procedure 9-5: Newborn Screening Test

Name: _____ Date: _____

Evaluated by: _____ Score: _____

Performance Objective

Outcome:	Collect a capillary blood specimen for a newborn screening test.
Conditions:	Using a pediatric training mannequin.
	Given the following: disposable gloves, infant heel or warm compress, antiseptic wipe, sterile gauze pad, sterile lancet, adhesive bandage, newborn screening test card, mailing envelope, and a biohazard sharps container.
Standards:	Time: 10 minutes. Student completed procedure in _____ minutes.
	Accuracy: Satisfactory score on the Performance Evaluation Checklist.

Performance Evaluation Checklist

Trial 1	Trial 2	Point Value	Performance Standards
		•	Sanitized hands.
		•	Assembled the equipment.
		•	Greeted the infant's parent and introduced yourself.
		•	Identified the infant and explained the procedure to the parent.
		•	Completed the information section of the newborn screening card.
		•	Selected an appropriate puncture site.
		•	Identified the sites that can be used for the heel puncture.
		▷	Explained what could occur if a different site is used.
		•	Warmed the puncture site.
		▷	Stated the purpose of warming the site.
		•	Cleaned the puncture site with an antiseptic wipe and allowed it to air-dry.
		•	Applied gloves and grasped the infant's foot around the puncture site.
		•	Punctured the heel using a sterile lancet, and disposed of the lancet.
		•	Wiped away the first drop of blood with a gauze pad.
		▷	Explained why the first drop of blood should be wiped away.
		•	Encouraged a large drop of blood to form by exerting gentle pressure on the heel.
		•	Did not excessively squeeze the heel.
		▷	Explained why the excessive squeezing should be avoided.
		•	Touched the drop of blood to the center of the first circle on the test card.
		•	Completely filled the circle on the test card with blood.

395

Trial 1	Trial 2	Point Value	Performance Standards
		•	Continued until all the circles are completely filled with blood.
		▷	Explained why each circle must be completely filled with blood.
		•	Did not touch the blood specimen with your gloved hand.
		▷	Stated why the specimen should not be touched.
		•	Held a gauze pad over the puncture site and applied pressure.
		•	Remained with the infant until bleeding stopped. Applied an adhesive bandage if needed.
		•	Removed gloves and sanitized hands.
		•	Allowed the test card to air-dry horizontally for 3 hours at room temperature.
		•	Did not allow the blood specimen to come in contact with any other surface and did not expose the test card to heat, moisture, or direct sunlight.
		•	Did not place the specimen in a plastic bag.
		▷	Explained what occurs if the specimen is placed in a plastic bag.
		•	Placed the test card in its protective envelope.
		•	Mailed the card to the laboratory within 48 hours.
		▷	Stated why the specimen must be mailed within 48 hours.
		•	Documented the procedure correctly.
		■	Demonstrated critical thinking skills.
		■	Demonstrated empathy for patients' concerns.
		■	Demonstrated tactfullness.
		★	Completed the procedure within 10 minutes.
			Totals

CHART	
Date	

Evaluation of Student Performance

<table>
<tr><th colspan="3">EVALUATION CRITERIA</th><th>COMMENTS</th></tr>
<tr><th>Symbol</th><th>Category</th><th>Point Value</th><td rowspan="8"></td></tr>
<tr><td>★</td><td>Critical Step</td><td>16 points</td></tr>
<tr><td>•</td><td>Essential Step</td><td>6 points</td></tr>
<tr><td>■</td><td>Affective Competency</td><td>6 points</td></tr>
<tr><td>▷</td><td>Theory Question</td><td>2 points</td></tr>
<tr><td colspan="3">Score calculation: 100 points
      −   points missed
          ___Score</td></tr>
<tr><td colspan="3">Satisfactory score: 85 or above</td></tr>
</table>

CAAHEP Competencies Achieved

Psychomotor (Skills)
☑ I. 2. c. Perform the following procedure: capillary puncture.
☑ III. 10. Demonstrate proper disposal of biohazardous material (a) sharps (b) regulated waste.

Affective (Behavior)
☑ A. 1. Demonstrate critical thinking skills.
☑ Demonstrate empathy for patients' concerns.
☑ A. 7. Demonstrate tactfullness.

ABHES Competencies Achieved

☑ 8. a. Practice standard precautions and perform disinfection/sterilization techniques.
☑ 9. c. Dispose of biohazardous materials.
☑ 9. d. Collect, label, and process specimens: (2) Perform capillary puncture.

Newborn Screening Test

USE BALL-
POINT PEN-
PRESS HARD

ALL
INFORMATION
MUST BE
PRINTED

Birth date: ___/___/___

Baby's name:
(last, first)

Hospital provider number:

Hospital of birth
or transfer:

Mom's name:
(last, first, initial)

Mom's address:

Mom's city: Ohio   Zip:

Mom's race: Mom's age:

Mom's phone: (   )   -

Mom's ID:

Specimen date ___/___/___   Time   :   (Use 24-hour time only)

Baby's physician:
(last name first)

Physician address:

City: Ohio   Zip   -

Physician phone: (   )   -   Physician
                                      provider number:

Time   :   (Use 24-hour time only)

Mom's SSN:

Mom's
county:

Baby's
ID:

1. SPECIMEN: ☐ FIRST ☐ SECOND
              ☐ other

2. BIRTH NUMBER/ SEX:
   ☐ SINGLE ☐ MULTIPLE
                A, B, C, etc.
   ☐ FEMALE ☐ MALE

3. BIRTH WEIGHT: _____ GRAMS

4. PREMATURE: ☐ YES ☐ NO

5. ANTIBIOTICS: ☐ YES ☐ NO

6. TRANSFUSION: ☐ YES ☐ NO

7. FEEDING: ☐ YES ☐ NO
   Type 1. Breast 2. Milk-base
   NO. 3. Soy 4. TPN 5. IV-only

8. SUBMITTER:
   ☐ HOSPITAL/BIRTH CENTER
   ☐ HEALTH DEPARTMENT
   ☐ PHYSICIAN
   ☐ HOME HEALTH CARE AGENCY
   ☐ CLINICAL LAB
   ☐ OTHER

   ☐ SPECIMEN REJECTED

10 Minor Office Surgery

CHAPTER ASSIGNMENTS

√ After Completing	Date Due	Study Guide Pages	STUDY GUIDE ASSIGNMENTS (CTA = Critical Thinking Activity)	Possible Points	Points You Earned
		403	⬚ Pretest	10	
			🔑Term Key Term Assessment		
		404	A. Definitions	26	
		405	B. Word Parts	9	
			(Add 1 point for each key term)		
		405-411	Evaluation of Learning questions	64	
		411-412	CTA A: Medical and Surgical Asepsis	10	
		412	CTA B: Violation of Surgical Asepsis	10	
		413-414	CTA C: Surgical Instruments (2 points each)	22	
			Evolve: It's Instrumental (Record points earned)		
			Evolve: Keep it Sterile (Record points earned)		
		415	CTA D: Pioneers in Surgical Asepsis (5 points each)	15	
		415-417	CTA E: Patient Instruction Sheet	20	
		419	CTA F: Crossword Puzzle	24	
			Evolve: Apply Your Knowledge questions	10	
			Evolve: Video Evaluation	70	
		403	⬚ Posttest	10	
			ADDITIONAL ASSIGNMENTS		
			Total points		

√ When Assigned By Your Instructor	Study Guide Pages	Practices Required	Laboratory Assignments (Procedure Number and Name)	Score*
	421-422	5	**Practice for Competency** 10-1: Applying and Removing Sterile Gloves	
	423-424		**Evaluation of Competency** 10-1: Applying and Removing Sterile Gloves	*
	421-422	5	**Practice for Competency** 10-2: Opening a Sterile Package	
	425-426		**Evaluation of Competency** 10-2: Opening a Sterile Package	*
	421-422	5	**Practice for Competency** 10-A: Adding a Sterile Article to a Sterile Field	
	427-428		**Evaluation of Competency** 10-A: Adding a Sterile Article to a Sterile Field	*
	421-422	3	**Practice for Competency** 10-3: Pouring a Sterile Solution	
	429-430		**Evaluation of Competency** 10-3: Pouring a Sterile Solution	*
	421-422	5	**Practice for Competency** 10-4: Changing a Sterile Dressing	
	431-433		**Evaluation of Competency** 10-4: Changing a Sterile Dressing	*
	421-422	Sutures: 3 Staples: 3	**Practice for Competency** 10-5: Removing Sutures and Staples	
	435-437		**Evaluation of Competency** 10-5: Removing Sutures and Staples	*
	421-422	3	**Practice for Competency** 10-6: Applying and Removing Skin Closure Tape	
	439-442		**Evaluation of Competency** 10-6: Applying and Removing Skin Closure Tape	*
	421-422	5	**Practice for Competency** 10-7: Assisting with Minor Office Surgery	

√ When Assigned By Your Instructor	Study Guide Pages	Practices Required	Laboratory Assignments (Procedure Number and Name)	Score*
	443-446		**Evaluation of Competency** 10-7: Assisting with Minor Office Surgery	*
	421-422	Each bandage turn: 3	**Practice for Competency** 10-B: Bandage Turns	
	447-449		**Evaluation of Competency** 10-B: Bandage Turns	*
			ADDITIONAL ASSIGNMENTS	

Name: _____ Date: _____

True or False

_____ 1. Surgical asepsis refers to practices that keep objects and areas free from all microorganisms.

_____ 2. Something that is sterile is contaminated, if it comes in contact with a pathogen.

_____ 3. Reaching over a sterile field is a violation of sterile technique.

_____ 4. An incision is a jagged tearing of the tissues.

_____ 5. The skin is the first line of defense of the body.

_____ 6. One of the local signs of inflammation is fever.

_____ 7. Sutures approximate the edges of a wound until proper healing occurs.

_____ 8. A biopsy is usually performed to determine, if a tumor is benign or malignant.

_____ 9. An ingrown toenail can be caused by shoes that are too tight.

_____10. One of the functions of a bandage is to hold a dressing in place.

📄 **POSTTEST**

True or False

_____ 1. Measuring a patient's temperature requires the use of surgical asepsis.

_____ 2. Hemostatic forceps are used to clamp off blood vessels.

_____ 3. An instrument with a ratchet should be kept in a closed position when not in use.

_____ 4. The provider would most likely order a tetanus booster for an abrasion.

_____ 5. Inflammation is the protective response of the body to trauma and the entrance of foreign substances.

_____ 6. A serous exudate is red in color.

_____ 7. Size 4-0 sutures have a smaller diameter than size 3 sutures.

_____ 8. Sebaceous cysts are commonly found on the palms of the hands.

_____ 9. Colposcopy is frequently used to evaluate lesions of the cervix.

_____10. Cryosurgery is used in the treatment of cervical cancer.

A. Definitions

Directions: Match each key term with its definition.

_____ 1. Abrasion

_____ 2. Abscess

_____ 3. Absorbable suture

_____ 4. Approximation

_____ 5. Bandage

_____ 6. Biopsy

_____ 7. Capillary action

_____ 8. Colposcope

_____ 9. Colposcopy

_____ 10. Contaminate

_____ 11. Contusion

_____ 12. Cryosurgery

_____ 13. Fibroblast

_____ 14. Forceps

_____ 15. Furuncle

_____ 16. Hemostasis

_____ 17. Incision

_____ 18. Infection

_____ 19. Inflammation

_____ 20. Laceration

_____ 21. Nonabsorbable suture

_____ 22. Puncture

_____ 23. Sterile

_____ 24. Surgery

_____ 25. Surgical asepsis

_____ 26. Wound

A. A protective response of the body to trauma and the entrance of foreign matter

B. To cause a sterile object or surface to become unsterile

C. A wound made by a sharp pointed object piercing the skin

D. The condition in which the body, or part of it, is invaded by a pathogen

E. A collection of pus in a cavity surrounded by inflamed tissue

F. The arrest of bleeding by natural or artificial means

G. Free of all living microorganisms and bacterial spores

H. A wound in which the tissues are torn apart, leaving ragged and irregular edges

I. A lighted instrument with a binocular magnifying lens used to examine the vagina and cervix

J. A localized staphylococcal infection that originates deep within a hair follicle; also known as a boil

K. An injury to the tissues under the skin that causes blood vessels to rupture, allowing blood to seep into the tissues

L. The surgical removal and examination of tissue from the living body

M. A wound in which the outer layers of the skin are damaged

N. The action that causes liquid to rise along a wick, a tube, or a gauze dressing

O. A two-pronged instrument for grasping and squeezing

P. Practices that keep objects and areas sterile or free from micro-organisms

Q. A break in the continuity of an external or internal surface caused by physical means

R. The therapeutic use of freezing temperatures to destroy abnormal tissue

S. The visual examination of the vagina and cervix using a lighted instrument with a magnifying lens

T. Suture material that is gradually digested and absorbed by the body

U. The process of bringing two parts, such as tissue, together through the use of sutures or other means

V. A strip of woven material used to wrap or cover a part of the body

W. A clean cut caused by a cutting instrument

X. Suture material that is not absorbed by the body

Y. An immature cell from which connective tissue can develop

Z. The branch of medicine that deals with operative and manual procedures for correction of deformities and defects, repair of injuries, and diagnosis and treatment of certain diseases

B. Word Parts

Directions: Indicate the meaning of each word part in the space provided. List as many medical terms as possible that incorporate the word part in the space provided.

Word Part	Meaning of Word Part	Medical Terms That Incorporate Word Part
1. bi/o		
2. -opsy		
3. colp/o		
4. -scope		
5. -scopy		
6. cry/o		
7. fibr/o		
8. hem/o		
9. -stasis		

EVALUATION OF LEARNING

Directions: Fill in each blank with the correct answer.

1. List the characteristics of a minor surgical procedure.

_____

_____

_____

2. List the responsibilities of the medical assistant during a minor surgical operation.

_____

_____

_____

_____

3. When must surgical asepsis be employed?

_____

_____

_____

4. What is the purpose of serrations found on some instruments?

_____

_____

5. What is the difference in function between mosquito hemostatic forceps and standard hemostatic forceps?

_____

_____

Chapter **10 Minor Office Surgery**

6. List five guidelines that should be followed in caring for instruments.

_____

_____

_____

_____

7. What is the difference between a closed and an open wound?

_____

_____

8. What is the difference between an incision and a laceration?

_____

_____

9. Why does a puncture wound encourage the growth of tetanus bacteria?

_____

_____

10. What is the purpose of inflammation?

_____

_____

11. List the four local signs that occur during inflammation.

_____

12. What occurs during the inflammatory phase of wound healing?

_____

_____

13. What occurs during the proliferative phase of wound healing?

_____

_____

14. What is the appearance of granulation tissue?

_____

_____

15. What occurs during the maturation phase of wound healing?

_____

16. What is an exudate?

_____

_____

17. What is the function of an exudate?

_____

_____

18. Describe the appearance of the following types of exudates:

a. Serous _____

b. Sanguineous _____

c. Purulent _____

d. Serosanguineous _____

e. Purosanguineous _____

19. What are the functions of a sterile dressing?

_____

_____

20. What are the most common methods of wound closure?

_____

_____

21. What is the purpose of wound closure?

_____

_____

22. The names and sizes of sutures are listed. In each set, circle the suture that has the smaller diameter:

a. 4-0 silk

2-0 silk

b. 0 chromic surgical gut

3-0 chromic surgical gut

c. 2-0 polypropylene

2 polypropylene

23. List five examples of materials used for nonabsorbable sutures.

_____

_____

24. What is a swaged needle? List advantages of using a swaged needle.

_____

_____

25. Why are sutures inserted in the head and neck generally removed sooner than other sutures?

_____

_____

407

26. List two advantages of using surgical skin staples to approximate a wound.

_____

_____

27. How do tissue adhesives work?

_____

_____

28. What types of wounds are tissue adhesives most commonly used to close?

_____

_____

29. What are the advantages of tissue adhesives?

_____

_____

30. What are the advantages of skin closure tape.

_____

_____

31. What are the disadvantages of skin closure tape?

_____

_____

32. What is the purpose of preparing the patient's skin before minor office surgery?

_____

33. What is the purpose of a fenestrated drape?

_____

_____

34. What are the characteristics of a local anesthetic?

_____

_____

35. What is the purpose of adding epinephrine to a local anesthetic?

_____

36. What is the name of the local anesthetic most frequently used in the medical office during minor office surgery?

_____

37. Explain how an instrument should be handed to the physician during minor office surgery.

_____

38. What is a sebaceous cyst, and what causes it to form?

_____

_____

39. Where do sebaceous cysts most frequently occur? Where do they not occur?

Most frequently occur: _____

Do not occur: _____

40. List reasons which may warrant the removal of a sebaceous cyst.

_____

_____

41. What is the purpose of using gauze packing or a rubber Penrose drain after incising a localized infection?

_____

42. What is the difference between congenital nevi and acquired nevi?

_____

_____

43. What are the characteristics of benign moles?

_____

_____

_____

44. What are skin tags? Where are they most frequently found on the body?

_____

_____

_____

45. Describe the appearance of dysplastic nevi. What concern exists with dysplastic nevi?

_____

_____

_____

46. List the characteristics of melanoma.

_____

_____

_____

47. What are the most common methods used to remove moles?

_____

48. What is the purpose of a biopsy?

_____

_____

409

49. What is the advantage of a needle biopsy?

_____

_____

50. What is an ingrown toenail?

_____

_____

51. List three causes of an ingrown toenail.

_____

_____

52. What are the postoperative instructions for ingrown toenail removal?

_____

_____

_____

53. List two reasons for performing a colposcopy.

_____

_____

54. What is the purpose of performing a cervical punch biopsy?

_____

_____

55. List the postoperative instructions that must be relayed to the patient after a cervical punch biopsy.

_____

_____

_____

56. List two uses of cervical cryosurgery.

_____

57. List the postoperative instructions that must be relayed to the patient after cervical cryosurgery.

_____

_____

_____

58. List three functions of a bandage.

_____

_____

59. List four guidelines to follow when applying a bandage.

_____

_____

_____

_____

60. List four signs that may indicate a bandage is too tight.

_____

_____

61. Why should the medical assistant be careful when applying an elastic bandage?

_____

62. What is the purpose of reversing the spiral during a spiral-reverse turn?

_____

_____

63. List two uses of the figure-eight bandage turn.

_____

64. What type of bandage turn is used to anchor a bandage?

_____

CRITICAL THINKING ACTIVITIES

A. Medical and Surgical Asepsis

Refer to Chapter 2 and describe the difference between medical asepsis and surgical asepsis.

_____

_____

_____

Which technique (medical asepsis or surgical asepsis) would be employed during the following procedures? For procedures requiring surgical asepsis, indicate which of the following reasons necessitate the use of surgical asepsis: caring for broken skin, penetrating a skin surface, or entering a body cavity that is normally sterile.

1. Administering oral medication

_____

2. Inserting sutures

_____

3. Measuring oral temperature

_____

4. Applying a bandage to the forearm

_____

5. Performing a needle biopsy

_____

411

6. Removing a sebaceous cyst

_____

7. Obtaining a Pap specimen

_____

8. Inserting a urinary catheter

_____

9. Incision and drainage of an abscess

_____

10. Applying a dressing to an open wound

_____

B. Violation of Surgical Asepsis

In the situations that follow, the principles of surgical asepsis have been violated. In the space provided, explain why the techniques should not be performed in this manner.

1. Placing a sterile 4 × 4 gauze pad within the 1-inch border around the sterile field

_____

2. Wearing rings during the application of sterile gloves

_____

3. Talking over a sterile field

_____

4. Reaching over a sterile field

_____

5. Holding sterile gauze below waist level

_____

6. Not palming the label when pouring an antiseptic solution

_____

7. Spilling an antiseptic solution on the sterile field

_____

8. Passing a soiled dressing over the sterile field

_____

9. Placing a vial of Xylocaine on the sterile field

_____

10. Using bare hands to arrange articles on the sterile field

_____

412

C. Surgical Instruments

In the space provided, state the name and use of each of the following types of surgical instruments. Identify any of the following parts present on each instrument by labeling the instrument: box lock, spring handle, ratchets, serrations, cutting edge, and teeth. <Insert Unn Fig 10-1>

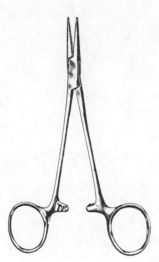

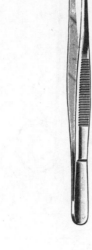

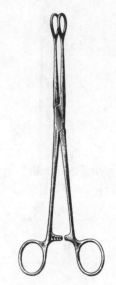

1. Name: _____

   Use _____

   _____

2. Name: _____

   Use _____

   _____

3. Name: _____

   Use _____

   _____

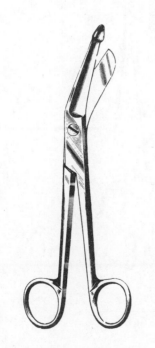

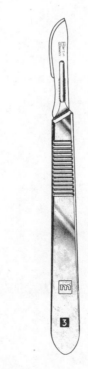

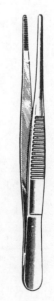

4. Name: _____

   Use _____

   _____

5. Name: _____

   Use _____

   _____

6. Name: _____

   Use _____

   _____

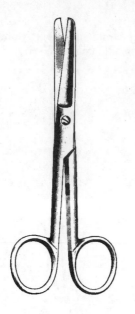

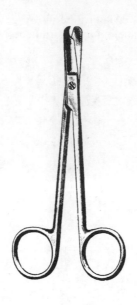

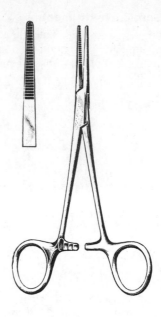

7. Name: _____

    Use _____

    _____

8. Name: _____

    Use _____

    _____

9. Name: _____

    Use _____

    _____

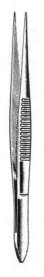

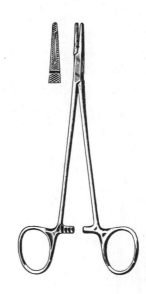

10. Name: _____

    Use _____

    _____

11. Name: _____

    Use _____

    _____

D. Pioneers in Surgical Asepsis

Using a reference source, describe the contributions the following men made to medicine, especially regarding surgical asepsis:

1. Ignaz Semmelweis

_____

_____

_____

2. Louis Pasteur

_____

_____

_____

3. Joseph Lister

_____

_____

_____

E Patient Instruction Sheet

1. You are working for a surgeon who would like you to develop a patient instruction sheet for minor surgery. Select one of the minor operations provided. Using the following instruction sheet, develop a sheet that would be informative and visually appealing to a patient. Be as creative as possible in designing your sheet.

2. Select a partner. Have your partner play the role of a patient who is going to have the minor surgery performed, and explain the information on the sheet. Ask the patient to sign the sheet, and witness the patient's signature.

Minor Office Operations

a. Sebaceous Cyst Removal
b. Mole Removal: Shave Excision
c. Mole Removal: Surgical Excision
d. Needle Biopsy
d. Ingrown Toenail Removal
e. Cervical Punch Biopsy
f. Cervical Cryosurgery

Notes

PATIENT INSTRUCTION SHEET

NAME OF THE PROCEDURE:

DESCRIPTION OF THE PROCEDURE:

PURPOSE OF THE PROCEDURE:

HOW TO PREPARE FOR THE PROCEDURE:

WHAT TO DO FOLLOWING THE PROCEDURE:

I have received and understand the above instructions:

Patient's Signature _____

Witness: _____ Date: _____

Notes

F. Crossword Puzzle: Minor Office Surgery

Directions: Complete the crossword puzzle using the clues presented below.

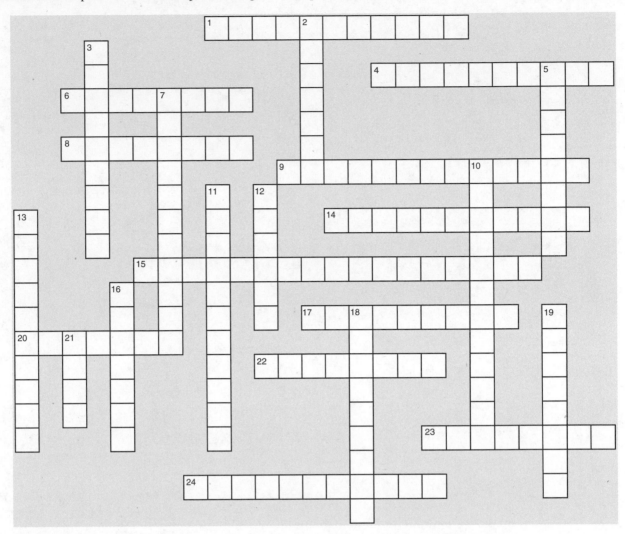

Across

1 Drape with a hole
4 Synthesizes collagen
6 Clean, smooth cut
8 Boil
9 Sac containing oil secretions
14 Pus formation
15 Clamps off blood vessels
17 Local anesthetic brand name
20 Pus in a cavity
22 Tetanus may grow here
23 A local sign of inflammation
24 Bring together

Down

2 Free of all MOs and spores
3 Bruise
5 Scrape
7 Exudate containing blood
10 Suture/needle combination
11 Tx for chronic cervicitis
12 Father of modern surgery
13 Ragged and irregular wound
16 Discovered penicillin
18 Position for colposcopy
19 Antiseptic brand name
21 Nonabsorbable suture material

Notes

PRACTICE FOR COMPETENCY

Sterile Technique

Procedure 10-1: Applying and Removing Sterile Gloves.

Apply and remove sterile gloves.

Procedure 10-2 and 10-A: Sterile Package

Open a sterile package. Add a sterile article to a sterile field using a commercially prepared peel-apart package. Practice each of the methods used to transfer articles to a sterile field as shown in Figure 10.4 of your textbook.

Procedure 10-3: Sterile Solution

Pour a sterile solution into a container on a sterile field.

Minor Surgical Procedures

Procedure 10-4: Sterile Dressing.

Change a sterile dressing and document the procedure in the chart provided.

Procedure 10-5: Suture and Staple Removal.

Practice the procedure for removing sutures and staples, and document the procedure in the chart provided.

Procedure 10-6: Skin Closure Tape.

Practice the procedure for applying and removing skin closure tape, and document the procedure in the chart provided.

Procedure 10-7: Assisting with Minor Office Surgery.

Obtain eight index cards. For each of the following minor office surgeries, indicate (on one side of the card) the equipment and supplies required for the side table. On the other side of the card, indicate the equipment and supplies required for the sterile tray setup. Set up a surgical tray for the procedures listed using your index cards. In the chart provided, document the instructions relayed to the patient following the surgery.

a. Suture insertion
b. Sebaceous cyst removal
c. Incision and drainage of a localized infection
d. Mole removal
e. Needle biopsy
f. Ingrown toenail removal
g. Colposcopy
h. Cervical punch biopsy
i. Cervical cryosurgery

Procedure 10-B: Bandage Turns.

Practice the following bandage turns:

a. Circular turn
b. Spiral turn
c. Spiral-reverse turn
d. Figure-eight turn
e. Recurrent turn

CHART	
Date	

Chapter **10 Minor Office Surgery**

Procedure 10-1: Applying and Removing Sterile Gloves

Name: _____   Date: _____

Evaluated by: _____   Score: _____

Performance Objective

Outcome:	Apply and remove sterile gloves.
Conditions:	Given the appropriate-sized sterile gloves. Using a clean flat surface.
Standards:	Time: 5 minutes. Student completed procedure in _____ minutes. Accuracy: Satisfactory score on the Performance Evaluation Checklist.

Performance Evaluation Checklist

Trial 1	Trial 2	Point Value	Performance Standards
			Application of gloves:
		•	Removed rings and washed hands with an antimicrobial soap.
		▷	Explained why the hands should be washed.
		•	Selected the appropriate-sized gloves.
		▷	Explained what may occur if the gloves are too small or too large.
		•	Placed the glove package on a clean flat surface.
		•	Opened the sterile glove package without touching the inside of the wrapper.
		•	Picked up the first glove on the inside of the cuff without contaminating.
		•	Did not touch the outside of the glove with the bare hand.
		•	Stepped back and pulled on glove and allowed the cuff to remain turned back on itself.
		•	Picked up the second glove by slipping sterile gloved fingers under its cuff and grasping the opposite side with the thumb.
		•	Pulled the glove on and turned back the cuff.
		•	Turned back the cuff of the first glove without contaminating it.
		•	Adjusted the gloves to a comfortable position.
		•	Inspected the gloves for tears.
		▷	Explained what should be done if a glove is torn.
			Removal of gloves:
		•	Grasped the outside of the right glove 1 to 2 inches from the top with the gloved left hand.

Trial 1	Trial 2	Point Value	Performance Standards
		•	Slowly pulled right glove off the hand.
		•	Pulled the right glove free and scrunched it into a ball with the gloved left hand.
		•	Placed index and middle fingers of the right hand on the inside of left glove.
		•	Did not allow the clean hand to touch the outside of the glove.
		•	Pulled the glove off the left hand, enclosing the balled-up right glove.
		•	Discarded both gloves in an appropriate waste container.
		▷	Stated how to discard gloves if they are visibly contaminated with blood.
		•	Sanitized hands.
		■	Demonstrated critical thinking skills.
		★	Completed the procedure within 5 minutes.
			Totals

Evaluation of Student Performance

EVALUATION CRITERIA			COMMENTS
Symbol	**Category**	**Point Value**	
★	Critical Step	16 points	
•	Essential Step	6 points	
■	Affective Competency	6 points	
▷	Theory Question	2 points	

Score calculation: 100 points

− _____ points missed

_____ Score

Satisfactory score: 85 or above

CAAHEP Competencies Achieved

Psychomotor (Skills)

☑ III. 2. Select appropriate barrier/personal protective equipment (PPE).

Affective (Behavior)

☑ A. 1. Demonstrate critical thinking skills.

ABHES Competencies Achieved

☑ 4. f. Comply with federal, state and local health laws as they relate to healthcare settings.
☑ 8. a. Practice standard precautions and perform disinfection/sterilization techniques.

EVALUATION OF COMPETENCY

Procedure 10-2: Opening a Sterile Package

Name: _____   Date: _____

Evaluated by: _____   Score: _____

Performance Objective

Outcome:	Open a sterile package.
Conditions:	Given a sterile package.
	Using a clean flat surface.
Standards:	Time: 5 minutes. Student completed procedure in _____ minutes.
	Accuracy: Satisfactory score on the Performance Evaluation Checklist.

Performance Evaluation Checklist

Trial 1	Trial 2	Point Value	Performance Standards
		•	Sanitized hands.
		•	Assembled the equipment.
		•	Checked pack to make sure it is not wet, torn, or opened.
		•	Checked the autoclave tape on the pack.
		▷	Stated the purpose of autoclave tape.
		•	Positioned the pack on the table so that the top flap of wrapper will open away from the body.
		•	Faced the sterile field at all times and did not talk, laugh, cough, or sneeze over the field.
		•	Removed the fastener on wrapped package and discarded it.
		•	Opened the first flap away from the body.
		•	Opened the left and right flaps without contaminating the contents.
		•	Opened the flap closest to the body.
		•	In all cases, touched only the outside of the wrapper.
		•	In all cases, did not reach over the sterile contents of the package.
		▷	Stated why the medical assistant should not reach over the contents of the package.
		•	Adjusted the sterile wrapper by the corners as needed.
		•	Checked the sterilization indicator on the inside of the pack.
		▷	Stated the reason for checking the sterilization indicator.
		★	Completed the procedure within 5 minutes.
			Totals

425

Evaluation of Student Performance

<table>
<tr><th colspan="3">EVALUATION CRITERIA</th><th>COMMENTS</th></tr>
<tr><th>Symbol</th><th>Category</th><th>Point Value</th><td rowspan="9"></td></tr>
<tr><td>★</td><td>Critical Step</td><td>16 points</td></tr>
<tr><td>•</td><td>Essential Step</td><td>6 points</td></tr>
<tr><td>■</td><td>Affective Competency</td><td>6 points</td></tr>
<tr><td>▷</td><td>Theory Question</td><td>2 points</td></tr>
<tr><td colspan="3">Score calculation: 100 points</td></tr>
<tr><td colspan="3" style="text-align:right">−   points missed</td></tr>
<tr><td colspan="3" style="text-align:right">___Score</td></tr>
<tr><td colspan="3">Satisfactory score: 85 or above</td></tr>
</table>

CAAHEP Competencies Achieved

Psychomotor (Skills)

☑ III. 6. Prepare a sterile field.
☑ III. 7. Perform within a sterile field.

ABHES Competencies Achieved

☑ 8. e. Perform specialty procedures including but not limited to pediatric care, minor surgery, cardiac, respiratory, OB-GYN, neurological, and gastroenterology.

EVALUATION OF COMPETENCY

10-A: Adding a Sterile Article to a Sterile Field

Name: _____   Date: _____

Evaluated by: _____   Score: _____

Performance Objective

Outcome:	Add a sterile article to a sterile field from a peel-apart package by ejecting its contents onto the field.
Conditions:	Given the following: peel-apart package and a sterile field.
Standards:	Time: 3 minutes. Student completed procedure in _____ minutes. Accuracy: Satisfactory score on the Performance Evaluation Checklist.

Performance Evaluation Checklist

Trial 1	Trial 2	Point Value	Performance Standards
		•	Sanitized hands.
		•	Grasped the two unsterile flaps of the peel-pack between thumbs.
		•	Pulled the package apart using a rolling-outward motion.
		▷	Stated what parts of the peel-pack must remain sterile.
		•	Stepped back slightly from the sterile field.
		▷	Explained the reason for stepping back.
		•	Gently ejected contents of the peel-pack onto the center of the sterile field.
		★	Completed the procedure within 3 minutes.
			Totals

Evaluation of Student Performance

EVALUATION CRITERIA			COMMENTS
Symbol	**Category**	**Point Value**	
★	Critical Step	16 points	
•	Essential Step	6 points	
■	Affective Competency	6 points	
▷	Theory Question	2 points	

Score calculation: 100 points

        − _____ points missed

        _____ Score

Satisfactory score: 85 or above

CAAHEP Competencies Achieved
Psychomotor (Skills)
☑ III. 7. Perform within a sterile field.

ABHES Competencies Achieved
☑ 8. e. Perform specialty procedures including but not limited to pediatric care, minor surgery, cardiac, respiratory, OB-GYN, neurological, and gastroenterology.

EVALUATION OF COMPETENCY

Procedure 10-3: Pouring a Sterile Solution

Name: _____   Date: _____

Evaluated by: _____   Score: _____

Performance Objective

Outcome:	Pour a sterile solution.
Conditions:	Given the following: sterile solution, sterile container, and a sterile towel.
Standards:	Time: 5 minutes. Student completed procedure in _____ minutes.
	Accuracy: Satisfactory score on the Performance Evaluation Checklist.

Performance Evaluation Checklist

Trial 1	Trial 2	Point Value	Performance Standards
		•	Checked the label of the solution to ensure it is the correct solution.
		•	Checked expiration date on the solution.
		▷	Explained why an outdated solution should not be used.
		•	Checked solution label a second time.
		•	Palmed the label of the bottle.
		▷	Explained why the label should be palmed.
		•	Removed cap and placed it on a flat surface with the open end up.
		▷	Stated why cap should be placed with the open end up.
		•	Rinsed the lip of the bottle.
		▷	Explained why the lip of the bottle should be rinsed.
		•	Poured the proper amount of solution into a sterile container at a height of 6 inches.
		•	Did not allow the neck of the bottle to come in contact with the sterile container.
		•	Did not allow any of the solution to splash onto the sterile field.
		▷	Explained why the sterile solution should not be allowed to splash onto the sterile field.
		•	Replaced cap on container without contaminating.
		•	Checked the label a third time.
		★	Completed the procedure within 5 minutes.
		Totals	

Evaluation of Student Performance

EVALUATION CRITERIA			COMMENTS
Symbol	**Category**	**Point Value**	
★	Critical Step	16 points	
•	Essential Step	6 points	
■	Affective Competency	6 points	
▷	Theory Question	2 points	

Score calculation: 100 points

       − _____ points missed

       _____ Score

Satisfactory score: 85 or above

CAAHEP Competencies Achieved

Psychomotor (Skills)

☑ III. 7. Perform within a sterile field.

ABHES Competencies Achieved

☑ 8. e. Perform specialty procedures including but not limited to pediatric care, minor surgery, cardiac, respiratory, OB-GYN, neurological, and gastroenterology.

Procedure 10-4: Changing a Sterile Dressing

Name: _____   Date: _____

Evaluated by: _____   Score: _____

Performance Objective

Outcome:	Change a sterile dressing.
Conditions:	Given the following: Mayo stand, biohazard waste container, clean and disposable gloves, antiseptic swabs, sterile gloves, plastic waste bag, surgical tape and scissors, sterile dressing, and thumb forceps.
Standards:	Time: 10 minutes. Student completed procedure in _____ minutes. Accuracy: Satisfactory score on the Performance Evaluation Checklist.

Performance Evaluation Checklist

Trial 1	Trial 2	Point Value	Performance Standards
		•	Washed hands with an antimicrobial soap.
		•	Assembled equipment.
		•	Set up the nonsterile items on a side table or counter.
		•	Positioned the plastic waste bag in a convenient location.
		•	Greeted the patient and introduced yourself.
		•	Identified patient and explained the procedure.
		•	Instructed patient not to move during procedure.
		•	Adjusted the light.
		•	Applied clean gloves.
		•	Loosened the tape and carefully removed soiled dressing by pulling it upward.
		•	Did not touch inside of dressing that was next to the wound.
		▷	Explained why the inside of the dressing should not be touched.
		▷	Described what to do if the dressing is stuck to the wound.
		•	Placed soiled dressing in the waste bag without touching outside of bag.
		•	Inspected the wound.
		▷	Stated what type of inspection should be performed.
		•	Opened the antiseptic swabs and placed the pouch in a convenient location or held the pouch in your hand.
		•	Applied the antiseptic to the wound.
		•	Used a new swab for each motion.
		•	Discarded each contaminated swab in the waste bag after use.

431

Chapter **10 Minor Office Surgery**

Trial 1	Trial 2	Point Value	Performance Standards
		•	Removed gloves and discarded them without contaminating.
		•	Sanitized hands and prepared the sterile field.
		•	Instructed patient not to talk, laugh, sneeze, or cough over the sterile field.
		•	Opened sterile glove package and applied sterile gloves.
		•	Picked up sterile dressing from the tray using sterile gloves or sterile forceps.
		•	Placed sterile dressing over the wound by lightly dropping it in place.
			Did not move dressing after dropping it in place.
		▷	Explained why the dressing should be dropped onto the wound and then not moved.
		•	Discarded gloves (and forceps) in the waste bag.
		•	Applied hypoallergenic tape to hold sterile dressing in place.
		•	Provided the patient with written wound care instructions.
		•	Instructed patient in wound care.
		▷	Described the wound care that should be relayed to the patient.
		•	Asked patient to sign instruction sheet.
		•	Witnessed the patient's signature.
		•	Gave a signed copy to the patient.
		•	Filed original in the patient's medical record.
		▷	Stated the purpose of filing original in patient's medical record.
		•	Returned equipment.
		•	Disposed of plastic bag in a biohazard waste container.
		•	Sanitized hands.
		•	Documented the procedure correctly.
		■	Demonstrated critical thinking skills.
		■	Reassured patients.
		■	Demonstrated empathy for patients' concerns.
		★	Completed the procedure within 10 minutes.
			Totals

CHART

Date	

Evaluation of Student Performance

EVALUATION CRITERIA			COMMENTS
Symbol	**Category**	**Point Value**	
★	Critical Step	16 points	
•	Essential Step	6 points	
■	Affective Competency	6 points	
▷	Theory Question	2 points	

Score calculation: 100 points

− _____ points missed

___Score

Satisfactory score: 85 or above

CAAHEP Competencies Achieved

Psychomotor (Skills)

☑ I. 8. Instruct and prepare a patient for a procedure or a treatment.
☑ III. 6. Prepare a sterile field.
☑ III. 7. Perform within a sterile field.
☑ III. 8. Perform wound care.
☑ III. 9. Perform dressing change.
☑ III. 10. Demonstrate proper disposal of biohazardous material: a. sharps b. regulated wastes.
☑ V. 3. Coach patient regarding: a. office policies; b. medical encounters.
☑ X. 3. Document patient care accurately in the medical record.

Affective (Behavior)

☑ A. 1. Demonstrate critical thinking skills.
☑ A. 2. Reassure patients.
☑ Demonstrate empathy for patients' concerns.

ABHES Competencies Achieved

☑ 4. a. Follow documentation guidelines.
☑ 7. g. Display professionalism through written and verbal communications.
☑ 8. e. Perform specialty procedures including but not limited to pediatric care, minor surgery, cardiac, respiratory, OB-GYN, neurological, and gastroenterology.
☑ 8. h. Teach self-examination, disease management and health promotion.
☑ 9. c. Dispose of biohazardous materials.

Notes

Procedure 10-5: Removing Sutures and Staples

Name: _____ Date: _____

Evaluated by: _____ Score: _____

Performance Objective

Outcome:	Remove sutures and staples.
Conditions:	Given the following: Mayo stand, antiseptic swabs, clean and disposable gloves, sterile 4 × 4 gauze, surgical tape, biohazard waste container, suture removal kit, and staple removal kit.
Standards:	Time: 10 minutes. Student completed procedure in _____ minutes. Accuracy: Satisfactory score on the Performance Evaluation Checklist.

Performance Evaluation Checklist

Trial 1	Trial 2	Point Value	Performance Standards
		•	Washed hands with an antimicrobial soap.
		•	Assembled equipment.
		•	Greeted the patient and introduced yourself.
		•	Identified patient and explained the procedure.
		•	Positioned the patient as required.
		•	Adjusted the light.
		•	Checked to make sure the sutures (or staples) were intact.
		•	Checked to make sure the incision line was approximated and free from infection.
		▷	Explained what to do if the incision line is not approximated.
		•	Opened the suture or staple removal kit.
		•	Applied clean gloves.
		•	Cleaned the incision line with antiseptic swabs using a new swab for each cleansing motion.
		•	Allowed the skin to dry.
		•	Informed the patient that he or she would feel a pulling sensation as each suture (or staple) is removed.
		Removed sutures as follows:	
		•	Picked up the knot of suture with thumb forceps.
		•	Placed curved tip of suture scissors under the suture.
		•	Cut suture below the knot on the side of suture closest to the skin.
		•	Gently pulled suture out of the skin, using a smooth, continuous motion.
		•	Did not allow any portion of suture previously on the outside to be pulled through the tissue lying beneath the incision line.

Trial 1	Trial 2	Point Value	Performance Standards
		•	Placed the suture on the gauze.
		•	Repeated above sequence until all sutures were removed.
			Removed staples as follows:
		•	Gently placed the jaws of the staple remover under the staple.
		•	Squeezed the staple handles until they were fully closed.
		•	Lifted the staple remover upward to remove the staple.
		•	Placed staple on gauze.
		•	Continued until all the staples were removed.
		•	Counted number of sutures or staples and checked number with the patient's medical record.
		•	Cleansed the site with an antiseptic swab.
		•	Applied skin closure tape, if directed by the provider.
		•	Applied DSD, if directed to do so by the provider.
		•	Disposed of sutures or staples and gauze in biohazard waste container.
		•	Removed gloves and sanitized hands.
		•	Documented the procedure correctly.
		■	Demonstrated critical thinking skills.
		■	Reassured patients.
		■	Demonstrated empathy for patients' concerns.
		★	Completed the procedure within 10 minutes.
			Totals

CHART	
Date	

Evaluation of Student Performance

EVALUATION CRITERIA			COMMENTS
Symbol	**Category**	**Point Value**	
★	Critical Step	16 points	
•	Essential Step	6 points	
■	Affective Competency	6 points	
▷	Theory Question	2 points	

Score calculation: 100 points

_ − _ points missed

_ ___Score

Satisfactory score: 85 or above

CAAHEP Competencies Achieved

Psychomotor (Skills)

- ☑ I. 8. Instruct and prepare a patient for a procedure or a treatment.
- ☑ III. 8. Perform wound care.
- ☑ III. 10. Demonstrate proper disposal of biohazardous material: a. sharps b. regulated wastes.
- ☑ V. 3. Coach patient regarding: a. office policies; b. medical encounters.
- ☑ X. 3. Document patient care accurately in the medical record.

Affective (Behavior)

- ☑ A. Demonstrate critical thinking skills.
- ☑ A. 2. Reassure patients.
- ☑ A. 3. Demonstrated empathy for patients' concerns.

ABHES Competencies Achieved

- ☑ 4. a. Follow documentation guidelines.
- ☑ 7. g. Display professionalism through written and verbal communications
- ☑ 8. e. Perform specialty procedures including but not limited to pediatric care, minor surgery, cardiac, respiratory, OB-GYN, neurological, and gastroenterology.
- ☑ 8. h. Teach self-examination, disease management and health promotion.
- ☑ 9. c. Dispose of biohazardous materials.

Notes

Procedure 10-6: Applying and Removing Skin Closure Tape

Name: _____ Date: _____

Evaluated by: _____ Score: _____

Performance Objective

Outcome:	Apply and remove skin closure tape.
Conditions:	Given the following: clean and disposable gloves, sterile gloves, antiseptic solution, surgical scrub brush, antiseptic swabs, tincture of benzoin, sterile cotton-tipped applicator, adhesive skin closure strips, sterile 4 × 4 gauze pads, surgical tape, and a biohazard waste container.
Standards:	Time: 10 minutes. Student completed procedure in _____ minutes. Accuracy: Satisfactory score on the Performance Evaluation Checklist.

Performance Evaluation Checklist

Trial 1	Trial 2	Point Value	Performance Standards
			Application of skin closure tape:
		•	Washed hands with an antimicrobial soap.
		•	Assembled equipment.
		•	Checked expiration date on the skin closure tape.
		•	Greeted patient and introduced yourself.
		•	Identified patient and explained the procedure.
		•	Positioned the patient as required.
		•	Adjusted the light.
		•	Applied clean gloves.
		•	Inspected the wound for redness, swelling, and drainage.
		•	Scrubbed the wound with an antiseptic solution.
		•	Allowed the skin to dry or patted dry with gauze pads.
		•	Applied antiseptic using a new swab for each motion.
		•	Allowed the skin to dry.
		▷	Explained why the skin must be completely dry.
		•	Applied tincture of benzoin without letting it touch the wound.
		▷	Stated the purpose of tincture of benzoin.
		•	Allowed the skin to dry.

Trial 1	Trial 2	Point Value	Performance Standards
		•	Removed gloves and washed hands.
		•	Opened the package of adhesive strips and laid them on a flat surface.
		•	Applied sterile gloves and tore the tab off the card of strips.
		•	Peeled a strip of tape off the card.
		•	Checked to make sure the skin surface was dry.
		•	Positioned the first strip over the center of the wound.
		•	Secured one end of the strip to the skin by pressing down firmly on the tape.
		•	Stretched the strip across the incision until the edges of the wound were approximated.
		•	Secured the strip to the skin on the other side of the wound.
		•	Applied the second strip on one side of center strip at an 1/8-inch interval.
		•	Applied a third strip at a 1/8-inch interval on the other side of the center strip.
		•	Continued applying the strips at 1/8-inch intervals until the edges of the wound were approximated.
		▷	Explained why the strips should be spaced at 1/8-inch intervals.
		•	Applied two closures approximately 1/2-inch from the ends of the strips.
		▷	Stated the purpose of applying a strip along each edge.
		•	Applied a sterile dressing over the strips if indicated by the provider.
		•	Removed gloves and sanitized hands.
		•	Provided patient with written wound care instructions.
		•	Explained the wound care instructions to the patient.
		•	Asked patient to sign instruction sheet and witnessed patient's signature.
		•	Gave a signed copy to the patient and filed original in the patient's medical record.
		•	Documented the procedure correctly.
			Removal of skin closure tape:
		•	Sanitized hands.
		•	Greeted patient and introduced yourself.
		•	Identified patient and explained the procedure.
		•	Positioned the patient as required.
		•	Adjusted the light.
		•	Checked to make sure the incision line was approximated and free from infection.
		•	Positioned a 4 × 4 gauze pad in a convenient location.

Trial 1	Trial 2	Point Value	Performance Standards
		•	Applied clean gloves.
		•	Peeled off each half of the strip from the outside toward the wound margin.
		•	Stabilized the skin with one finger.
		•	Gently lifted the strip up and away from the wound and placed it on the gauze.
		•	Continued until all closures were removed.
		•	Cleansed the site with an antiseptic swab.
		•	Applied a sterile dressing if indicated by the provider.
		•	Disposed of strips and gauze in a biohazard waste container.
		•	Removed gloves and sanitized hands.
		•	Documented the procedure correctly.
		■	Demonstrated critical thinking skills.
		■	Reassured patients.
		■	Demonstrated empathy for patients' concerns.
		★	Completed the procedure within 10 minutes.
			Totals

CHART

Date	

Evaluation of Student Performance

EVALUATION CRITERIA			COMMENTS
Symbol	**Category**	**Point Value**	
★	Critical Step	16 points	
•	Essential Step	6 points	
■	Affective Competency	6 points	
▷	Theory Question	2 points	

Score calculation: 100 points

     − ____ points missed

     ____Score

Satisfactory score: 85 or above

CAAHEP Competencies Achieved

Psychomotor (Skills)

☑ I. 8. Instruct and prepare a patient for a procedure or a treatment.
☑ III. 8. Perform wound care.
☑ V. 03. Coach patient regarding: a. office policies; b. medical encounters.
☑ X. 3. Document patient care accurately in the medical record.

Affective (Behavior)

☑ A. 1. Demonstrate critical thinking skills.
☑ A. 2. Reassure patients.
☑ A. 3. Demonstrate empathy for patients' concerns.

ABHES Competencies Achieved

☑ 4. a. Follow documentation guidelines.
☑ 7. g. Display professionalism through written and verbal communications.
☑ 8. e. Perform specialty procedures including but not limited to minor surgery, cardiac, respiratory, OB-GYN, neurological, gastroenterology.
☑ 8. h. Teach self-examination, disease management and health promotion.
☑ 9. c. Dispose of biohazardous materials.

Procedure 10-7: Assisting with Minor Office Surgery

Name: _____   Date: _____

Evaluated by: _____   Score: _____

Performance Objective

Outcome:	Set up the surgical tray and assist with minor office surgery.
Conditions:	Given a Mayo stand, biohazard waste container, and the instruments and supplies required for a specific minor office surgery as designed by the instructor.
Standards:	Time: 15 minutes. Student completed procedure in _____ minutes. Accuracy: Satisfactory score on the Performance Evaluation Checklist.

Performance Evaluation Checklist

Trial 1	Trial 2	Point Value	Performance Standards
		•	Determined the type of minor office surgery to be performed.
		•	Prepared examining room.
		•	Sanitized hands.
		•	Set up articles required that are not sterile on a side table or counter.
		•	Labeled the specimen container (if included in the setup).
		•	Washed hands with an antimicrobial soap.
		•	Set up the minor office surgery tray on a clean, dry, flat surface, using the principles of surgical asepsis.
		Prepackaged sterile setup	
		•	Selected the appropriate package from supply shelf and placed it on a flat surface.
		•	Opened the setup using the inside of wrapper as the sterile field.
		•	Checked the sterilization indicator on inside of pack.
		•	Added any additional articles required for the surgery and covered tray setup with a sterile towel.
		Transferring articles to a sterile field:	
		•	Placed sterile towel on a flat surface by two corner ends, making sure not to contaminate it.
		•	Transferred sterile articles to the field from wrapped or peel-apart packages.
		•	Applied sterile glove.
		•	Arranged articles neatly on the sterile field with sterile glove.
		•	Checked to make sure all articles were available on the sterile field.
		•	Covered the tray setup with a sterile towel without allowing arms to pass over the sterile field.

Trial 1	Trial 2	Point Value	Performance Standards
			Prepared the patient:
		•	Greeted the patient and introduced yourself.
		•	Identified patient, explained the procedure, and reassured the patient.
		•	Asked patient if he or she needs to void before the surgery.
		•	Instructed patient on clothing removal.
		•	Instructed patient not to move during procedure or to talk, laugh, sneeze, or cough over the sterile field.
		•	Positioned patient as required for the type of surgery to be performed.
		•	Adjusted the light so that it was focused on the operative site.
			Prepared the patient's skin:
		•	Applied clean disposable gloves.
		•	Shaved skin (if required).
		•	Cleansed skin with an antiseptic solution.
		•	Rinsed and dried the area.
		•	Applied antiseptic using antiseptic swabs.
		•	Allowed the skin to dry.
		•	Removed gloves and sanitized hands.
		•	Checked to make sure that everything was ready and informed provider.
			Assisted the provider:
		•	Uncovered the tray setup.
		•	Opened the outer glove wrapper for provider.
		•	Held the vial while the provider withdrew the local anesthetic.
		•	Adjusted the light as required.
		•	Restrained patient (e.g., child).
		•	Relaxed and reassured patient.
		•	Handed instruments and supplies to provider. Sterile gloves required.
		•	Kept the sterile field neat and orderly. Sterile gloves required.
		•	Held basin for provider to deposit soiled instruments and supplies. Clean gloves required.
		•	Retracted tissue. Sterile gloves required.
		•	Sponged blood from operative site. Sterile gloves required.

444

Trial 1	Trial 2	Point Value	Performance Standards
		•	Added instruments and supplies as necessary to the sterile field.
		•	Held specimen container to accept specimen. Clean gloves required.
		•	Cut ends of suture material after insertion by the provider Sterile gloves required.
			After surgery:
		•	Applied sterile dressing to the surgical wound if ordered by provider.
		•	Stayed with patient as a safety precaution.
		•	Assisted and instructed patient as required.
		•	Verified that patient understood postoperative instructions.
		•	Provided patient with verbal and written wound care instructions.
		▷	Stated the patient instructions that should be relayed for wound and suture care.
		•	Asked patient to sign instruction sheet and witnessed the patient's signature.
		•	Gave a signed copy to the patient and filed original in patient's medical record.
		•	Relayed information regarding the return visit
		•	Assisted patient off table.
		•	Instructed patient to get dressed.
		•	Prepared any specimens collected for transfer to the laboratory with a completed biopsy request.
		•	Documented correctly.
		•	Cleaned examining room.
		•	Discarded disposable contaminated articles in a biohazard waste container.
		•	Sanitized and sterilized instruments.
		■	Demonstrated critical thinking skills.
		■	Reassured patients.
		■	Demonstrated empathy for patients' concerns.
		★	Completed the procedure within 15 minutes.
			Totals

CHART

Date	

Evaluation of Student Performance

EVALUATION CRITERIA			COMMENTS
Symbol	**Category**	**Point Value**	
★	Critical Step	16 points	
•	Essential Step	6 points	
■	Affective Competency	6 points	
▷	Theory Question	2 points	

Score calculation: 100 points

− _____ points missed

_____Score

Satisfactory score: 85 or above

CAAHEP Competencies Achieved

Psychomotor (Skills)
- ☑ I. 8. Instruct and prepare a patient for a procedure or a treatment.
- ☑ III. 6. Prepare a sterile field.
- ☑ III. 7. Perform within a sterile field.
- ☑ III. 10. Demonstrate proper disposal of biohazardous material: regulated wastes: a. sharps; b. regulates wastes.
- ☑ V. 3. Coach patient regarding: a. office policies; b. medical encounters.
- ☑ X. 3. Document patient care accurately in the medical record.

Affective (Behavior)
- ☑ A. 1. Demonstrate critical thinking skills.
- ☑ Reassure patients.
- ☑ A. 3. Demonstrate empathy for patients' concerns.

ABHES Competencies Achieved

- ☑ 4. a. Follow documentation guidelines.
- ☑ 7. g. Display professionalism through written and verbal communications.
- ☑ 8. d. Assist provider with specialty examination including pediatric care, cardiac, respiratory, OB-GYN, neurological, and gastroenterology procedures.
- ☑ 8. e. Perform specialty procedures including but not limited to pediatric care, minor surgery, cardiac, respiratory, OB-GYN, neurological, and gastroenterology.
- ☑ 8. g. Recognize and respond to medical office emergencies.
- ☑ 8. h. Teach self-examination, disease management and health promotion.
- ☑ 8. j. Accommodate patients with special needs.
- ☑ 9. c. Dispose of biohazardous materials.

Procedure 10-B: Bandage Turns

Name: _____   Date: _____

Evaluated by: _____   Score: _____

Performance Objective

Outcome:	Apply the following bandage turns: circular, spiral, spiral-reverse, figure-eight, and recurrent.
Conditions:	Given the following: a roller bandage and an elastic bandage.
Standards:	Time: 15 minutes. Student completed procedure in _____ minutes. Accuracy: Satisfactory score on the Performance Evaluation Checklist.

Performance Evaluation Checklist

Trial 1	Trial 2	Point Value	Performance Standards
			Circular turn:
		•	Placed the end of a bandage on a slant.
		•	Encircled the body part while allowing the corner of the bandage to extend.
		•	Turned down corner of bandage.
		•	Made another circular turn around the body part.
		▷	Stated a use of the circular turn.
			Spiral turn:
		•	Anchored bandage using a circular turn.
		•	Encircled the body part while keeping bandage at a slant.
		•	Carried each spiral turn upward at a slight angle.
		•	Overlapped each previous turn by one half to two thirds of the width of the bandage.
		▷	Stated a use of the spiral turn.
			Spiral-reverse turn:
		•	Anchored bandage using a circular turn.
		•	Encircled the body part while keeping bandage at a slant.
		•	Reversed the spiral turn using the thumb or index finger.
		•	Directed bandage downward and folded it on itself.
		•	Kept bandage parallel to the lower edge of the previous turn.
		•	Overlapped each previous turn by two thirds the width of the bandage.
		▷	Stated a use of the spiral-reverse turn.
			Figure-eight turn:
		•	Anchored bandage using a circular turn.

447

Trial 1	Trial 2	Point Value	Performance Standards
		•	Slanted bandage turns to alternately ascend and descend around the body part.
		•	Crossed the turns over one another in the middle to resemble a figure eight
		•	Overlapped each previous turn by two thirds of the width of the bandage.
		▷	Stated a use of the figure-eight turn.
			Recurrent turn:
		•	Anchored bandage using two circular turns.
		•	Passed bandage back and forth over the tip of the body part being bandaged.
		•	Overlapped each previous turn by two thirds of the width of the bandage.
		▷	Stated a use of the recurrent turn.
		■	Demonstrated critical thinking skills.
		★	Completed the procedure within 15 minutes.
			Totals
CHART			
Date			

Evaluation of Student Performance

EVALUATION CRITERIA			COMMENTS
Symbol	**Category**	**Point Value**	
★	Critical Step	16 points	
•	Essential Step	6 points	
■	Affective Competency	6 points	
▷	Theory Question	2 points	

Score calculation: 100 points

      −   points missed

          ___Score

Satisfactory score: 85 or above

CAAHEP Competencies Achieved

Psychomotor (Skills)

☑ I. 8. Instruct and prepare a patient for a procedure or a treatment.
☑ V. 3. Coach patient regarding: a. office policies; b. medical encounters.

Affective (Behavior)

☑ A. 1. Demonstrate critical thinking skills.

ABHES Competencies Achieved

☑ 8. h. Teach self-examination, disease management and health promotion.
☑ 8. j. Accommodate patients with special needs (psychological or physical limitations).

11 Administration of Medication and Intravenous Therapy

√ After Completing	Date Due	Study Guide Pages	STUDY GUIDE ASSIGNMENTS (CTA = Critical Thinking Activity)	Possible Points	Points You Earned
		457	?≣ Pretest	10	
			🔑Term Key Term Assessment		
		458	A. Definitions	26	
		459	B. Word Parts	13	
			(Add 1 point for each key term)		
		459-466	📝 Evaluation of Learning questions	78	
		466-469	CTA A: Drug Package Insert	32	
		469	CTA B: Drug Classifications (3 points each)	30	
			Evolve: Road to Recovery. Drug Classifications		
			Evolve: Road to Recovery: Abbreviations		
		470	CTA C: Medication Record	20	
		471	CTA D: Seven Rights of Medication Administration	35	
			Evolve: Script It! (Record points earned)		
		472	CTA E: Liquid Measurement	11	
		472	CTA F: Parts of a Needle and Syringe	11	
			Evolve: Take the Plunge (Record points earned)		
		473	CTA G: Hypodermic Syringe Calibrations	10	
			Evolve: Which Needle? (Record points earned)		
		473	CTA H: Insulin Syringe Calibrations	20	
		474	CTA I: Tuberculin Syringe Calibrations	14	

451

√ After Completing	Date Due	Study Guide Pages	STUDY GUIDE ASSIGNMENTS (CTA = Critical Thinking Activity)	Possible Points	Points You Earned
			Evolve: Draw It Up! (Record points earned)		
		474	CTA J: Syringe and Needle Labels (3 points each)	12	
		475	CTA K: Angle of Insertion for Injections	3	
		475-476	CTA L: Preparing and Administering Parenteral Medication	18	
		477	CTA M: Measuring Mantoux Test Reactions	5	
		478	CTA N: Interpreting Mantoux Skin Test Reactions	11	
		478-479	CTA O: Anaphylactic Reaction	20	
		480-495	CTA P: Researching Drugs (5 points per drug researched)	325	
		496	CTA Q: Crossword Puzzle	37	
			Evolve: Math Review (Record points earned)		
			Evolve: Apply Your Knowledge questions	10	
			Evolve: Video Evaluation	59	
		457	? Posttest	10	
			ADDITIONAL ASSIGNMENTS		
			Total points		

√ After Completing	Date Due	Study Guide Pages	STUDY GUIDE ASSIGNMENTS Drug Dosage Calculation: Supplemental Education for Chapter 11	Possible Points	Points You Earned
		533	Unit 1: The Metric System A. Units of Measurement	10	
		533	Unit 1: The Metric System B. Metric Abbreviations	6	
		534	Unit 1: The Metric System C. Metric Notation	15	
		534	Unit 2: The Household System A. Units of Measurements	4	
		535	Unit 3: Medication Orders A. Medical Abbreviations	25	
		536-537	Unit 3: Medication Orders B. Interpreting Medication Orders (3 points each)	30	
		537-538	Unit 4: Converting Units of Measurement A. Using Conversion Tables (2 points each)	38	
		538-540	Unit 4: Converting Units of Measurement B. Converting Units Within the Metric System (2 points each)	40	
		540-542	Unit 4: Converting Units of Measurement C. Converting Units Within the Household System (2 points each)	20	
		542-544	Unit 5: Ratio and Proportion A. Ratio and Proportion Guidelines (6 points each)	48	
		545-546	Unit 5: Ratio and Proportion B. Converting Units Using Ratio and Proportion (2 points each)	20	
		546-552	Unit 6: Determining Drug Dosage A. Oral Administration (2 points each)	30	
		552-555	Unit 6: Determining Drug Dosage B. Parenteral Administration (2 points each)	20	

√ After Completing	Date Due	Study Guide Pages	STUDY GUIDE ASSIGNMENTS Drug Dosage Calculation: Supplemental Education for Chapter 11	Possible Points	Points You Earned
			ADDITIONAL ASSIGNMENTS		
			Total points		

√ When Assigned by Your Instructor	Study Guide Pages	Practices Required	LABORATORY ASSIGNMENTS (Procedure Number and Name)	Score*
	497	5	**Practice for Competency** 11-1: Administering Oral Medication	
	503-505		**Evaluation of Competency** 11-1: Administering Oral Medication	*
	497	Vial: 5 Ampule: 5	**Practice for Competency** 11-2: Preparing an Injection	
	507-509		**Evaluation of Competency** 11-2: Preparing an Injection	*
	497	3	**Practice for Competency** 11-3: Reconstituting Powdered Drugs	
	511-512		**Evaluation of Competency** 11-3: Reconstituting Powdered Drugs	*
	497-498	5	**Practice for Competency** 11-4: Administering a Subcutaneous Injection	
	513-515		**Evaluation of Competency** 11-4: Administering a Subcutaneous Injection	*
	499	5	**Practice for Competency** 11-A: Locating Intramuscular Injection Sites	
	517-519		**Evaluation of Competency** 11-A: Locating Intramuscular Injection Sites	*
	499	5	**Practice for Competency** 11-5: Administering an Intramuscular Injection	
	521-523		**Evaluation of Competency** 11-5: Administering an Intramuscular Injection	*
	499	5	**Practice for Competency** 11-6: Z-Track Intramuscular Injection Technique	
	525-527		**Evaluation of Competency** 11-6: Z-Track Intramuscular Injection Technique	*
	499-501	5	**Practice for Competency** 11-7: Administering an Intradermal Injection	

√ When Assigned by Your Instructor	Study Guide Pages	Practices Required	LABORATORY ASSIGNMENTS (Procedure Number and Name)	Score*
	529-532		**Evaluation of Competency** 11-7: Administering an Intradermal Injection	*
			ADDITIONAL ASSIGNMENTS	

Name _____ Date _____

True or False

_____ 1. A drug is a chemical that is used for treatment, prevention, or diagnosis of disease.

_____ 2. The brand name of a drug is assigned by the pharmaceutical manufacturer that markets a drug.

_____ 3. The Rx symbol comes from the Latin word recipe and means "take."

_____ 4. An anaphylactic reaction can be life threatening.

_____ 5. The deltoid site is the most common site for administering injections in infants.

_____ 6. A subcutaneous injection is given into muscle tissue.

_____ 7. The gauge of the needle used depends upon the viscosity of the medication being administered.

_____ 8. The Mantoux tuberculin skin test is administered through a subcutaneous injection.

_____ 9. The peripheral veins of the arm and hand are used most often for administering IV therapy.

_____ 10. Chemotherapy is the use of chemicals to treat disease.

? POSTTEST

True or False

_____ 1. OSHA is responsible for determining whether drugs are safe before release for human use.

_____ 2. An enteric-coated tablet does not dissolve until it reaches the intestines.

_____ 3. The apothecary system is most often used to administer medication in the medical office.

_____ 4. The parenteral route of administering medications is used when the patient is allergic to the oral form of the drug.

_____ 5. Hypodermic syringes are calibrated in milliliters.

_____ 6. The maximum amount of medication that can be administered through the subcutaneous route is 2 mL.

_____ 7. A patient with latent tuberculosis infection has a negative reaction to a TB test.

_____ 8. A tuberculin skin test result should be read 15 to 20 minutes after administration.

_____ 9. The administration of fluids, medications, or nutrients through the IV route is known as an infusion.

_____ 10. The administration of blood through the IV route is known as an IV push.

Chapter **11** **Administration of Medication and Intravenous Therapy**

A. Definitions

Directions: Match each key term with its definition.

_____ 1. Adverse reaction

_____ 2. Allergen

_____ 3. Allergy

_____ 4. Ampule

_____ 5. Anaphylactic reaction

_____ 6. Chemotherapy

_____ 7. Controlled drug

_____ 8. Dose

_____ 9. Drug

_____ 10. Gauge

_____ 11. Induration

_____ 12. Infusion

_____ 13. Inhalation administration

_____ 14. Intradermal injection

_____ 15. Intramuscular injection

_____ 16. Intravenous therapy

_____ 17. Oral administration

_____ 18. Parenteral

_____ 19. Pharmacology

_____ 20. Prescription

_____ 21. Subcutaneous injection

_____ 22. Sublingual administration

_____ 23. Topical administration

_____ 24. Transfusion

_____ 25. Vial

_____ 26. Wheal

A. Application of a drug to a particular spot, usually for a local action
B. Introduction of medication into the dermal layer of the skin
C. A small, sealed glass container that holds a single dose of medication
D. An order from a licensed provider authorizing the dispensing of a drug by a pharmacist.
E. An unintended and undesirable effect produced by a drug
F. An abnormal hypersensitivity of the body to substances that are ordinarily harmless
G. The administration of a liquid agent directly into a patient's vein, where it is distributed throughout the body by way of the circulatory system
H. A tense, pale raised area of the skin
I. Introduction of medication beneath the skin, into the subcutaneous or fatty layer of the body
J. An abnormally raised hardened area of the skin with clearly defined margins
K. A closed glass container with a rubber stopper that holds medication
L. The administration of medication by way of air or other vapor being drawn into the lungs
M. A serious allergic reaction that requires immediate treatment
N. Administration of medication by mouth
O. A drug that has restrictions placed on it by the federal government because of its potential for abuse
P. Introduction of medication into the muscular layer of the body
Q. Administration of medication by placing it under the tongue
R. The quantity of a drug to be administered at one time
S. A substance that is capable of causing an allergic reaction
T. A chemical used for the treatment, prevention, or diagnosis of disease
U. The diameter of the lumen of a needle used to administer medication
V. Administration of medication by injection
W. The study of drugs
X. The use of chemicals to treat disease; most often refers to the treatment of cancer using antineoplastic medications
Y. The administration of fluids, medications, or nutrients into a vein
Z. The administration of whole blood or blood products through the intravenous route

B. Word Parts

Directions: Indicate the meaning of each word part in the space provided. List as many medical terms as possible that incorporate the word part in the space provided.

Word Part	Meaning of Word Part	Medical Terms That Incorporate Word Part
1. chem/o		
2. -therapy		
3. intra-		
4. derm/o		
5. muscul/o		
6. -ar		
7. ven/o		
8. -ous		
9. pharmac/o		
10. sub-		
11. cutane/o		
12. lingu/o		
13. trans-		

EVALUATION OF LEARNING

Directions: Fill in each blank with the correct answer.

Administration of Medication

1. What is the difference between administering, prescribing, and dispensing medication at the medical office?

Administering: _____

Prescribing: _____

Dispensing: _____

2. What is the brand name of a drug?

_____

_____

3. What is a liniment?

_____

_____

4. What is a spray?

_____

_____

5. What is a syrup?

_____

_____

6. What is a tablet?

_____

7. What is the purpose of scoring a tablet?

_____

8. List two drugs that come in the form of chewable tablets.

_____

9. List two reasons for enterically coating a tablet.

_____

_____

10. What is a capsule?

_____

11. Why must a suppository have a cylindrical or conical shape?

_____

12. What is a transdermal patch?

_____

13. Why is the metric system used most often to administer medication?

_____

14. Define the term volume.

_____

15. Describe the use of the household system of measurement for administering medication.

_____

16. When is conversion required?

_____

_____

17. What is a controlled drug?

_____

18. In what forms can a prescription be authorized?

_____

_____

19. What requirements must be followed when issuing a prescription for a schedule II drug?

_____

_____

_____

20. List five brand names of schedule II analgesics.

_____

_____

21. What requirements must be followed when issuing a prescription for a schedule III drug?

_____

_____

22. What is a schedule IV drug?

_____

_____

23. List two brand names of schedule IV analgesics.

_____

24. List three brand names of schedule IV antianxiety agents.

_____

25. What is included in each of the following parts of a prescription?
    a. Superscription: _____
    b. Inscription: _____
    c. Subscription: _____
    d. Signatura: _____

26. Why is it important for the patient's age to be indicated on a prescription?

_____

_____

27. What functions can be performed by an EHR prescription program?

_____

_____

_____

28. What types of medications should be documented on a medication record form?

_____

29. List and describe factors that affect the action of drugs in the body.

_____

_____

_____

_____

30. Why is it so important to ask the patient what medications he or she is taking and document this information in the medical record?

_____

_____

31. What are the symptoms and treatment of an anaphylactic reaction?

Symptoms:

_____

Treatment: _____

32. Why is it important to administer the proper dose of a drug?

_____

_____

33. Where does the absorption of oral medication take place in the body?

_____

_____

34. What are the advantages and disadvantages of using the parenteral route of medication administration?

_____

_____

_____

35. How do safety-engineered syringes reduce the risk of a needlestick injury?

_____

36. What is the purpose of using a filter needle when withdrawing medication from an ampule?

_____

37. Why do some medications require reconstitution?

_____

38. What sites are used most frequently to administer a subcutaneous injection?

_____

_____

39. What type of tissue should not be used as a site for a subcutaneous injection?

_____

_____

40. What is the maximum amount of medication that can be administered through the subcutaneous route?

_____

41. List three medications commonly administered through a subcutaneous injection.

_____

_____

42. Why is medication absorbed faster through the intramuscular route than through the subcutaneous route?

_____

_____

43. Why is irritating medication often administered through the intramuscular route?

_____

_____

44. What needle length is typically used to administer an intramuscular injection to the following individuals? Explain why the needle varies in length depending on the size of the individual.

   a. Average-sized adult: _____

   b. Thin adult or child: _____

   c. Obese adult: _____

45. List the four intramuscular (IM) injection sites, and explain why these sites must be used to administer an IM injection.

_____

_____

_____

46. What types of medications are given using the Z-track technique?

_____

_____

47. What sites are used most frequently to administer an intradermal injection?

_____

48. What is the most frequent use of an intradermal injection?

_____

49. What are the symptoms of active pulmonary tuberculosis?

_____

_____

Chapter **11** **Administration of Medication and Intravenous Therapy**

50. What is latent tuberculosis infection?

_____

_____

51. What are examples of categories of individuals who should have a tuberculin test?

_____

_____

_____

52. Why might a person who was recently infected with tuberculosis have a negative tuberculin skin test result?

_____

_____

53. What is induration, and what causes it?

_____

_____

54. What procedures are performed if a patient has a positive reaction to a tuberculin skin test?

_____

_____

55. Who should have a two-step tuberculin skin test?

_____

_____

56. What does it mean if the first test of a two-step tuberculin skin test is negative and the second test is positive? What does it mean if both tests are negative?

_____

_____

_____

57. What are the advantages of the IGRA tests for tuberculosis?

_____

_____

_____

_____

58. How can allergens enter the body?

_____

_____

59. What are 10 examples of common allergens?

_____

_____

_____

_____

60. What are the different forms in which allergies appear in individuals?

_____

_____

61. What is the general treatment for allergies?

_____

62. Why must a patient discontinue the use of an antihistamine for 3 days before skin testing?

_____

_____

63. What is the purpose of patch testing?

_____

_____

64. What is the purpose of skin-prick testing?

_____

_____

65. How long does it take for a reaction to occur with a skin-prick test?

_____

66. Explain what is meant by each of the following intradermal skin test reactions.

a. ± 1 _____

b. + 2 _____

c. + 3 _____

d. + 4 _____

67. How does intradermal skin testing compare to skin-prick testing?

_____

68. What are the advantages of in vitro blood testing over direct skin testing?

_____

_____

_____

465

Intravenous Therapy

1. What is intravenous therapy?

   _____

2. Which veins are most often used for IV therapy?

   _____

3. What types of liquid agents are administered through IV therapy?

   _____

4. What is the difference between an infusion and a transfusion?

   _____

   _____

5. List examples of outpatient ambulatory sites in which IV therapy may be administered.

   _____

   _____

6. List five reasons for administering IV therapy in an outpatient setting.

   _____

   _____

   _____

7. What are the advantages of outpatient IV therapy?

   _____

   _____

8. What requirements must be met before an entry-level medical assistant can perform IV therapy at a medical office?

   _____

   _____

9. What must be determined by the provider before prescribing outpatient IV therapy?

   _____

   _____

10. What instructions should the MA relay to a patient scheduled for outpatient IV therapy?

    _____

    _____

CRITICAL THINKING ACTIVITIES

A. Drug Package Insert

1A. Using Figure 11.1 in your textbook as a reference, indicate under which heading you would look to find the following information in a drug package insert.

1. Conditions the drug is approved by the FDA to treat

   _____

2. Information to relay to the patient to ensure safe and effective use of the drug

   _____

3. Route of administration

   _____

4. Symptoms associated with an overdose of the drug

   _____

5. Diseased states or situations that require special consideration when the drug is being taken

   _____

6. Generic name of the drug

   _____

7. How the drug functions in the body to produce its therapeutic effect

   _____

8. Situations in which the drug should not be used

   _____

9. Recommended adult dosage and duration of treatment

   _____

10. How to pronounce the brand name of the drug

    _____

11. Handling and storage conditions

    _____

12. Serious adverse reactions that may occur with the drug

    _____

13. The dosage forms in which the drug is available

    _____

14. Unintended and undesirable effects that may occur with the use of the drug

    _____

15. Modification of dosage needed for children

    _____

16. Laboratory tests that may be affected when taking the drug

    _____

Chapter **11** **Administration of Medication and Intravenous Therapy**

17. Interactions of the drug that may occur with other drugs

_____

2A. Obtain a package insert for a prescription drug, and answer the following questions:

1. What is the brand name of the drug?

_____

2. What is the generic name of the drug?

_____

3. What is the drug category of this drug?

_____

4. What are the dosage forms for this drug?

_____

5. What is the route of administration of this drug?

_____

6. What are the indications and usage for this drug?

_____

_____

_____

7. What are the contraindications for this drug?

_____

_____

_____

8. List the warnings for this drug.

_____

_____

_____

9. What are the general precautions for this drug?

_____

_____

_____

10. What information should be relayed to patients regarding this drug?

_____

_____

_____

11. What laboratory tests may be affected when taking this drug?

   _____

12. What are the adverse reactions for this drug?

   _____

   _____

   _____

13. What are the symptoms associated with an overdose of this drug?

   _____

14. What is the dosage and administration for this medication?

   _____

   _____

15. How should this drug be stored?

   _____

   _____

B. Drug Classifications

Inspect the package labels of 10 drugs (or use other means) to assess the classification of each drug based on preparation and action. List the name of each drug along with its appropriate category in the spaces provided. Compare results. Example: drug: Tylenol elixir; classification based on preparation: elixir; classification based on action: analgesic, antipyretic.

		Classification Based On	
	Drug	Preparation	Action
1.	_____	_____	_____
2.	_____	_____	_____
3.	_____	_____	_____
4.	_____	_____	_____
5.	_____	_____	_____
6.	_____	_____	_____
7.	_____	_____	_____
8.	_____	_____	_____
9.	_____	_____	_____
10.	_____	_____	_____

C. Medication Record

Complete the following medication record form using yourself as the patient. Make sure to include all prescription medications and OTC medications, including vitamin supplements and herbal products. Use Figure 11.5 in your textbook as a guide in completing this form.

							MEDICATION RECORD				

Patient _____

Birth date _____

ALLERGY

DATE	MEDICATION AND DOSAGE	FREQUENCY	RX	OTC	REFILLS			STOP

D. Seven Rights of Medication Administration

You are the office manager at a large clinic. Six new MAs were just hired. Your provider asks you to design an illustrated poster portraying the seven rights of medication administration to remind the new employees of the importance of following these guidelines. Use the diagram below to design your poster.

Follow the Seven Rights	
Right Drug	Right Dose
Right Time	Right Patient
Right Route	Right Technique
Right Documentation	

Chapter **11** **Administration of Medication and Intravenous Therapy**

E. Liquid Measurement

Obtain a medicine cup that is graduated into the metric (milliliters), apothecary (drams and ounces), and household (teaspoons and tablespoons) systems. Complete the following:

1. What is its capacity?

_____ ounces

_____ milliliters

_____ tablespoons

_____ drams

2. Practice pouring oral liquid medication by pouring the following amounts of water into the medicine cup. Place a check mark by each amount after it has been properly poured.

20 mL _____

4 drams _____

1 ounce _____

10 mL _____

$^1/_2$ ounce _____

1 tablespoon _____

2 drams _____

F. Parts of a Needle and Syringe

Obtain a needle and syringe. Locate the following parts of each and explain their function.

Needle   **Function**

1. Hub _____

2. Shaft _____

3. Lumen _____

4. Point _____

5. Bevel _____

6. What is the gauge of the needle? _____

7. What is the length of the needle? _____

Syringe   **Function**

8. Barrel _____

9. Flange _____

10. Plunger _____

11. What is the capacity of the syringe? _____

472

G. Hypodermic Syringe Calibrations

1. Obtain a 3-mL syringe that is divided into tenths of a milliliter. Locate the following calibrations on the syringe. Place a check mark in the blank next to each calibration after it has been correctly located.

Calibration (mL)

0.5 mL _____

1.0 mL _____

1.2 mL _____

2.5 mL _____

2.7 mL _____

2. Locate each calibration (listed in the previous question) on the illustration of the hypodermic syringe by placing an arrow on the correct calibration line and labeling it with the calibration.

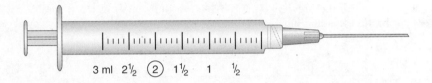

H. Insulin Syringe Calibrations

1. Obtain a U-100 insulin syringe. Locate the following calibrations (units) on the syringe, and place a check mark in the blank next to each calibration after it has been correctly located.

Calibration (units)

10 _____

16 _____

20 _____

44 _____

60 _____

68 _____

70 _____

86 _____

90 _____

100 _____

2. Locate each calibration (listed in the previous question) on the illustration of the insulin syringe by placing an arrow on the correct calibration line and labeling it with the calibration.

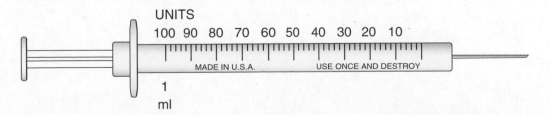

Chapter **11 Administration of Medication and Intravenous Therapy**

I. Tuberculin Syringe Calibrations

1. Obtain a 1-mL tuberculin syringe that is divided into tenths and hundredths of a milliliter. Locate the following calibrations on the syringe. Place a check mark in the blank next to each calibration after it has been correctly located.

Calibration (mL)

0.05 mL _____

0.10 mL _____

0.15 mL _____

0.34 mL _____

0.52 mL _____

0.75 mL _____

0.92 mL _____

2. Locate each calibration (listed in the previous question) on the illustration of the tuberculin syringe by placing an arrow on the correct calibration line and labeling it with the calibration.

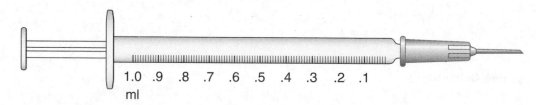

J. Syringe and Needle Labels

Refer to Figure 11.8 in your textbook and indicate the following information for each syringe and needle starting at the top of the illustration: the syringe capacity and the gauge and length of the needle.

a. _____

b. _____

c. _____

d. _____

K. Angle of Insertion for Injections

In the diagram that follows, draw three lines indicating the angle of insertion into the correct body tissue for an intradermal, a subcutaneous, and an intramuscular injection. Label the lines.

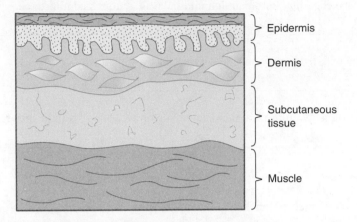

L. Preparing and Administering Parenteral Medication

For each of the following situations involving the preparation and administration of medication, write **C** if the technique is correct and **I** if it is incorrect. If the technique is correct, state the principle underlying the technique. If the technique is incorrect, explain what might happen if it were performed.

_____ 1. The expiration date of the medication is checked before administering the medication.

_____

_____ 2. The MA is unfamiliar with the drug to be administered, so he or she looks it up in a drug reference.

_____

_____ 3. The MA compares the medication label with the provider's instructions three times: as it is taken from the shelf, before preparing the medication, and after preparing the medication.

_____

_____ 4. The rubber stopper of the multidose vial is cleansed with an antiseptic wipe before withdrawing the medication.

_____

_____ 5. Air is not injected into the multidose vial before withdrawing the medication.

_____

_____ 6. A filter needle is used to withdraw medication from an ampule.

_____

_____ 7. Air bubbles are present in the medication in the syringe that has been withdrawn from an ampule.

_____

_____ 8. The injection sites are not rotated when repeated injections are given.

_____

_____ 9. The antiseptic is not allowed to dry before administering an injection.

_____

_____10. The skin is stretched taut before an intramuscular injection is administered.

_____

_____11. The needle is inserted slowly and steadily for an IM injection.

_____

_____12. An IM injection is given in the deltoid site to a patient who has a tight sleeve.

_____

_____ 13. An IM injection is given into the ventrogluteal site when the site is not fully exposed.

_____ 14. The medication is injected quickly for an IM injection.

_____

_____ 15. The needle is withdrawn quickly and at the same angle as for insertion.

_____

_____ 16. The intradermal needle is inserted with the bevel facing downward.

_____

_____ 17. The MA does not aspirate when giving an intradermal injection.

_____

_____ 18. Pressure is applied to the injection site after the administration of a tuberculin skin test.

_____

M. Measuring Mantoux Test Reactions

Measure the diameter of the following circles, which represent induration from a Mantoux tuberculin skin test. A millimeter ruler is provided below. Cut it out and use it to measure the tuberculin reactions. Document results in the chart provided.

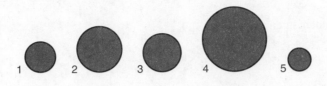

1   2   3   4   5

TB Skin Testing
(mm ruler)
0   10   20

CHART	
Date	

N. Interpreting Mantoux Skin Test Reactions

Tuberculin skin test reactions are listed for various individuals. Using Box 11.3 in your textbook as a reference, determine if the individual's test results are positive or negative, and indicate your answer in the space provided.

_____ a. 2 mm of induration; an individual who is caring for a parent with active TB

_____ b. 7 mm of induration; a student attending college

_____ c. 12 mm of induration; an individual who is 12% below ideal body weight

_____ d. 8 mm of induration; an HIV-infected individual

_____ e. Erythema that is 6 mm wide (no induration); an individual with rheumatoid arthritis on Enbrel

_____ f. 16 mm of induration; a dietitian working in a nursing home

_____ g. 12 mm of induration; an individual who recently traveled to Canada

_____ h. 5 mm of induration; a child living with a parent who has active TB

_____ i. 6 mm of induration; an individual with diabetes mellitus

_____ j. 11 mm of induration; a recent immigrant from Africa

_____ k. 9 mm of induration; an individual working in a home and garden center

O. Anaphylactic Reaction

Create a profile of an individual who is experiencing an anaphylactic reaction following these guidelines:

1. Using the next page and colored pencils, crayons, or markers, draw a figure of an individual exhibiting the symptoms of an anaphylactic reaction. Be as creative as possible.

2. Do not use any text on your drawing other than to label items you have drawn in your picture. (A picture is worth a thousand words!)

3. Try to include as many of the symptoms of an anaphylactic reaction as possible.

4. In the classroom, find a partner, and trade drawings. Identify the symptoms in your partner's drawing. With your partner, discuss what causes an anaphylactic reaction and how to prevent it. Also discuss the method of treatment for an anaphylactic reaction.

ANAPHYLACTIC REACTION

P. Researching Drugs

Obtain a drug reference book, and look up the following information for each of the drugs listed on the Pharmacology Drug Sheets: generic name and drug classification, indications, and patient teaching. Document this information in the appropriate space on the Pharmacology Drug Sheets.

Pharmacology Drug Sheet

Name: _____

Generic Name and Drug Classification	Indications	Patient Teaching
Abilify		
Accupril		
Adderall		
Adrenalin		

Pharmacology Drug Sheet

Name: _____

Generic Name and Drug Classification	Indications	Patient Teaching
Advair Diskus		
Ambien		
Amoxil		
Aricept		

Chapter **11** **Administration of Medication and Intravenous Therapy**

Pharmacology Drug Sheet

Generic Name and Drug Classification	Indications	Patient Teaching
Ativan		
Bentyl		
Cardizem		
Catapres		

Pharmacology Drug Sheet

Name: _____

Generic Name and Drug Classification	Indications	Patient Teaching
Celebrex		
Cipro		
Coumadin		
Cozaar		

Pharmacology Drug Sheet

Name: _____

Generic Name and Drug Classification	Indications	Patient Teaching
Crestor		
Cymbalta		
Depo-Medrol		
Depo-Provera		

Pharmacology Drug Sheet

Name: _____

Generic Name and Drug Classification	Indications	Patient Teaching
Detrol		
Diflucan		
Dilantin		
Flagyl		

Pharmacology Drug Sheet

Name: _____

Generic Name and Drug Classification	Indications	Patient Teaching
Flexeril		
Flonase		
Fosamax		
Glucotrol XL		

Pharmacology Drug Sheet

Name: _____

Generic Name and Drug Classification	Indications	Patient Teaching
Humulin		
Imitrex		
InFeD		
Keflex		

Pharmacology Drug Sheet

Name: _____

Generic Name and Drug Classification	Indications	Patient Teaching
Lamisil		
Lanoxin		
Lasix		
Lipitor		

Pharmacology Drug Sheet

Name: _____

Generic Name and Drug Classification	Indications	Patient Teaching
Loestrin Fe		
Lomotil		
Lyrica		
Macrobid		

489

Name: _____

Generic Name and Drug Classification	Indications	Patient Teaching
Mexate		
Nitro-Bid		
Norvasc		
Percocet		

Pharmacology Drug Sheet

Name: _____

Generic Name and Drug Classification	Indications	Patient Teaching
Phenergan		
Plavix		
Premarin		
Prevacid		

Pharmacology Drug Sheet

Name: _____

Generic Name and Drug Classification	Indications	Patient Teaching
Prinivil		
Prozac		
Requip		
Rocephin		

492

Chapter **11 Administration of Medication and Intravenous Therapy**

Pharmacology Drug Sheet

Name: _____

Generic Name and Drug Classification	Indications	Patient Teaching
Singulair		
Synthroid		
Tessalon		
Toprol XL		

Pharmacology Drug Sheet

Name: _____

Generic Name and Drug Classification	Indications	Patient Teaching
Valium		
Valtrex		
Viagra		
Vicodin		

Pharmacology Drug Sheet

Name: _____

Generic Name and Drug Classification	Indications	Patient Teaching
Xanax		
Zithromax		
Zybanww		
Zyloprim		
Zyrtec		

Chapter **11** **Administration of Medication and Intravenous Therapy**

Q. Crossword Puzzle: Administration of Medication

Directions: Complete the crossword puzzle using the clues provided.

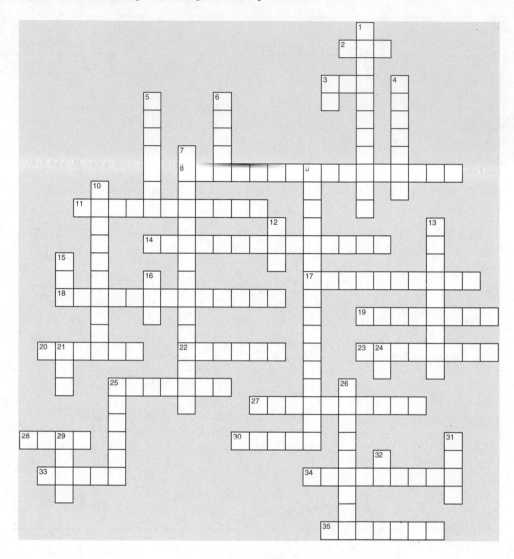

Across

2 Tuberculin is made of this
3 As needed
8 Runny and inflamed nose
11 Conditions a drug is approved to treat
14 Calibrated in units
17 Where an enteric-coated drug dissolves
18 Drug to d/c before allergy testing
19 Causes house dust allergy
20 Most aggressive Hymenoptera
22 Sym: wheezing and dyspnea
23 Allergy to molds and pollen
25 Discovered penicillin
27 This drug may cause an allergic reaction
28 Blood test for allergies
30 Needle opening
33 Ranges between 18 and 27
34 Hives
35 No need to aspirate for this

Down

1 Used to treat anaphylactic reaction
3 By mouth
4 Max of 1 mL into this IM site
5 Name assigned by USAN Council
6 Slant of the needle
7 Best IM site for infants
9 Do not use this drug!
10 Present with a + Mantoux
12 Aspirin
13 Rx requirement for controlled drug
15 Approves drugs
16 Three times per day
21 Available w/o a Rx
24 Before meals
25 Prevents syringe from rolling
26 Medication label info
29 Immediately!
31 Metric weight unit
32 1 mL = 1 _____

PRACTICE FOR COMPETENCY

Prerequisite. Complete the Drug Dosage Calculation: Supplemental Education for Chapter 11 (pp. pp. 505-528 in this manual).

Procedure 11-1: Oral Medication

Administer oral solid and liquid medication, and document the procedure in the chart provided.

Procedure 11-2: Preparing the Injection

Prepare an injection from an ampule and a vial.

Procedure 11-3: Reconstituting Powdered Drugs

Reconstitute a powdered drug for parenteral administration.

Procedure 11-4: Subcutaneous Injection

Administer an allergy injection, and document the procedure in the allergy injection form provided.

CHART	
Date	

ALLERGY INJECTION (IMMUNOTHERAPY) RECORD

Name_____

Date of Birth_____

ADMINISTRATION GUIDELINES:

Allergy injections are administered weekly. The allergy extract should be increased by 0.05 mL per week until symptomatic improvement is achieved or until a maximum dosage of 0.5 mL is reached.

The patient should remain in the office for 20 minutes following the injection, and the reaction should be noted. If no reaction occurs, the abbreviation NR should be recorded. If a reaction occurs, it should be recorded in mm.

Do not administer the allergy injection in the following situations:
   a. The patient is ill with a temperature that is greater than 101° F
   b. The patient is having an acute asthma attack
   c. The patient is experiencing shortness of breath

Vial Number: **Vial Expiration Date:** _____
   _____1
   _____2
   _____3
   _____4

DATE	DOSAGE (mL)	Left Arm	Right Arm	REACTION (mm)	ADMINISTERED BY:

Procedure 11-A: Intramuscular Injection Sites

Locate the following intramuscular injection sites: deltoid, vastus lateralis, ventrogluteal, and dorsogluteal.

Procedure 11-5: Intramuscular Injection

Administer an intramuscular injection, and document the procedure in the chart provided.

Procedure 11-6: Z-Track Method

Administer an intramuscular injection using the Z-track method. Document the procedure in the chart provided.

Procedure 11-7: Intradermal Injection

Administer an intradermal injection, and document the procedure in the chart provided. Read and interpret the test results, and document them in the chart. Complete three TB test record cards located on the following page.

CHART	
Date	

499

Notes

CHART	
Date	

TUBERCULOSIS TEST RECORD

Name	Date Admin: / /
	Date Read: / /
MANTOUX TEST	RESULT
	____ mm

Logan Family Practice
401 St. George St.
St. Augustine, FL 32084
(904) 555-3933

Performed by _____

TUBERCULOSIS TEST RECORD

Name	Date Admin: / /
	Date Read: / /
MANTOUX TEST	RESULT
	____ mm

Logan Family Practice
401 St. George St.
St. Augustine, FL 32084
(904) 555-3933

Performed by _____

TUBERCULOSIS TEST RECORD

Name	Date Admin: / /
	Date Read: / /
MANTOUX TEST	RESULT
	____ mm

Logan Family Practice
401 St. George St.
St. Augustine, FL 32084
(904) 555-3933

Performed by _____

Chapter **11** **Administration of Medication and Intravenous Therapy**

Procedure 11-1: Administering Oral Medication

Name: _____   Date: _____

Evaluated by: _____   Score: _____

Performance Objective

Outcome:	Administer oral solid and liquid medication.
Conditions:	Given the following: appropriate medication, medication order, medicine cup, and a medication tray.
Standards:	Time: 5 minutes. Student completed procedure in _____ minutes.
	Accuracy: Satisfactory score on the Performance Evaluation Checklist.

Performance Evaluation Checklist

Trial 1	Trial 2	Point Value	Performance Standards
		•	Sanitized hands.
		•	Assembled the equipment.
		•	Worked in a quiet, well-lit atmosphere.
		•	Selected the correct medication from the shelf.
		•	Compared the medication with the provider's instructions.
		•	Checked the drug label.
		•	Checked the expiration date.
		•	Calculated the correct dose to be given, if needed.
		•	Removed the bottle cap.
		•	Checked the drug label and poured the medication.
		Solid medication	
		★	Poured the correct number of capsules or tablets into the bottle cap.
		▷	Explained why the medication is poured into the bottle cap.
		•	Transferred the medication to a medicine cup.
		Liquid medication	
		•	Placed lid of bottle on a flat surface with the open end facing up.
		•	Palmed the surface of the drug label.
		▷	Explained why the medication label should be palmed.
		•	Placed thumbnail at the proper calibration on the medicine cup.
		•	Held the medicine cup at eye level.
		★	Poured the correct amount of medication and read the dose at the lowest level of the meniscus.

Chapter **11** **Administration of Medication and Intravenous Therapy**

Trial 1	Trial 2	Point Value	Performance Standards
		•	Replaced the bottle cap.
		•	Checked the drug label and returned the medication to its storage location.
		•	Greeted the patient and introduced yourself.
		•	Identified the patient by full name and date of birth and explained the procedure.
		•	Handed the medicine cup to the patient along with a glass of water.
		▷	Stated one instance when water should not be offered.
		•	Remained with the patient until the medication was swallowed.
		•	Sanitized hands.
		•	Documented the procedure correctly.
		■	Demonstrated critical thinking skills.
		■	Demonstrated empathy for patients' concerns.
		★	Completed the procedure within 10 minutes.
			Totals

CHART

Date	

Evaluation of Student Performance

EVALUATION CRITERIA			COMMENTS
Symbol	**Category**	**Point Value**	
★	Critical Step	16 points	
•	Essential Step	6 points	
■	Affective Competency	6 points	
▷	Theory Question	2 points	

Score calculation: 100 points

−   points missed

___ Score

Satisfactory score: 85 or above

CAAHEP Competencies Achieved

Psychomotor (Skills)
- ☑ I. 4. Verify the rules of medication administration: (a) right patient (b) right medication (c) right dose (d) right route (e) right time (f) right documentation.
- ☑ I. 6. Administer oral medications.
- ☑ II. 1. Calculate proper dosages of medication for administration.
- ☑ X. 3. Document patient care accurately in the medical record.
- ☑ II. 4. Apply mathematical computations to solve equations.
- ☑ II. 5. Convert among measurement systems.

Affective (Behavior)
- ☑ A. 1. Demonstrate critical thinking skills.
- ☑ A. 3. Demonstrate empathy for patient's concerns.

ABHES Competencies Achieved

- ☑ 4. a. Follow documentation guidelines.
- ☑ 6. b. Calculate proper dosages for medication administration.
- ☑ 8. f. Prepare and administer oral and parenteral medications and monitor intravenous (IV) infusions.

Notes

Procedure 11-2: Preparing an Injection

Name: _____   Date: _____

Evaluated by: _____   Score: _____

Performance Objective

Outcome:	Prepare an injection from an ampule and a vial.
Conditions:	Given the following: medication ordered by the provider, mediation order, needle and syringe, antiseptic wipe, and medication tray.
Standards:	Time: 10 minutes. Student completed procedure in _____ minutes.
	Accuracy: Satisfactory score on the Performance Evaluation Checklist.

Performance Evaluation Checklist

Trial 1	Trial 2	Point Value	Performance Standards
		•	Sanitized hands.
		•	Assembled the equipment.
		•	Worked in a quiet, well-lit atmosphere.
		★	Selected the proper medication from its storage location.
		•	Compared the medication with the provider's instructions.
		•	Checked the expiration date.
		★	Calculated the correct dose to be given, if needed.
		•	Opened syringe and needle packages.
		•	Assembled the needle and syringe, if necessary.
		•	Made sure that the needle is attached firmly to the syringe and moved the plunger back and forth.
		•	Checked the drug label a second time.
		•	If required, mixed the medication.
			Withdrew medication from a vial
		•	Removed the metal or plastic cap, if vial is new.
		•	Cleansed the rubber stopper of the vial with an antiseptic wipe and allowed it to dry.
		•	Placed the vial in an upright position on a flat surface.
		•	Removed the needle guard.
		•	Drew air into the syringe equal to the amount of medication to be withdrawn.
		•	Inserted the needle through the rubber stopper until it reached the empty space between the stopper and the fluid level.
		•	Pushed down on the plunger to inject air into the vial.

Trial 1	Trial 2	Point Value	Performance Standards
		•	Kept the needle above the fluid level.
		▷	Explained why air must be injected into the vial.
		•	Inverted the vial while holding onto the syringe and plunger.
		★	Held the syringe at eye level and withdrew the proper amount of medication.
		•	Kept the needle opening below the fluid level.
		▷	Explained why the needle opening must be kept below the fluid level.
		•	Removed any air bubbles in the syringe by tapping the barrel with the fingertips.
		▷	Explained why air bubbles should be removed from the syringe.
		•	Removed any air remaining at the top of the syringe by pushing the plunger forward.
		•	Held the syringe at eye level and checked to make sure the proper amount of medication had been drawn up.
		•	Removed the needle from the rubber stopper and replaced the needle guard.
		•	If required, removed the needle and replaced it with a new needle.
		•	Checked the drug label a third time and returned the medication to its storage location.
			Withdrew medication from an ampule
		•	Removed the regular needle from the syringe and attached a filter needle.
		▷	Stated the purpose of a filter needle.
		•	Cleansed the neck of the vial with an antiseptic wipe.
		•	Tapped the stem of the ampule lightly to remove any medication in the neck of the ampule.
		•	Checked the medication label a second time.
		•	Placed a piece of gauze around the neck of the ampule.
		•	Broke off the stem by snapping it quickly and firmly away from the body.
		•	Discarded the stem and gauze in a biohazard sharps container.
		•	Placed the ampule on a flat surface.
		•	Removed the needle guard.
		•	Inserted the needle opening below the fluid level.
		★	Withdrew the proper amount of medication.
		•	Kept the needle opening below the fluid level.
		▷	Explained why the needle opening must be kept below the fluid level.
		•	Held the syringe at eye level and checked to make sure the proper amount of medication had been drawn up.
		•	Removed the needle from the ampule and replaced the needle guard.
		•	Checked the drug label for a third time.

Trial 1	Trial 2	Point Value	Performance Standards
		•	Discarded the ampule in a biohazard sharps container.
		•	Removed the filter needle and reapplied the regular needle (and guard) to the syringe.
		•	Tapped the syringe to remove air bubbles.
		•	Removed the needle guard and expelled air remaining at the top of the syringe.
		•	Replaced the needle guard.
		■	Demonstrated critical thinking skills.
		★	Completed the procedure within 10 minutes.
			Totals

Evaluation of Student Performance

EVALUATION CRITERIA			COMMENTS
Symbol	**Category**	**Point Value**	
★	Critical Step	16 points	
•	Essential Step	6 points	
■	Affective Competency	6 points	
▷	Theory Question	2 points	

Score calculation: 100 points

    −   points missed

          Score

Satisfactory score: 85 or above

CAAHEP Competencies Achieved

Psychomotor (Skills)
☑   I. 4. Verify the rules of medication administration: (a) right patient (b) right medication (c) right dose (d) right route (e) right time (f) right documentation.
☑   II. 1. Calculate proper dosages of medication for administration.
☑   II. 4. Apply mathematical computations to solve equations.
☑   II. 5. Convert among measurement systems.

Affective (Behavior)
☑   A. 1. Demonstrate critical thinking skills.

ABHES Competencies Achieved

☑   6. b. Calculated proper dosages for medication administration.
☑   8. f. Prepare and administer oral and parenteral medications and monitor the patient.

         Chapter **11** **Administration of Medication and Intravenous Therapy**

Notes

Procedure 11-3: Reconstituting Powdered Drugs

Name: _____   Date: _____

Evaluated by: _____   Score: _____

Performance Objective

Outcome:	Reconstitute a powdered drug for parenteral administration.
Conditions:	Given the following: vial containing the powdered drug, reconstituting liquid, mediation order, needle and syringe, antiseptic wipe, and mediation tray.
Standards:	Time: 5 minutes.　　　Student completed procedure in _____ minutes.
	Accuracy: Satisfactory score on the Performance Evaluation Checklist.

Performance Evaluation Checklist

Trial 1	Trial 2	Point Value	Performance Standards
		•	Sanitized hands.
		•	Assembled the equipment.
		★	Selected the proper medication from its storage location.
		•	Checked the drug label.
		•	Compared the medication with the provider's instructions.
		•	Checked the expiration date.
		★	Calculated the correct dose to be given, if needed.
		•	Opened the syringe and needle packages.
		•	Assembled the needle and syringe, if necessary.
		•	Made sure that the needle is attached firmly to the syringe and moved the plunger back and forth.
		•	Checked the drug label a second time.
		•	Withdrew an amount of air equal to the amount of liquid to be injected into the vial from the vial containing the powdered drug.
		•	Injected the air into the vial of diluent.
		★	Inverted the diluent vial and withdrew the proper amount of liquid into the syringe.
		•	Removed air bubbles from the syringe.
		•	Held the syringe at eye level and checked to make sure the proper amount of diluent had been drawn up.
		•	Removed the needle from the vial.
		•	Inserted the needle into the powdered drug vial.
		•	Injected the diluent into the vial.
		•	Removed the needle from the vial and discarded the syringe and needle in a biohazard sharps container.

　　　　　Chapter **11** **Administration of Medication and Intravenous Therapy**

Trial 1	Trial 2	Point Value	Performance Standards
☐	☐	•	Rolled the vial between the hands to mix it.
☐	☐	•	Labeled multiple-dose vials with the date of preparation and your initials.
☐	☐	•	Prepared the injection and administered the medication.
☐	☐	•	Stored multiple-dose vials as indicated in the manufacturer's instructions.
☐	☐	▷	Explained the importance of checking the date of preparation of a reconstituted multiple-dose vial before administering it.
☐	☐	■	Demonstrated critical thinking skills.
☐	☐	★	Completed the procedure within 5 minutes.
☐	☐		**Totals**

Evaluation of Student Performance

EVALUATION CRITERIA			COMMENTS
Symbol	**Category**	**Point Value**	
★	Critical Step	16 points	
•	Essential Step	6 points	
■	Affective Competency	6 points	
▷	Theory Question	2 points	

Score calculation: 100 points

−   points missed

_____

__ Score

Satisfactory score: 85 or above

CAAHEP Competencies Achieved

Psychomotor (Skills)
- ☑ I. 4. Verify the rules of medication administration: (a) right patient (b) right medication (c) right dose (d) right route (e) right time (f) right documentation.
- ☑ II. 1. Calculate proper dosages of medication for administration.
- ☑ II. 4. Apply mathematical computations to solve equations.
- ☑ II. 5. Convert among measurement systems.

Affective (Behavior)
- ☑ A. 1. Demonstrate critical thinking skills.

ABHES Competencies Achieved

- ☑ 6. b. Calculate proper dosages for medication administration.
- ☑ 8. f. Prepare and administer oral and parenteral medications and monitor the patient.

Procedure 11-4: Administering a Subcutaneous Injection

Name: _____   Date: _____

Evaluated by: _____   Score: _____

Performance Objective

Outcome:	Administer a subcutaneous injection.
Conditions:	Given the following: appropriate medication, medication order, needle and syringe, antiseptic wipe, 2 × 2 gauze pad, disposable gloves, and a biohazard sharps container.
Standards:	Time: 5 minutes. Student completed procedure in _____ minutes. Accuracy: Satisfactory score on the Performance Evaluation Checklist.

Performance Evaluation Checklist

Trial 1	Trial 2	Point Value	Performance Standards
		•	Sanitized hands.
		•	Prepared the injection.
		•	Greeted the patient and introduced yourself.
		•	Identified the patient and explained the procedure and purpose of the injection.
		•	Selected an appropriate subcutaneous injection site.
		▷	Stated the sites that can be used to administer a subcutaneous injection.
		•	Cleansed the injection site with an antiseptic wipe and allowed it to dry completely.
		▷	Explained why the site should be allowed to dry.
		•	Did not touch the site after cleansing it.
		•	Applied gloves.
		•	Removed the needle guard.
		•	Properly positioned the nondominant hand on the area surrounding the injection site.
		▷	Explained when the area should be grasped and when it should be held taut.
		•	Inserted needle to the hub at a 45-degree or 90-degree angle (depending on the length of the needle) with a quick, smooth motion.
		▷	Explained how needle length determines the angle of insertion for a subcutaneous injection.
		•	Removed the hand from the skin.
		▷	Explained why the hand should be removed from the skin.
		▷	Explained why aspiration of a subcutaneous injection is not necessary.
		•	Injected the medication slowly and steadily while holding the syringe steady.
		▷	Described what would happen if the medication were injected rapidly.

513

Trial 1	Trial 2	Point Value	Performance Standards
		•	Placed a gauze pad gently over the injection site and removed needle quickly at the same angle as insertion.
		▷	Explained why the needle should be removed quickly and at the angle of insertion.
		•	Applied gentle pressure to the injection site.
		▷	Stated why the site should not be vigorously massaged.
		•	Activated the safety feature on the syringe.
		•	Properly disposed of needle and syringe.
		•	Removed gloves and sanitized hands.
		•	Documented the procedure correctly.
		•	Remained with the patient to make sure there were no unusual reactions.
		▷	Stated the steps to follow, if the patient has been given an allergy injection.
		■	Demonstrated critical thinking skills.
		■	Reassured patients.
		■	Demonstrated empathy for patients' concerns.
		★	Completed the procedure within 5 minutes.
			Totals

CHART

Date	

Evaluation of Student Performance

EVALUATION CRITERIA			COMMENTS
Symbol	**Category**	**Point Value**	
★	Critical Step	16 points	
•	Essential Step	6 points	
■	Affective Competency	6 points	
▷	Theory Question	2 points	

Score calculation: 100 points

      −   points missed

          __Score

Satisfactory score: 85 or above

Chapter **11** **Administration of Medication and Intravenous Therapy**

CAAHEP Competencies Achieved

Psychomotor (Skills)
- ☑ I. 4. Verify the rules of medication administration: (a) right patient (b) right medication (c) right dose (d) right route (e) right time (f) right documentation.
- ☑ I. 5. Select proper sites for administering parenteral medication.
- ☑ I. 7. Administer parenteral (excluding IV) medications.
- ☑ III. 2. Select appropriate barrier/personal protective equipment.
- ☑ III. 10. Demonstrate proper disposal of biohazardous material: (a) sharps (b) regulated waste.
- ☑ V. 1. Respond to nonverbal communication.
- ☑ X. 3. Document patient care accurately in the medical record.

Affective (Behavior)
- ☑ A. 1. Demonstrate critical thinking skills.
- ☑ A. 2. Reassure patients.
- ☑ A. 3. Demonstrate empathy for patients' concerns.

ABHES Competencies Achieved

- ☑ 4. a. Follow documentation guidelines.
- ☑ 8. f. Prepare and administer oral and parenteral medications and monitor the patient.
- ☑ 9. c. Dispose of biohazardous materials.

Notes

Procedure 11-A: Locating Intramuscular Injection Sites

Name: _____   Date: _____

Evaluated by: _____.   Score: _____

Performance Objective

Outcome:	Locate intramuscular injection sites.
Conditions:	None required.
Standards:	Time: 5 minutes. Student completed procedure in _____ minutes.
	Accuracy: Satisfactory score on the Performance Evaluation Checklist.

Performance Evaluation Checklist

Trial 1	Trial 2	Point Value	Performance Standards
			DELTOID SITE
		•	Placed the patient in a sitting position.
		•	Pulled up the patient's sleeve or removed the sleeve from the arm.
		▷	Explained why a tight sleeve should be avoided.
		•	Ensured that the entire arm was exposed.
		•	Palpated the lower edge of the acromion process.
		•	Placed 4 fingers horizontally across the deltoid muscle with the top finger along the acromion process.
		•	Explained that the injection site is located 2 to 3 finger-widths below the acromion process (approximately 1–2 inches below the acromion process).
		▷	Identified the maximum amount of medication that can be administered into this site.
			VASTUS LATERALIS SITE
			Adult:
		•	Placed the patient in a supine or sitting position.
		•	Located the midanterior thigh (on the front of the leg).
		•	Located the midlateral thigh (on the side of the leg).
		•	Located the proximal boundary by coming down a hand's breadth from the greater trochanter.
		•	Located the distal boundary by coming up a hand's breadth from the knee.
		•	Stated that the injection is administered within the boundaries identified above.
			Infants and Children:
		•	Placed the infant or child in a supine position or asked the parent to hold the infant in a sitting position on his or her lap.
		•	Located the midanterior thigh (on the front of the leg).

517

Trial 1	Trial 2	Point Value	Performance Standards
		•	Located the midlateral thigh (on the side of the leg).
		•	Located the greater trochanter through palpation.
		•	Located the knee joint through palpation.
		•	Divided the area between the greater trochanter and knee joint into thirds and made a mental note of the middle third of the divided area.
		•	Stated that the injection is administered within the boundaries identified above.
		▷	Explained why this site is commonly used with children younger than 3 years of age.
			VENTROGLUTEAL SITE
		•	Placed the patient in a prone position or lying on one side.
		•	Located the greater trochanter through palpation.
		•	Located the anterior superior iliac spine and the iliac crest through palpation.
			For an injection being administered into the left side:
		•	Placed the palm of the right hand on the greater trochanter.
		•	Placed the index finger on the anterior superior iliac spine.
		•	Spread the middle finger posteriorly as far as possible away from the index finger to touch the iliac crest.
		•	Stated that the injection is administered into the triangle formed by the fingers.
			For an injection being administered into the right side:
		•	Placed the palm of the left hand on the greater trochanter.
		•	Placed the index finger on the anterior superior iliac spine.
		•	Spread the middle finger posteriorly as far as possible away from the index finger to touch the iliac crest.
		•	Stated that the injection is administered into the triangle formed by the fingers.
			DORSOGLUTEAL SITE
			Method 1:
		•	Asked the patient to lie on the abdomen with the toes pointed inward.
		•	Made sure the injection site was fully exposed.
		▷	Stated why the injection site should be fully exposed.
		•	Located the greater trochanter through palpation.
		•	Located the posterior superior iliac spine through palpation.
		•	Draw an imaginary line between these two points.
		•	Stated that the injection is administered above and outside this area.
			Method 2:
		•	Asked the patient to lie on the abdomen with the toes pointed inward.

Trial 1	Trial 2	Point Value	Performance Standards
		•	Made sure the injection area was fully exposed.
		•	Divided the buttocks into quadrants.
		•	Stated that the injection is administered into the upper outer quadrant approximately 2 to 3 inches below the iliac crest.
		▷	Explained why it is important to maintain proper boundary lines.
		■	Demonstrated critical thinking skills.
		★	Completed the procedure within 5 minutes.
			Totals

Evaluation of Student Performance

EVALUATION CRITERIA			COMMENTS
Symbol	**Category**	**Point Value**	
★	Critical Step	16 points	
•	Essential Step	6 points	
■	Affective Competency	6 points	
▷	Theory Question	2 points	

Score calculation:

100 points

−   points missed

_____

____ Score

Satisfactory score: 85 or above

CAAHEP Competencies Achieved

Psychomotor (Skills)
☑ I. 4. Verify the rules of medication administration: (a) right patient (b) right medication (c) right dose (d) right route (e) right time (f) right documentation.
☑ I. 5. Select proper sites for administering parenteral medication.

Affective (Behavior)
☑ A. 1. Demonstrate critical thinking skills.

ABHES Competencies Achieved

☑ 8. f. Prepare and administer oral and parenteral medications and monitor the patient.

Notes

Chapter **11** **Administration of Medication and Intravenous Therapy**

Procedure 11-5: Administering an Intramuscular Injection

Name: _____   Date: _____

Evaluated by: _____   Score: _____

Performance Objective

Outcome:	Administer an intramuscular injection.
Conditions:	Given the following: appropriate medication, medication order, needle and syringe, antiseptic wipe, 2 × 2 gauze pad, disposable gloves, and a biohazard sharps container.
Standards:	Time: 5 minutes. Student completed procedure in _____ minutes.
	Accuracy: Satisfactory score on the Performance Evaluation Checklist.

Performance Evaluation Checklist

Trial 1	Trial 2	Point Value	Performance Standards
		•	Sanitized hands.
		•	Prepared the injection.
		•	Greeted the patient and introduced yourself.
		•	Identified the patient and explained the procedure and purpose of the injection.
		★	Located the appropriate intramuscular injection site.
		▷	Stated what tissue layer of the body the medication will be injected into.
		•	Cleansed area with an antiseptic wipe and allowed it to dry completely.
		•	Did not touch the injection site after cleansing it.
		•	Applied gloves.
		•	Removed the needle guard.
		•	Stretched the skin taut over the injection site.
		▷	Explained why the skin should be stretched taut.
		•	Held the barrel of the syringe like a dart and inserted the needle quickly at a 90-degree angle to the patient's skin with a firm motion.
		•	Inserted the needle to the hub.
		▷	Explained why the needle should be inserted at a 90-degree angle and to the hub.
		★	If needed, aspirated to make sure that the needle was not in a blood vessel.
		▷	Identified an IM medication that does not require aspirating.
		•	Injected the medication slowly and steadily.
		▷	Described what would happen if the medication was injected rapidly.
		•	Placed a gauze pad gently over the injection site and removed the needle quickly at the same angle as insertion.

Trial 1	Trial 2	Point Value	Performance Standards
		•	Applied gentle pressure to the injection site.
		▷	Stated the reason for applying pressure to the injection site.
		•	Activated the safety feature on the syringe.
		•	Properly disposed of the needle and syringe.
		•	Removed gloves and sanitized hands.
		•	Documented the procedure correctly.
		▷	Stated the purpose of the lot number on the medication vial.
		•	Remained with the patient to make sure there were no unusual reactions.
		■	Demonstrated critical thinking skills.
		■	Reassured patients.
		■	Demonstrated empathy for patients' concerns.
		★	Completed the procedure within 5 minutes.
			Totals

CHART	
Date	

Evaluation of Student Performance

EVALUATION CRITERIA			COMMENTS
Symbol	**Category**	**Point Value**	
★	Critical Step	16 points	
•	Essential Step	6 points	
■	Affective Competency	6 points	
▷	Theory Question	2 points	

Score calculation:

       100 points

−   points missed
_____

       Score

Satisfactory score: 85 or above

CAAHEP Competencies Achieved

Psychomotor (Skills)

☑ I. 4. Verify the rules of medication administration: (a) right patient (b) right medication (c) right dose (d) right route (e) right time (f) right documentation.

☑ I. 5. Select proper sites for administering parenteral medication.

☑ I. 7. Administer parenteral (excluding IV) medications.

☑ III. 2. Select appropriate barrier/personal protective equipment.

☑ III. 10. Demonstrate proper disposal of biohazardous material: (a) sharps (b) regulated waste.

☑ V. 1. Respond to nonverbal communication.

☑ X. 3. Document patient care accurately in the medical record.

Affective (Behavior)

☑ A. 1. Demonstrate critical thinking skills.

☑ A. 2. Reassure patients.

☑ A. 3. Demonstrate empathy for patients' concerns.

ABHES Competencies Achieved

☑ 4. a. Follow documentation guidelines.

☑ 8. f. Prepare and administer oral and parenteral medications and monitor the patient.

☑ 9. c. Dispose of biohazardous materials.

Notes

EVALUATION OF COMPETENCY

Procedure 11-6: Z-Track Intramuscular Injection Technique

Name: _____ Date: _____

Evaluated by: _____ Score: _____

Performance Objective

Outcome:	Administer an intramuscular injection using the Z-track method.
Conditions:	Given the following: appropriate medication, medication order, needle and syringe, antiseptic wipe, disposable gloves, and a biohazard sharps container.
Standards:	Time: 5 minutes. Student completed procedure in _____ minutes.
	Accuracy: Satisfactory score on the Performance Evaluation Checklist.

Performance Evaluation Checklist

Trial 1	Trial 2	Point Value	Performance Standards
		•	Sanitized hands.
		•	Prepared the injection.
		•	Greeted the patient and introduced yourself.
		•	Identified the patient and explained the procedure and purpose of the injection.
		•	Selected and properly located the intramuscular injection site.
		•	Cleansed the area with an antiseptic wipe and allowed it to dry completely.
		•	Applied gloves.
		•	Removed the needle guard.
		•	Pulled the skin away laterally from the injection site with the nondominant hand approximately 1 to 1 $\frac{1}{2}$ inches.
		•	Inserted the needle quickly and smoothly at a 90-degree angle.
		★	If needed, aspirated to make sure that the needle was not in a blood vessel.
		•	Injected the medication slowly and steadily.
		•	Waited 10 seconds before withdrawing the needle.
		▷	Explained why there should be a 10-second waiting period.
		•	Withdrew the needle quickly at the same angle as that of insertion.
		•	Released the traction on the skin.
		▷	Described what occurs when the skin traction is released.
		•	Did not apply pressure to the injection site.
		▷	Stated why pressure should not be applied to the injection site.
		•	Activated the safety feature on the syringe.
		•	Properly disposed of the needle and syringe.

Trial 1	Trial 2	Point Value	Performance Standards
		•	Removed gloves and sanitized hands.
		•	Documented the procedure correctly.
		•	Remained with the patient to make sure there were no unusual reactions.
		■	Demonstrated critical thinking skills.
		■	Reassured patients.
		■	Demonstrated empathy for patients' concerns.
		★	Completed the procedure within 5 minutes.
			Totals

CHART	
Date	

Evaluation of Student Performance

EVALUATION CRITERIA			COMMENTS
Symbol	Category	Point Value	
★	Critical Step	16 points	
•	Essential Step	6 points	
■	Affective Competency	6 points	
▷	Theory Question	2 points	

Score calculation: 100 points
−   points missed
___ Score

Satisfactory score: 85 or above

CAAHEP Competencies Achieved

Psychomotor (Skills)

☑ I. 4. Verify the rules of medication administration: (a) right patient (b) right medication (c) right dose (d) right route (e) right time (f) right documentation.

☑ I. 5. Select proper sites for administering parenteral medication.

☑ I. 7. Administer parenteral (excluding IV) medications.

☑ III. 2. Select appropriate barrier/personal protective equipment.

☑ III. 10. Demonstrate proper disposal of biohazardous material: (a) sharps (b) regulated waste.

☑ V. 1. Respond to nonverbal communication.

☑ X. 3. Document patient care accurately in the medical record.

Affective (Behavior)

☑ A. 1. Demonstrate critical thinking skills.

☑ A. 2. Reassure patients.

☑ A. 3. Demonstrate empathy for patients' concerns.

ABHES Competencies Achieved

☑ 4. a. Follow documentation guidelines.

☑ 8. f. Prepare and administer oral and parenteral medications and monitor the patient.

☑ 9. c. Dispose of biohazardous materials.

Notes

Procedure 11-7: Administering an Intradermal Injection

Name: _____   Date: _____

Evaluated by: _____   Score: _____

Performance Objective

Outcome:	Administer an intradermal injection and read the test results.
Conditions:	Given the following: skin testing solution, mediation order, needle and syringe, antiseptic wipe, 2 × 2 gauze pad, disposable gloves, millimeter ruler, TB skin test record card, and a biohazard sharps container.
Standards:	Time: 5 minutes. Student completed procedure in _____ minutes.
	Accuracy: Satisfactory score on the Performance Evaluation Checklist.

Performance Evaluation Checklist

Trial 1	Trial 2	Point Value	Performance Standards
		•	Sanitized hands.
		•	Prepared the injection.
		•	Greeted the patient and introduced yourself.
		•	Identified the patient and explained the procedure and purpose of the injection.
		•	Selected an appropriate intradermal injection site.
		▷	Stated the recommended sites for an intradermal injection.
		•	Cleansed the area with an antiseptic wipe and allowed it to dry completely.
		•	Did not touch the injection site after cleansing it.
		•	Applied gloves.
		•	Removed needle guard.
		•	Stretched the skin taut at the site of administration.
		▷	Explained why the skin is held taut.
		•	Inserted the needle at an angle of 10 to 15 degrees and with the bevel upward.
		•	The bevel of the needle just penetrated the skin.
		▷	Stated why the bevel should face upward.
		•	Released the stretched skin and injected the medication slowly and steadily, ensuring that a wheal formed (approximately 6–10 mm in diameter).
		▷	Explained what to do if a wheal does not form.
		•	Placed a gauze pad gently over the injection site and removed the needle quickly at the same angle as that of insertion.
		•	Did not apply pressure to the injection site.
		▷	Explained why pressure should not be applied to the site.

Trial 1	Trial 2	Point Value	Performance Standards
		•	Activated the safety feature on the syringe.
		•	Properly disposed of the needle and syringe.
		•	Removed gloves and sanitized hands.
		•	Remained with the patient to make sure that there were no unusual reactions.
			Allergy skin tests
		•	Read the test results within 20 to 30 minutes.
		•	Inspected and palpated the site of the skin tests.
		•	Interpreted the skin test results.
		•	Documented the procedure correctly.
			Mantoux tuberculin test
		•	Informed the patient to return in 48 to 72 hours to have the results read.
		▷	Stated what must be done if the patient does not return to have the results read.
		•	Instructed the patient in the care of the test site.
		▷	Stated the instructions that must be relayed to the patient.
		•	Documented the procedure correctly.
			Reading Mantoux TST results
		•	Greeted the patient and introduced yourself.
		•	Identified the patient and explained the procedure.
		•	Worked in a quiet, well-lit atmosphere.
		•	Checked the patient's medical record to determine the site of administration of the test.
		•	Sanitized hands and applied gloves.
		•	Positioned the patient's arm on a firm surface with the arm flexed at the elbow.
		•	Located the application site.
		•	Gently rubbed the fingertip over the test site to palpate for the presence of induration.
		•	If induration is present, rubbed the area lightly, going from the area of normal skin to the indurated area to assess the size of the indurated area.
		•	Measured the diameter of the induration with a millimeter ruler.
		★	The measurement was documented in millimeters and was identical to the evaluator's measurement.
		•	Removed gloves and sanitized hands.
		•	Documented the results correctly.

Trial 1	Trial 2	Point Value	Performance Standards
		•	Completed a TB test record card and gave it to the patient.
		■	Demonstrated critical thinking skills.
		■	Reassured patients.
		■	Demonstrated empathy for patients' concerns.
		★	Completed the procedure within 10 minutes.
			Totals

CHART

Date	

Evaluation of Student Performance

EVALUATION CRITERIA			COMMENTS
Symbol	**Category**	**Point Value**	
★	Critical Step	16 points	
•	Essential Step	6 points	
■	Affective Competency	6 points	
▷	Theory Question	2 points	

Score calculation: 100 points

–   points missed
_____

___ Score

Satisfactory score: 85 or above

CAAHEP Competencies Achieved

Psychomotor (Skills)

- ☑ I. 4. Verify the rules of medication administration: (a) right patient (b) right medication (c) right dose (d) right route (e) right time (f) right documentation.
- ☑ I. 5. Select proper sites for administering parenteral medication.
- ☑ I. 7. Administer parenteral (excluding IV) medications.
- ☑ III. 2. Select appropriate barrier/personal protective equipment.
- ☑ III. 10. Demonstrate proper disposal of biohazardous material: (a) sharps (b) regulated waste.
- ☑ V. 2. Respond to nonverbal communication.
- ☑ X. 3. Document patient care accurately in the medical record.

Affective (Behavior)

- ☑ A. 1. Demonstrate critical thinking skills.
- ☑ A. 2. Reassure patients.
- ☑ A. 3. Demonstrate empathy for patients' concerns.

ABHES Competencies Achieved

- ☑ 4. a. Follow documentation guidelines.
- ☑ 8. f. Prepare and administer oral and parenteral medications and monitor the patient.
- ☑ 9. c. Dispose of biohazardous materials.

This section is designed as supplemental education for Chapter 11 (Administration of Medication) in your textbook. Completion of these exercises will enable you to calculate drug dosage effectively and accurately, which is essential for administering the proper amount of medication to patients and preventing medication errors. Because each unit builds on the next one, you should become completely familiar with each step before proceeding to the next.

LEARNING OBJECTIVES

After completing this chapter, you should be able to:
1. Identify metric abbreviations.
2. Indicate dose quantity using metric notation guidelines.
3. Identify common medical abbreviations used in writing medication orders.
4. Interpret medication orders.
5. Convert units of measurement within the following systems: metric and household.
6. Convert units of measurement using ratio and proportion.
7. Convert units of measurement between the metric and household systems.
8. Determine oral drug dosage.
9. Determine parenteral drug dosage.

UNIT 1: THE METRIC SYSTEM

A. Units of Measurement: Practice Problems

The basic units of measurement in the metric system are the gram, liter, and meter. The gram is a unit of weight used to measure solids, the liter is a unit volume used to measure liquids, and the meter is a unit of length used to measure distance. In the space provided, indicate whether each of the following metric units of measurement is a unit of weight (W), volume (V), or length (L).

_____ 1. milligram

_____ 2. cubic centimeter

_____ 3. meter

_____ 4. kilogram

_____ 5. liter

_____ 6. milliliter

_____ 7. kiloliter

_____ 8. millimeter

_____ 9. microgram

_____ 10. gram

B. Metric Abbreviations: Practice Problems

Review the metric abbreviations in your textbook before completing these problems. In the space provided, indicate the correct abbreviation for each of the metric units of measurement.

_____ 1. milligram

_____ 2. gram

_____ 3. kilogram

_____ 4. liter

_____ 5. microgram

_____ 6. milliliter

533

C. Metric Notation: Practice Problems

To read prescriptions and medication orders, to record medication administration, and to avoid medication errors, the MA must be able to use metric notation guidelines. Review the Metric Notation Guidelines in Box 11.1 of your textbook before completing the following practice problems. In the space provided, use metric notation guidelines to indicate the dose quantities.

_____ 1. 25 milligrams

_____ 2. 5 grams

_____ 3. 11/2 liters

_____ 4. 10 milliliters

_____ 5. 1/2 gram

_____ 6. 50 milligrams

_____ 7. 4 milliliters

_____ 8. 2 kilograms

_____ 9. 120 milliliters

_____ 10. 4 gram

_____ 11. 250 milligrams

_____ 12. 1/2 liter

_____ 13. 500 milliliters

_____ 14. 5 kilograms

_____ 15. $2^1/_2$ grams

UNIT 2: THE HOUSEHOLD SYSTEM

The household system is a more complicated and less accurate method for administering medication than the metric system. However, most individuals are familiar with this system because of its frequent use in the United States. This system of measurement may be the only one the patient can fully relate to and therefore may safely use to administer liquid medication at home.

A. Units of Measurement: Practice Problems

Volume is the only household unit of measurement used to administer medication. The basic unit of liquid volume is the drop. The remaining units, in order of increasing volume, are the teaspoon, tablespoon, ounce, cup, and glass. In the space provided, indicate the correct abbreviation for each of the household units of measurement listed.

_____ 1. drop

_____ 2. teaspoon

_____ 3. tablespoon

_____ 4. ounce

A. Medical Abbreviations: Practice Problems

To safely administer medication, the MA must be completely familiar with common medical abbreviations. Review Table 11.5 in your textbook before completing the following practice problems. In the space provided, write the meaning of the following medical abbreviations.

_____ 1. NPO

_____ 2. prn

_____ 3. tab

_____ 4. ac

_____ 5. DAW

_____ 6. pc

_____ 7. qid

_____ 8. c̄

_____ 9. -s

_____ 10. bid

_____ 11. tid

_____ 12. qh

_____ 13. gtts

_____ 14. q4h

_____ 15. qs

_____ 16. IM

_____ 17. caps

_____ 18. po

_____ 19. ad lib

_____ 20. aa

_____ 21. OTC

_____ 22. subcut

_____ 23. per

_____ 24. SL

_____ 25. STAT

B. Interpreting Medication Orders: Practice Problems

To safely administer medication and instruct patients on administering medication at home, the medical assistant must be able to interpret medication orders. Interpret the following medication orders, and using a drug reference, indicate the drug category based on action and a brand name for each medication.

1. Tetracycline 250 mg po qid × 10 days

   _____

   Drug category: _____

   Brand name: _____

2. Lansoprazole 30 mg po every day ac

   _____

   Drug category: _____

   Brand name: _____

3. Alprazolam 0.25 mg po tid

   _____

   Drug category: _____

   Brand name: _____

4. Diltiazem 50 mg po q4h

   _____

   Drug category: _____

   Brand name: _____

5. Ciprofloxacin 500 mg q12h

   Drug category: _____

   Brand name: _____

6. Hydrocodone/acetaminophen 5 mg q4h prn

   _____

   Drug category: _____

   Brand name: _____

7. Furosemide 40 mg po q AM

   _____

   Drug category: _____

   Brand name: _____

8. Paroxetine 20 mg po every day in AM

   _____

   Drug category: _____

   Brand name: _____

9. Cetirizine 5 mg po every day

_____

   Drug category: _____

   Brand name: _____

10. Cyclobenzaprine 10 mg po tid × 1 wk

_____

   Drug category: _____

   Brand name: _____

UNIT 4: CONVERTING UNITS OF MEASUREMENT

A. Using Conversion Tables

Changing from one unit of measurement to another is known as *conversion*. Conversion is required when medication is ordered in one unit of measurement and the medication label expresses the drug strength in a different unit. The dose quantity must be mathematically translated or converted to the unit of measurement of the medication on hand. For example, if the provider orders 5 grams of an oral solid medication and the medication label expresses the drug strength in milligrams, the medical assistant must convert the grams into milligrams to know how much medication to administer. Converting units of measurement can be classified as follows:

1. Conversion of units within a measurement system
2. Conversion of units from one measurement system to another

Converting units within a measurement system allows a quantity to be expressed in a different but equal unit of measurement within the same system. An example of converting between units of weight within the metric system is as follows: 1 gram is equal to 1000 milligrams.

Converting from one measurement system to another allows a quantity to be expressed in a unit of measurement of another system. An example of a conversion between the household and metric systems is as follows: 1 ounce (household system) is equivalent to 30 milliliters (metric system). Methods used to convert units of measurement are presented in this unit and in Unit 5.

Conversion requires the use of a conversion table to indicate the equivalent values between units of measurement. The practice problems that follow can assist you in attaining competency in using conversion tables.

Conversion Tables: Practice Problems

Refer to the conversion tables at the end of this chapter. Locate and document the equivalent value for each of the units of measurement listed.

			ANSWER	
1.	1 g	=	_____	mg
2.	1 ounce	=	_____	mL
3.	1 tablespoon	=	_____	teaspoons
4.	1 mg	=	_____	mcg
5.	1 liter	=	_____	mL
6.	1 kiloliter	=	_____	liters
7.	1 teacup	=	_____	ounces
8.	1 teaspoon	=	_____	drops
9.	1 mL	=	_____	cc

ANSWER

10. 1 cup = _____ ounces

11. 1 drop = _____ mL

12. 1 kg = _____ g

13. 1 mL = _____ drops

14. 1 teaspoon = _____ mL

15. 1 ounce = _____ tablespoons

16. 1 tablespoon = mL

17. 1 ounce = _____ teaspoons

18. 1 glass = _____ mL

19. 1 glass = _____ ounces

B. Converting Units Within the Metric System

Drug administration often requires conversion within the metric system to prepare the correct dose. Metric conversion involves converting a larger unit to a smaller unit (e.g., grams to milligrams) or converting a smaller unit to a larger unit (e.g., milliliters to liters). Methods used to convert one metric unit to another are described in the next sections.

Converting a Larger Unit to a Smaller Unit

Converting a larger unit to a smaller unit within the metric system can be accomplished using one of three methods. The method chosen is based on personal preference and the level of difficulty of the conversion problem. For example, more difficult problems require the use of ratio and proportion as the method of conversion. Examples of converting a larger unit to a smaller unit are as follows:

1. Grams to milligrams
2. Liters to milliliters
3. Kilograms to grams

Methods of Conversion: To convert a larger unit to a smaller unit within the metric system, use one of the following:
   Method 1: Multiply the unit to be changed by 1000.
   Method 2: Move the decimal point of the unit to be changed three places to the right.
   Method 3: Ratio and proportion (see Unit 5).
Guideline: When converting a larger unit to a smaller unit, expect the quantity to become larger. Use this guideline to assist in making accurate conversions. The problems illustrate this guideline.

EXAMPLES

PROBLEM   2 L = _____ mL
Method 1:   Multiply the unit to be changed by 1000.
             2 × 1000 = 2000 mL
Method 2:   Move the decimal point of the unit to be changed three places to the right.
             2.0 0 0. = 2000 mL

Answer   2 L = 2000 mL

538

PROBLEM   4 g = _____ mg
Method 1:   Multiply the unit to be changed by 1000.
                      $4 \times 1000 = 4000$ mg
Method 2:   Move the decimal point of the unit to be changed three places to the right.
                      4.0 0 0. = 4000 mL

Answer	4 g = 4000 mg

Converting a Smaller Unit to a Larger Unit

Converting a smaller unit to a larger unit within the metric system can be accomplished using one of three methods of conversion as outlined below. Examples of converting a smaller unit to a larger unit are as follows:

1. Milligrams to grams
2. Milliliters to liters
3. Grams to kilograms

> ***Methods of Conversion:*** To convert a smaller unit to a larger unit within the metric system, use one of the following:
>   *Method 1*: Divide the unit to be changed by 1000.
>   *Method 2*: Move the decimal point of the unit to be changed three places to the left.
>   *Method 3*: Ratio and proportion (see Unit 5).
> ***Guideline:*** When converting a smaller unit to a larger unit, expect the quantity to become smaller. The problems illustrate this guideline.

EXAMPLES

PROBLEM   250 mg = _____ g
Method 1:   Divide the unit to be changed by 1000.
                      $250 \div 1000 = 0.25$ g
Method 2:   Move the decimal point of the unit to be changed three places to the left.
                      .2 5 0. = 0.25 g

Answer	250 mg = 0.25 g

PROBLEM   1500 mL = _____ L
Method 1:   Divide the unit to be changed by 1000.
                      $1500 \div 1000 = 1.5$ L
Method 2:   Move the decimal point of the unit to be changed three places to the left.
                      1.5 0 0. = 1.5 L

Answer	1500 mL = 1.5 L

Converting Units Within the Metric System: Practice Problems

Directions: Convert the following metric units of measurement using Method 1 or Method 2. In the space provided, indicate if the conversion is going from a larger to smaller unit (L→S) or smaller to larger unit (S→L).

			ANSWER		CONVERSION
1.	1 g	=	_____ mg		_____
2.	750 mg	=	_____ g		_____
3.	2 kg	=	_____ g		_____
4.	1000 g	=	_____ kg		_____

Chapter **11** **Administration of Medication and Intravenous Therapy**

			ANSWER		CONVERSION
5.	1.5 L	=	_____	mL	_____
6.	250 mL	=	_____	L	_____
7.	5 g	=	_____	mg	_____
8.	0.25 kg	=	_____	g	_____
9.	1000 mg	=	_____	g	_____
10.	2.5 g	=	_____	mg	_____
11.	475 mL	=	L		_____
12.	0.05 g	=	_____	mg	_____
13.	0.5 L	=	_____	mL	_____
14.	1000 mL	=	_____	L	_____
15.	500 g	=	_____	kg	_____
16.	50 mg	=	_____	g	_____
17.	1 L	=	_____	mL	_____
18.	40 g	=	_____	mg	_____
19.	50 mL	=	_____	L	_____
20.	1 kg	=	_____	g	_____

C. Converting Units Within the Household System

Household system conversion involves converting a larger unit to a smaller unit (e.g., tablespoons to teaspoons) or converting a smaller unit to a larger unit (e.g., tablespoons to ounces). Methods used to convert one unit to another are described.

Converting a Larger Unit to a Smaller Unit

Converting a larger unit to a smaller unit within the household system is accomplished using the equivalent value method or the ratio and proportion method. The method chosen is based on personal preference and on the level of difficulty of the conversion problem. Examples of converting a larger unit to a smaller unit follow:

Volume:
teaspoons to drops
tablespoons to teaspoons
ounces to teaspoons
ounces to tablespoons
teacup to ounces
glass to ounces

Method of Conversion: To convert a larger unit to a smaller unit within the household system, use one of the following:
  Method 1:
  a. Look at Table 11.2 (Household Conversion) at the end of this chapter to determine the equivalent value between the two units of measurement.
  b. Multiply the equivalent value by the number next to the larger unit of measurement.
  Method 2: Ratio and proportion (see Unit 5).

PROBLEM 2 tablespoons = _____ teaspoons

Method 1:

  a. Look at the conversion table to determine the equivalent value:

      1 tablespoon = 3 teaspoons

      3 = the equivalent value

  b. Multiply the equivalent value by the number next to the larger unit of measurement:

      $2 \times 3 = 6$

Answer	2 tablespoons = 6 teaspoons

PROBLEM ½ teaspoon = _____ drops

Method 1:

  a. Look at the conversion table to determine the equivalent value:

      1 teaspoon = 60 drops

      60 = the equivalent value

  b. Multiply the equivalent value by the number next to the larger unit of measurement:

      $\frac{1}{2} \times 60 = 30$ drops

Answer	$^1/_2$ tablespoon = 30 drops

Converting a Smaller Unit to a Larger Unit

Converting a smaller unit to a larger unit within the household system is accomplished using the equivalent value method or the ratio and proportion method. Examples of converting from a smaller unit to a larger unit follow:

Volume

drops to teaspoons

teaspoons to tablespoons

teaspoons to ounces

tablespoons to ounces

ounces to teacups

ounces to glasses

Method of Conversion: To convert a smaller unit to a larger unit within the household system, use one of the following:

  Method 1:

  a. Look at Table 11.2 (Household Conversion) at the end of this chapter to determine the equivalent value between the two units of measurement.

  b. Divide the equivalent value into the number next to the smaller unit of measurement.

  Method 2: Ratio and proportion (see Unit 5).

PROBLEM 4 tablespoons = _____ ounces

Method 1:

  a. Look at the conversion table to determine the equivalent value:

      1 ounce = 2 tablespoons

      2 = the equivalent value

  b. Divide the equivalent value into the number next to the smaller unit of measurement:

      $4 \div 2 = 2$

Answer	4 tablespoons = 2 ounces

PROBLEM 24 ounces = _____ glasses
Method 1:
a. Look at the conversion table to determine the equivalent value:
1 glass = 8 ounces
8 = the equivalent value
b. Divide the equivalent value into the number next to the smaller unit of measurement:
24 ÷ 8 = 3 glasses

Answer	24 ounces = 3 glasses

Converting Units Within the Household System: Practice Problems

Directions: Convert the following household units of measurement using the equivalent value method of conversion. In the space provided, indicate the equivalent value for each problem.

		ANSWER		EQUIVALENT VALUE
1. 12 teaspoons	=	_____ ounces		_____
2. 4 ounces	=	_____ glasses		_____
3. 90 drops	=	_____ teaspoons		_____
4. ½ ounce	=	_____ tablespoons		_____
5. 6 teaspoons	=	_____ tablespoons		_____
6. 3 tablespoons	=	_____ ounces		_____
7. 18 ounces	=	_____ teacups		_____
8. ½ ounce	=	_____ teaspoons		_____
9. 3 tablespoons	=	_____ teaspoons		_____
10. ½ teaspoon	=	_____ drops		_____

UNIT 5: RATIO AND PROPORTION

Ratio and proportion are used to convert units of measurement. This method of conversion has the advantage of clarifying the mathematical rationale for the methods of conversion previously presented. It is also useful in converting units of measurement that are more difficult to calculate, such as converting between systems—for example, when converting a metric unit of measurement to a household unit of measurement.

A. Ratio and Proportion Guidelines

Some guidelines must be followed when using ratio and proportion:

1. A **ratio** is composed of two related numbers separated by a colon. It indicates the relationship between two quantities or numbers. The ratio example shows a relationship between milligrams and grams (i.e., 1000 mg = 1 g).

    EXAMPLE   1000 mg : 1 g

2. A proportion shows the relationship between two equal ratios. The proportion consists of two ratios separated by an equal sign (=), which indicates that the two ratios are equal. This proportion example shows the relationship between two equal ratios of milligrams and grams.

    EXAMPLE   1000 mg : 1 g = 2000 mg : 2 g

3. The units of measurement in the two ratios of a proportion must be expressed in the same sequence. The correct sequencing in the proportion example is mg : g = mg : g, not mg : g = g : mg.

   EXAMPLE   *Correct:*   1000 mg : 1 g = 2000 mg : 2 g

                Incorrect: 1000 mg : 1 g = 2g : 2000 mg

4. The numbers on the ends of a proportion are called the extremes, and the numbers in the middle of the proportion are known as the means. In this example, the means consist of 1 g and 2000 mg, and the extremes are 1000 mg and 2 g.

   EXAMPLE   1000 mg : 1 g = 2000 mg : 2g
                  └─── means ───┘
                  └──── extremes ────┘

5. The product of the means equals the product of the extremes. The calculation of the product of the means in the example is 1 × 2000 = 2000. The calculation of the product of the extremes is 1000 × 2 = 2000. The product of the means equals the product of the extremes, or 2000 = 2000.

   EXAMPLE   1000 mg : 1 g = 2000 mg : 2 g
                            1 × 2000 = 1000 × 2
                            2000 = 2000

6. In setting up a proportion, one side of the equation consists of the known quantities, and the other side of the equation consists of the unknown quantity. The letter x is commonly used to express the unknown quantity. To be consistent, the known quantities are indicated on the left side of the equation, and the unknown quantity is indicated on the right side of the equation. Using the previous proportion example, but inserting an unknown quantity, or x, the equation is set up as follows:

   EXAMPLE   1000 mg : 1 g   = x mg : 2 g
                        (known quantities)   (unknown quantity)

Ratio and Proportion: Practice Problems
Answer the following questions.

1. What is a ratio?

   _____

2. In the space provided, place a check mark next to each correct example of a ratio.

   _____ a.   1000 mg × 10 grams

   _____ b.   1000 mL = 1 L

   _____ c.   1 mg : 1000 mcg

   _____ d.   1000 mg/1 gram

   _____ e.   1 tablespoon : 1 ounce

   _____ f.   1 mL : 1 cc

3. What is a proportion?

   _____

   _____

   _____

Chapter **11** **Administration of Medication and Intravenous Therapy**

4. In the space provided, place a check mark next to each correct example of a proportion.

_____ a. 1 mL : 1 cc

_____ b. 2 tablespoons : 1 ounce = 4 tablespoons : 2 ounces

_____ c. $2x = 60$ mg

_____ d. 1000 mL : 1 L = 500 mL : 0.5 L

_____ e. 1000 mg : 1 gram = 1000 mL : 1 L

5. In the space provided, place a check mark next to each proportion that has correct sequencing for the units of measurement.

_____ a. 1000 g : 1 kg = 1500 g : 1.5 kg

_____ b. 3 teaspoons : 1 tablespoon = 2 tablespoons : 6 teaspoons

_____ c. 1000 mg : 1 g = 2000 mg : x g

6. Circle the means and underline the extremes in each of the following proportions:

a. 1000 mg : 1 g = 500 mg : 0.5 g

b. 8 ounces : 1 glass = 16 ounces : 2 glasses

c. 1 mL : 1 cc = 2 mL : 2cc

7. In each of the following proportions, what is the product of the means, and what is the product of the extremes?

a. 1000 g : 1 kg = 1500 g : 1.5 kg

_____ product of the means

_____ product of the extremes

b. 60 drops : 1 teaspoon = 120 drops : 2 teaspoons

_____ product of the means

_____ product of the extremes

c. 1 ounce : 30 mL = 4 ounces : 120 mL

_____ product of the means

_____ product of the extremes

8. In each of the following proportions, circle the known quantities and underline the unknown quantity.

a. 1000 mg : 1 g = 500 mg : x g

b. 2 tablespoons : 1 ounce = 6 tablespoons : x ounces

c. 1000 mL : 1 L = x mL : 2 L

B. Converting Units Using Ratio and Proportion

Units can be converted using ratio and proportion.

> **Method of Conversion:**
>
> To convert a unit of measurement using ratio and proportion, use the following steps:
> a. Look at the appropriate conversion table at the end of this chapter to determine what is known about the two units of measurement (equivalent value).
> b. State the known quantities as a ratio.
> c. Determine the unknown quantity.
> d. State the unknown quantity as a ratio.
> e. Set up the proportion with the known quantities on the left side and the unknown quantity on the right side of the equation.
> f. To solve the equation, multiply the product of the means and the product of the extremes. Divide the equation by the number before the x.
> g. Include the unit of measure corresponding to x in the original equation with the answer.

EXAMPLES

PROBLEM   2 g = _____ mg
  a. Look at Table 11.1 (Metric Conversion) to determine what is known about the two units of measurement:
     1000 mg = 1 g
  b. State the known quantities as a ratio:
     1000 mg : 1 g
  c. Determine the unknown quantity:
     2 g = x mg
  d. State the unknown quantity as a ratio using the correct unit of measurement sequencing:
     x mg : 2 g
  e. Set up the proportion with the known quantities on the left side and the unknown quantity on the right side of the equation:
     1000 mg : 1 g = x mg : 2 g
  f. Solve the equation by multiplying the product of the means and the product of the extremes and dividing the equation by the number before the x:
     1000 mg : 1 g = x mg : 2 g
     $1 \times x = 1000 \times 2$
     1x = 2000
     x = 2000
  g. Include the unit of measure corresponding to x in the original equation with the answer:
     x = 2000 mg

Answer	2 g = 2000 mg

PROBLEM   4 ounces = _____ mL
The steps previously outlined are followed here. However, they are combined as they would be in working an actual conversion problem.
   1 ounce : 30 mL = 4 ounces : x mL
   $30 \times 4 = 1 \times x$
   120 = 1x
   x = 120 mL

Answer	4 ounces = 120 mL

Converting Units Using Ratio and Proportion: Practice Problems

Directions: Use ratio and proportion to convert between the metric and household systems by completing the problems below. In the space at the right, indicate what is known regarding the two units of measurement.

			ANSWER	KNOWN QUANTITIES
1.	30 drops	=	_____ mL	_____
2.	2 ounces	=	_____ mL	_____
3.	90 mL	=	_____ ounces	_____
4.	2 glasses	=	_____ mL	_____
5.	360 mL	=	_____ teacups	_____
6.	10 mL	=	_____ teaspoons	_____
7.	60 drops	=	_____ mL	_____
8.	60 mL	=	_____ tablespoons	_____
9.	3 teaspoons	=	_____ mL	_____
10.	5 mL	=	_____ drops	_____

UNIT 6: DETERMINING DRUG DOSAGE

A. Oral Administration

Dosage refers to the amount of medication to be administered to the patient. Each medication has a certain dosage range, or range of quantities that produce therapeutic effects. It is important to administer the exact drug dosage. If a dose is too small, it will not produce a therapeutic effect, whereas too large a dose could harm or even kill the patient. The steps to follow in determining drug dosage depend on the unit of measurement in which the drug is ordered and the unit of measurement of the drug you have available, or the dose on hand.

1. If the dose on hand is the same as that ordered, no calculation is required. In this example, the dose ordered and the dose on hand are in the same unit of measurement, and one tablet is administered to the patient.

> EXAMPLE   The provider orders 50 mg of a medication po.
> The drug label reads 50 mg/tablet.

2. If the dosage ordered is in the same unit of measurement as that indicated on the medication label, only one calculation step is required. In this example, the dose ordered and the dose on hand are in the same unit of measurement, or milligrams. The calculation determines the number of tablets to administer to the patient.

> EXAMPLE   The provider orders 500 mg of a medication po.
> The drug label reads 250 mg/tablet.

3. If the dosage ordered is in a different unit of measurement than indicated on the drug label, two calculation steps are required to determine the amount of medication to administer to the patient. In this example, the dose ordered and the dose on hand are stated in different units of measurement, or in grams and milligrams. The first step requires conversion of the dose ordered to the unit of measurement of the dose on hand; in this example, grams must be converted to milligrams. The second step is to determine the number of tablets to administer to the patient.

> EXAMPLE   The provider orders 1 g of a medication po.
> The drug label reads 500 mg/tablet.

A detailed discussion of determining drug dosage for administration of oral medication follows. The method used to calculate drug dosage when the units of measurement are the same is presented first, followed by the method used when the units of measurement are different.

Determining Drug Dosage with the Same Units of Measurement

Determining the correct drug dosage to be administered when the units of measurement are the same requires the use of a drug dosage formula.

Drug Dosage Formula

$$\frac{D(dose\ ordered)}{H(on\ hand)} \times V\ (vehicle) = x\ (amount\ of\ medication\ to\ be\ administered)$$

D (*dose ordered*): This is the amount of medication ordered by the provider.
H (*drug strength on hand*): This is the dosage strength available as indicated on the medication label or the dose on hand.
V (*vehicle*): The vehicle refers to the type of preparation containing the dose on hand (e.g., tablet, capsule, liquid).
x: The letter x is used to express the unknown quantity or the amount of medication to be administered.

Guidelines

1. The units of measurement must be included when setting up the problem.
2. The values for D and H must be in the same unit of measurement.
3. The value of x is expressed in the same unit as V.
4. When determining the drug dosage for oral liquid medication, the vehicle must also include the amount of liquid in which the available drug is contained. For example, if the medication label reads 250 mg/5 mL, the value of V is 5 mL.

The method to follow to determine drug dosage using this formula is outlined in the following examples. The first problem illustrates determining the dosage for solid medication taken orally.

EXAMPLES

PROBLEM   *Oral solid medication:*
               The provider orders 50 mg of a medication po.
               The medication label reads 25 mg/tablet.
               How much medication should be administered to the patient?

Drug dosage formula:

$$\frac{D}{H} \times V = x$$

a. Identify the dose ordered.
   D = 50 mg

b. Identify the strength of the drug on hand.
   H = 25 mg

c. Determine the vehicle containing the dose on hand.
   V = 1 tablet

Chapter **11** **Administration of Medication and Intravenous Therapy**

d. Calculate the amount of medication to administer to the patient. The units of measurement must be included when setting up the problem, and the values for D and H must be in the same unit of measurement. The value of x is expressed in the same unit as V; in this problem V = 1 tablet.

$$\frac{50 \text{ mg}}{25 \text{ mg}} \times 1 \text{ tablet} = x$$

$(50 \div 25 = 2) \times 1 \text{ tablet} = x$

$2 \times 1 \text{ tablet} = x$

$x = 2 \text{ tablets}$

Answer	2 tablets administered to the patient

The next problem illustrates the determination of drug dosage for liquid medication taken orally. The steps previously outlined are followed; however, they are combined as should be done when working out drug dosage problems. Remember, with oral liquid medication, the vehicle must also include the amount of liquid in which the available drug is contained; in the following problem, V = 5 mL.

PROBLEM   *Oral liquid medication:*
The provider orders 500 mg of a medication.
The medication label reads 250 mg/5 mL.
How much medication should be administered to the patient?

$$\frac{D}{H} \times 1 \text{ tablet} = x$$

$$\frac{500 \text{ mg}}{250 \text{ mg}} \times 1 \text{ tablet} = x$$

$(500 \div 250 = 2) \times 5 \text{ mL} = x$

$2 \times 5 \text{ mL} = x$

$x = 10 \text{ mL}$

Answer	A dose of 10 mL of medication is administered to the patient.

Determining Drug Dosage with Different Units of Measurement

Sometimes, the medication ordered is in a different unit of measurement than indicated on the drug label. In this case, the desired dose quantity must be converted to the unit of measurement of the dose on hand before the drug dosage is determined. The method chosen to convert a unit of measurement is based on personal preference. Refer to Units 4 and 5 to review methods of conversion before completing this section.

The following steps are required to determine drug dosage when the units of measurement are different:
Step 1: Convert the dose quantities to the same unit of measurement. For consistency, it is best to convert to the unit of measurement of the drug on hand.
Step 2: Determine the amount of medication to administer to the patient, using the drug dosage formula.

EXAMPLES

PROBLEM   *Oral solid medication:*
The provider orders 0.5 gram of medication po.
The medication label reads 250 mg/tablet.
How much medication should be administered to the patient?

Step 1: The dosage ordered must be converted to the unit of measurement of the medication on hand. In this problem, 0.5 gram must be converted to milligrams. The ratio and proportion method of conversion is used to make the conversion.

1 gram = _____ mg
1 gram : 1000 mg = 0.5 gram : x mg
$500 = 1x$
$x = 500$ mg

Answer	0.5 gram = 500 mg

548

The medication ordered is in the same unit of measurement as the medication on hand.

Step 2: Determine the amount of medication to administer to the patient using the drug dosage formula.

$$\frac{D}{H} \times V = x$$

$$\frac{500 \text{ mg}}{250 \text{ mg}} \times 1 \text{ tablet}$$

$(500 \div 250 = 2) \times 1 \text{ tablet} = x$

$2 \times 1 \text{ tablet} = x$

$x = 2 \text{ tablets}$

Answer	A dose of 2 tablets is administered to the patient.

PROBLEM

Oral liquid medication:
The provider orders 0.5 gram of a medication po.
The medication label reads 125 mg/5 mL.
How much medication should be administered to the patient?

Step 1: Convert 0.5 gram to milligrams using ratio and proportion:

0.5 gram = _____ mg

1 gram : 1000 mg = 0.5 gram : x mg

$1x = 500 \text{ mg}$

$x = 500 \text{ mg}$

Answer	0.5 gram = 500 mg

Step 2: Determine the amount of medication to administer to the patient using the drug dosage formula.

$$\frac{D}{H} \times V = x$$

$$\frac{500 \text{ mg}}{125 \text{ mg}} \times 5 \text{ mL} = x$$

$(500 \div 125 = 4) \times 5 \text{ mL} = x$

$4 \times 5 \text{ mL} = x$

$x = 20 \text{ mL}$

Answer	A dose of 20 mL of medication is administered to the patient.

Oral Administration: Practice Problems

Directions: Determine the drug dosage to be administered for each of the following oral medication orders, and document your answer below. In the space provided, indicate the drug category based on action for each medication using a drug reference.

Oral Solid Medications

1. The provider orders Inderal 160 mg po.

   Medication label:

Inderal
propranolol
80 mg/capsule

   How much medication should be administered? _____

   Drug category: _____

2. The provider orders Tagamet 600 mg po.

   Medication label:

Tagamet cimetidine 300 mg/tablet

   How much medication should be administered? _____

   Drug category: _____

3. The provider orders Amoxil 0.5 g po.

   Medication label:

Amoxil amoxicillin 250 mg/capsule

   How much medication should be administered? _____

   Drug category: _____

4. The provider orders Lasix 80 mg po.

   Medication label:

Lasix furosemide 40 mg/tablet

   How much medication should be administered? _____

   Drug category: _____

5. The provider orders Lomotil 5 mg po.

   Medication label:

Lomotil diphenoxylate/atropine 2.5 mg/tablet

   How much medication should be administered? _____

   Drug category: _____

6. The provider orders Zithromax 0.5 g po.

   Medication label:

Zithromax azithromycin 250 mg/tablet

   How much medication should be administered? _____

   Drug category: _____

7. The provider orders Calan 120 mg po.

   Medication label:

Calan
verapamil
40 mg/tablet

   How much medication should be administered? _____

   Drug category: _____

8. The provider orders Xanax 0.5 mg po.

   Medication label:

Xanax
alprazolam
0.25 mg/tablet

   How much medication should be administered? _____

   Drug category: _____

9. The provider orders Phenergan 25 mg po.

   Medication label:

Phenergan
promethazine
12.5 mg/tablet

   How much medication should be administered? _____

   Drug category: _____

10. The provider orders Procardia XL 30 mg po.

    Medication label:

Procardia
nifedipine
10 mg/tablet

    How much medication should be administered? _____

    Drug category: _____

Oral Liquid Medications

1. The provider orders Sumycin Suspension 250 mg po.

   Medication label:

Sumycin Suspension
tetracycline
125 mg/5 mL

   How much medication should be administered? _____

   Drug category: _____

551

2. The provider orders Tagamet liquid 300 mg po.
   Medication label:

Tagamet
cimetidine liquid
300 mg/5 mL

   How much medication should be administered? _____

   Drug category: _____

3. The provider orders Tylenol Elixir 60 mg po.
   Medication label:

Tylenol Elixir
acetaminophen
120 mg/5 mL

   How much medication should be administered? _____

   Drug category: _____

4. The provider orders Amoxil Suspension 0.5 g po.
   Medication label:

Amoxil Suspension
amoxicillin
125 mg/5 mL

   How much medication should be administered? _____

   Drug category: _____

5. The provider orders Gantanol Suspension 1 g po.
   Medication label:

Gantanol Suspension
sulfamethoxazole
500 mg/5 mL

   How much medication should be administered? _____

   Drug category: _____

B. Parenteral Administration

Medications for parenteral administration must be suspended in solution. The medication label indicates the amount of the drug contained in each milliliter of solution. For example, if a medication label reads 10 mg/mL, there are 10 mg of medication for each 1 mL of liquid volume. Some medications, such as penicillin, insulin, and heparin, are ordered and measured in units (e.g., 300,000 units/mL). This refers to their biologic activity in animal tests or the amount of the drug that is required to produce a particular response.

Parenteral medication is available in several dispensing forms, including ampules, single-dose vials, and multiple-dose vials. After the proper drug dosage has been determined, the medication is drawn into a syringe from the dispensing unit. Most syringes are calibrated in milliliters (mL).

Determining drug dosage for parenteral administration is calculated in a similar manner as that for oral liquid medication. The first problem illustrates the determination of drug dosage when the medication is ordered in a different unit of measurement from the dose on hand, requiring two calculation steps.

EXAMPLES

PROBLEM The provider orders 0.5 g of a medication IM.
The medication label reads 250 mg/2 mL.
How much medication should be administered?

Step 1: Convert 0.5 gram to milligrams.
0.5 gram = _____ mg
1000 mg : 1 g = x mg : 0.5 g
$1x = 500$
$x = 500$ mg

Answer	0.5 mg = 500 mg

Step 2: Determine the amount of medication to administer to the patient:

$$\frac{D}{H} \times V = x$$

$$\frac{500 \text{ mg}}{250 \text{ mg}} \times 2 \text{ mL} = x$$

$(500 \div 250 = 2) \times 2 \text{ mL} = x$
$2 \times 2 \text{ mL} = x$
$x = 4 \text{ mL}$

Answer	A dose of 4 mL of medication is administered to the patient.

The next problem illustrates the determination of drug dosage with a medication ordered in units. Notice that the dose ordered and the dose on hand are in the same unit of measurement; therefore, conversion of units of measurement is not necessary.

PROBLEM The provider orders 600,000 units of a medication IM.
The medication label reads 300,000 units/mL.
How much medication should be administered?

$$\frac{D}{H} \times V = x$$

$$\frac{600,000 \text{ units}}{300,000 \text{ units}} \times 1 \text{ mL} = x$$

$(600,000 \div 300,000 = 2) \times 1 \text{ mL} = x$
$x = 2 \text{ mL}$

Answer	A dose of 2 mL of medication is administered to the patient.

Parenteral Administration: Practice Problems

Determine the drug dosage to be administered for each of the following parenteral medication orders, and document your answer. In the space provided, indicate the drug category based on action using a drug reference.

1. The provider orders Vistaril 75 mg IM.
   Medication label:

Vistaril
hydroxyzine injection
50 mg/mL

   How much medication should be administered? _____

   Drug category: _____

553

2. The provider orders Cobex (vitamin B$_{12}$) 200 mcg IM.
   Medication label:

   > Cobex
   > cyanocobalamin injection
   > 100 mcg/mL

   How much medication should be administered? _____

   Drug category: _____

3. The provider orders Depo-Medrol 40 mg IM.
   Medication label:

   > Depo-Medrol
   > methylprednisolone injection
   > 80 mg/mL

   How much medication should be administered? _____

   Drug category: _____

4. The provider orders Wycillin 600,000 units IM.
   Medication label:

   > Wycillin
   > porcine penicillin G injection
   > 300,000 units/mL

   How much medication should be administered? _____

   Drug category: _____

5. The provider orders Rocephin 1000 mg IM.
   Medication label:

   > Rocephin
   > ceftriaxone injection
   > 1 g/mL

   How much medication should be administered? _____

   Drug category: _____

6. The provider orders INFeD 100 mg IM.
   Medication label:

   > INFeD
   > iron dextran injection
   > 50 mg/mL

   How much medication should be administered? _____

   Drug category: _____

7. The provider orders Bicillin 1.2 million units IM.
   Medication label:

   > Bicillin
   > benzathine penicillin G injection
   > 600,000 units/mL

   How much medication should be administered? _____

   Drug category: _____

8. The provider orders Depo-Provera 150 mg IM.
   Medication label:

Depo-Provera medroxyprogesterone 150 mg/mL

   How much medication should be administered? _____

   Drug category: _____

9. The provider orders Pronestyl 0.25 g IM.
   Medication label:

Pronestyl procainamide injection 500 mg/mL

   How much medication should be administered? _____

   Drug category: _____

10. The provider orders Compazine 7 mg IM.
    Medication label:

Compazine prochlorperazine injection 5 mg/mL

    How much medication should be administered? _____

    Drug category: _____

Table 11.1 Metric System Conversion of Equivalent Values

WEIGHT
1000 micrograms = 1 milligram
1000 milligrams = 1 gram
1000 grams = 1 kilogram

VOLUME
1000 milliliters = 1 liter
1000 liters = 1 kiloliter
1 milliliter = 1 cubic centimeter

Table 11.2 Household System: Conversion of Equivalent Values

ABBREVIATIONS
drop: gtt
teaspoon: tsp
tablespoon: T
ounce: oz
cup: c

VOLUME
60 drops = 1 teaspoon
3 teaspoons = 1 tablespoon
6 teaspoons = 1 ounce
2 tablespoons = 1 ounce
6 ounces = 1 teacup
8 ounces = 1 glass
8 ounces = 1 cup

Table 11.3 Conversion Chart for Household and Metric Equivalents (Volume)

Household		Metric
1 drop	=	0.06 mL
15 drops	=	1 mL (cc)
1 teaspoon	=	5 (4) mL
1 tablespoon	=	15 mL
2 tablespoons	=	30 mL
1 ounce	=	30 mL
1 teacup	=	180 mL
1 glass	=	240 mL

12 Cardiopulmonary Procedures

√ After Completing	Date Due	Study Guide Pages	STUDY GUIDE ASSIGNMENTS (CTA = Critical Thinking Activity)	Possible Points	Points You Earned
		561	📋 Pretest	10	
		562-563	🔑Term Key Term Assessment A. Definitions B. Word Parts (Add 1 point for each key term)	21 15	
		563-571	📝 Evaluation of Learning questions	67	
			Evolve: Find That Lead (Record points earned)		
		571	CTA A: ECG Cycle	10	
			Evolve: It's a Cycle (Record points earned)		
			Evolve: It's an Artifact (Record points earned)		
		571-572	CTA B: ECG Artifacts (2 points each)	20	
		572-574	CTA C: Myocardial Infarction	20	
		575-576	CTA D: Peak Flow Chart	20	
		577	CTA E: Crossword Puzzle	30	
			Evolve: Apply Your Knowledge questions	12	
			Evolve: Video Evaluation	33	
		561	📋 Posttest	10	
			ADDITIONAL ASSIGNMENTS		
			Total points		

√ When Assigned by Your Instructor	Study Guide Pages	Practices Required	LABORATORY ASSIGNMENTS (Procedure Number and Name)	Score*
	578	3	**Practice for Competency** 12-1: Running a 12-Lead, Three-Channel Electrocardiogram	
	580-582		**Evaluation of Competency** 12-1: Running a 12-Lead, Three-Channel Electrocardiogram	*
	578	3	**Practice for Competency** 12-2: Applying a Holter Monitor	
	583-585		**Evaluation of Competency** 12-2: Applying a Holter Monitor	*
	579	3	**Practice for Competency** 12-3: Spirometry Testing	
	587-589		**Evaluation of Competency** 12-3: Spirometry Testing	*
	579	3	**Practice for Competency** 12-4: Measuring Peak Flow Rate	
	591-593		**Evaluation of Competency** 12-4: Measuring Peak Flow Rate	*
			ADDITIONAL ASSIGNMENTS	

Notes

Name: _____   Date: _____

True or False

_____ 1. The cardiac cycle represents one complete heartbeat.

_____ 2. The portion of the ECG between two waves is known as a segment.

_____ 3. A standard electrocardiogram consists of 10 leads.

_____ 4. An electrolyte facilitates the transmission of electrical impulses.

_____ 5. Leads V_1 through V_6 are known as the augmented leads.

_____ 6. Electrodes that are too loose can cause a 60-cycle interference artifact.

_____ 7. When running an ECG, the medical assistant should work on the left side of the patient.

_____ 8. An electrocardiographic (ECG) result that is within normal limits is said to have a normal sinus rhythm.

_____ 9. The purpose of a pulmonary function test is to assess cardiac functioning.

_____ 10. During a severe asthma attack, the bronchial tubes constrict, swell, and become clogged with mucus.

?≡ **POSTTEST**

True or False

_____ 1. An electrocardiogram is a recording of the electrical activity of the heart.

_____ 2. The amplifier is a device placed on the skin that picks up electrical impulses released by the heart.

_____ 3. The P wave represents the contraction of the ventricles.

_____ 4. If the electrocardiograph is properly standardized, the standardization mark will be 20 mm high.

_____ 5. A muscle artifact can be identified by its fuzzy, irregular baseline.

_____ 6. A spirometer measures how much air is exhaled from the lungs and how fast it is exhaled.

_____ 7. Spirometry can be used to assess a patient with emphysema.

_____ 8. Quick-relief asthma medication is used to prevent asthma symptoms.

_____ 9. The amount of supplemental oxygen prescribed for a patient is known as the flow rate.

_____ 10. A nasal cannula interferes with a patient's ability to talk, eat, and drink.

A. Definitions

Directions: Match each key term with its definition.

_____ 1. Artifact

_____ 2. Atherosclerosis

_____ 3. Baseline

_____ 4. Cardiac cycle

_____ 5. Dysrhythmia

_____ 6. ECG cycle

_____ 7. Electrocardiogram

_____ 8. Electrocardiograph

_____ 9. Electrode

_____ 10. Electrolyte

_____ 11. Flow rate

_____ 12. Hypoxemia

_____ 13. Hypoxia

_____ 14. Interval

_____ 15. Ischemia

_____ 16. Normal sinus rhythm

_____ 17. Oxygen therapy

_____ 18. Peak flow rate

_____ 19. Segment

_____ 20. Spirometer

_____ 21. Wheezing

A. A chemical substance that promotes conduction of an electrical current
B. The flat, horizontal line that separates the various waves of the ECG cycle
C. The instrument used to record the electrical activity of the heart
D. Additional electrical activity picked up by the electrocardiograph that interferes with the normal appearance of the ECG cycles
E. Refers to an electrocardiogram that is within normal limits
F. One complete heartbeat
G. The graphic representation of the electrical activity of the heart
H. The length of one or more waves and a segment
I. The graphic representation of a heartbeat
J. A conductor of electricity, which is used to promote contact between the body and the electrocardiograph
K. The portion of the ECG between two waves
L. Deficiency of blood in a body part
M. An instrument for measuring air taken into and expelled from the lungs
N. Buildup of fibrous plaques of fatty deposits and cholesterol on the inner walls of an artery that causes narrowing, obstruction, and hardening of the artery
O. An irregular heart rate or rhythm
P. The number of liters of oxygen per minute that come out of an oxygen delivery system
Q. A decrease in the oxygen saturation of the blood
R. A reduction in the oxygen supply to the tissues of the body
S. The administration of supplemental oxygen at concentrations greater than room air to treat or prevent hypoxemia
T. The maximum volume of air that can be exhaled when a patient blows into a peak flow meter as forcefully and as rapidly as possible
U. A continuous, high-pitched whistling musical sound heard particularly during exhalation and sometimes during inhalation

B. Word Parts

Directions: Indicate the meaning of each word part in the space provided. List as many medical terms as possible that incorporate the word part in the space provided.

Word Part	Meaning of Word Part	Medical Terms That Incorporate Word Part
1. ather/o		
2. -sclerosis		
3. cardi/o		
4. electr/o		
5. dys-		
6. -gram		
7. -graph		
8. hypo-		
9. ox/I		
10. -emia		
11. -ia		
12. isch/o		
13. spir/o		
14. -meter		
15. -metry		

EVALUATION OF LEARNING

Directions: Fill in each blank with the correct answer.

1. List 5 reasons for performing electrocardiography.

_____

_____

_____

2. Trace the path blood takes through the heart, starting with the right atrium.

_____

_____

_____

3. What are the coronary arteries and what is the function of the coronary arteries?

_____

_____

4. What is the SA node and what is the function of the SA node?

_____

_____

5. Why is the impulse initiated by the SA node delayed momentarily by the AV node?

_____

6. What is the cardiac cycle and what events occur in one cardiac cycle?

_____

7. Label the following on the ECG cycle.

   P wave   P–R segment

   QRS complex   S–T segment

   T wave   P–R interval

   Q–T interval

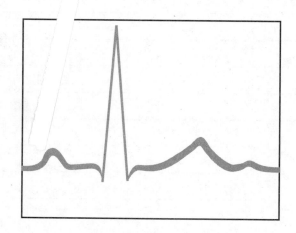

8. Explain what each component of the ECG cycle represents.

   P wave _____

   QRS complex _____

   T wave _____

   P–R segment _____

   S–T segment _____

   P–R interval _____

   Q–T interval _____

9. Why is the R wave taller than the P wave on the ECG graph cycle?

   _____

   _____

10. Why does atrial repolarization not appear as a separate wave on the ECG cycle?

   _____

   _____

11. Why is the baseline flat following the U wave?

_____

_____

12. What changes can occur on an ECG due to the following?

   a. Myocardial ischemia: _____

   b. Myocardial infarction: _____

13. What is the purpose of standardizing the electrocardiograph?

_____

_____

14. How high should the standardization mark be when the electrocardiograph is standardized?

_____

15. What is a lead, and what information does it provide?

_____

_____

16. How many "electrical photographs" of the heart are recorded by the electrocardiograph?

_____

17. What is the purpose of the right leg lead wire?

_____

18. What is the function of an electrode?

_____

_____

19. What is the function of each of the following parts of an electrocardiograph?

   a. Amplifier: _____

   b. Output device: _____

_____

20. Why must an electrolyte be used when recording an electrocardiogram?

_____

_____

21. Why should the expiration date on an electrode pouch be checked before use?

_____

22. How should electrodes be stored?

_____

_____

23. Diagram the bipolar leads on the following illustration:

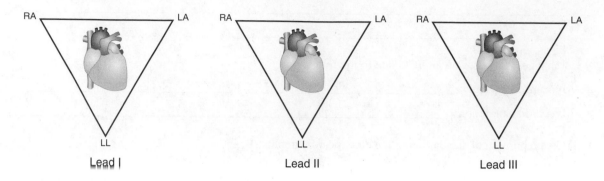

Lead I　　　　　　　Lead II　　　　　　　Lead III

24. Locate and label the locations of the chest electrodes on the following illustration:

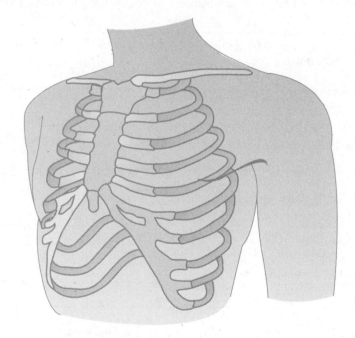

25. What patient preparation is required for an ECG?

_____

_____

26. What is the difference between a single-channel and a three-channel electrocardiograph?

_____

_____

_____

27. What is the purpose of each of the following electrocardiograph capabilities?

a. Interpretive capability

_____

_____

b. EHR connectivity

_____

_____

c. Teletransmission

_____

_____

28. Why should artifacts be eliminated, if they occur in an ECG recording?

_____

_____

_____

29. What causes muscles artifacts on an ECG?

_____

_____

30. What causes wandering baseline artifacts on an ECG?

_____

_____

31. What causes 60-cycle interference artifacts on an ECG?

_____

_____

32. What causes an interrupted baseline artifact to occur on an ECG?

_____

_____

33. List four uses of Holter monitor electrocardiography.

_____

_____

_____

34. List five guidelines that should be relayed to a patient undergoing Holter monitor electrocardiography.

_____

_____

_____

_____

567

35. Explain the use of the patient diary in Holter monitor electrocardiography.

_____

_____

36. List the distinguishing characteristics of each of the following cardiac arrhythmias.

   a. Paroxysmal supraventricular tachycardia

_____

_____

   b. Atrial fibrillation

_____

_____

   c. Premature ventricular contraction

_____

_____

   d. Ventricular fibrillation

_____

_____

37. What is the purpose of a pulmonary function test?

_____

38. What are the indications for performing spirometry?

_____

_____

_____

39. What patient preparation is required for spirometry?

_____

_____

_____

40. What is the purpose of postbronchodilator spirometry?

_____

_____

41. What are the characteristics of asthma?

_____

_____

42. What are five examples of allergens that may trigger an asthma attack?

_____

_____

43. What are five examples of environmental irritants, activities, or events that may trigger an asthma attack?

_____

_____

44. What happens to the bronchial tubes during an asthma attack?

_____

45. What is the purpose of long-term-control asthma medication?

_____

_____

46. What is the purpose of quick-relief asthma medication?

_____

_____

47. What is the purpose of a peak flow meter?

_____

_____

48. What is the difference between a low-range and a full-range peak flow meter?

_____

_____

49. What information is provided by a peak flow measurement?

_____

_____

50. What is the purpose of a peak flow chart?

_____

_____

51. What is an asthma action plan?

_____

_____

52. What information is included in an asthma action plan?

_____

_____

_____

53. Why is oxygen needed by the body?

_____

_____

569

54. What is the purpose of the regulator and flow meter on an oxygen cylinder?

_____

55. What occurs when the body cannot maintain an adequate oxygen level?

_____

_____

56. What conditions may require home oxygen therapy?

_____

_____

57. What information is included on a prescription for home oxygen therapy?

_____

_____

58. What are the advantages and disadvantages of compressed oxygen gas?

   a. Advantages:

_____

_____

   b. Disadvantages:

_____

_____

59. What is liquid oxygen?

_____

_____

60. What are the advantages and disadvantages of liquid oxygen?

   a. Advantages:

_____

_____

   b. Disadvantages:

_____

_____

61. What is an oxygen concentrator?

_____

_____

62. What is the advantage of using a nasal cannula to administer oxygen?

_____

570

63. List two reasons for using a face mask to administer oxygen therapy.

_____

_____

64. What are the symptoms of a low oxygen level in the body?

_____

_____

65. How much tubing should be used with an oxygen delivery system and why?

_____

_____

66. What occurs if oxygen comes in contact with a fire?

_____

_____

67. How should oxygen be stored?

_____

_____

CRITICAL THINKING ACTIVITIES

A. ECG Cycle

Attach part of an ECG from a recording. Identify and label the various waves, intervals, and segments making up an ECG cycle on two of the leads.

B. ECG Artifacts

When recording ECGs, the following situations occur (outlined below). In the space provided, indicate the **type of artifact** that usually occurs with each situation and the **action to take** to eliminate the artifact.

1. An electrode becomes loose during the recording.

Type: _____

Action: _____

2. The lead wires are not following body contour.

   Type: _____

   Action: _____

3. The room temperature is too cold for the patient causing the patient to shiver.

   Type: _____

   Action: _____

4. The patient is fearful of being hooked up to wires for the procedure.

   Type: _____

   Action: _____

5. The electrolyte gel on the upper arm electrodes becomes dried out during the recording.

   Type: _____

   Action: _____

6. There are numerous electrical devices plugged into outlets in the room where an ECG is to be recorded.

   Type: _____

   Action: _____

7. The patient moves continuously during the recording.

   Type: _____

   Action: _____

8. The metal tip of a lead wire becomes detached during the recording.

   Type: _____

   Action: _____

9. The patient has Parkinson's disease.

   Type: _____

   Action: _____

10. The patient is wearing lotion on the upper arms and the electrodes will not adhere to the skin.

    Type: _____

    Action: _____

C. Myocardial Infarction

You are working for a cardiologist. Your provider is concerned about the increase in the numbers of patients having heart attacks. He asks you to design a colorful, creative, and informative brochure on heart attacks using the brochure provided on the following page. This brochure will be published and placed in the waiting room to provide patients with education about heart attacks. Heart disease Internet sites can be used to complete this activity.

FAQ
ON:

Q: A:

Q: A:

Q: A:

Q: A:

Q:

A:

Q:

A:

Illustration

Q:

A:

Q:

A:

D. Peak Flow Chart

Nancy Collins, 27 years of age, is at your medical office for an asthma check-up. At her last visit, your provider asked Nancy to measure her peak flow rate once a day in the morning before taking her asthma medication and to document her results on a peak flow chart. Nancy says she is not sure how to record results on the chart. She asks you to record her results and provides you with two weeks of measurements. Nancy also asks you to help her understand how to record her peak flow results. Complete the following:

1. Using the peak flow chart provided, record Nancy's peak flow results.
2. Using a classmate as a patient, explain how to document peak flow results.

Date	Peak Flow Results
10/1	410
10/2	440
10/3	440
10/4	430
10/5	420
10/6	410
10/7	390
10/8	380
10/9	360
10/10	350
10/11	370
10/12	400
10/13	420
10/14	430

PEAK FLOW CHART

Name _____

DATE																
TIME																
800																
750																
700																
650																
600																
550																
500																
450																
400																
350																
300																
250																
200																
150																
100																
50																
Peak Flow Number																

E. Crossword Puzzle: Cardiopulmonary Procedures

Directions: Complete the crossword puzzle using the clues provided.

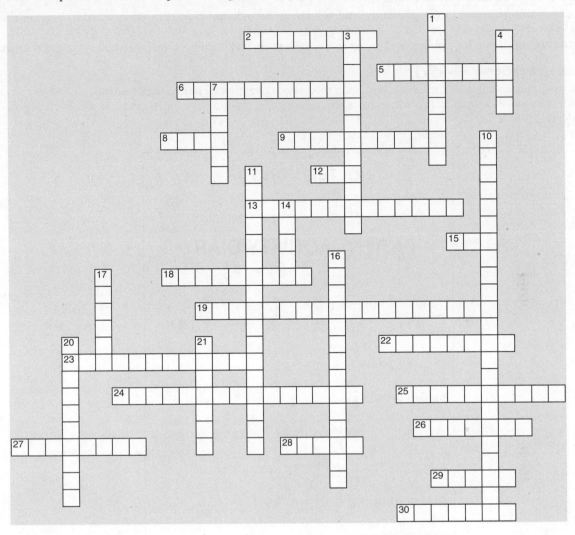

Across

2 Flat horizontal ECG line
5 Not enough blood
6 Irregular heart rhythm
8 Fourth intercostal to the left
9 Heart muscle layer
12 ECG std mark in mm
13 Drug for angina
15 Take a deep breath and blow it all out!
18 Asthma trigger
19 Separates O_2 out of air
22 Keep this blanket away from a Holter
23 Inflammation of heart's lining
24 Artery plaque condition
25 Lower heart chambers
26 Delivers asthma med
27 High-pitched whistling sound
28 Mighty big artery
29 Upper heart chambers
30 Primary cause of COPD

Down

1 Damaged alveoli disease
3 O_2 administration device
4 Atria contract
7 Pacemaker of the heart
10 Most serious dysrhythmia
11 "Too loose" electrodes cause this artifact
14 The ventricles are recovering
16 Drug that widens air passages
17 Not with a Holter on
20 "How well can you breathe" test
21 Leads I, II, III

Procedure 12-1: 12-Lead Electrocardiogram

1. Practice locating the six chest leads on five individuals. Select individuals of both genders and of varying ages and body contours.
2. Practice the procedure for running a 12-lead electrocardiogram, and document the procedure in the chart provided.

Procedure 12-2: Holter Monitor

1. Activity diary. Complete the patient information section on the Holter Activity Diary below.
2. Holter monitor. Practice the procedure for applying a Holter monitor, and document the procedure in the chart provided.

HOLTER MONITOR

PATIENT ACTIVITY DIARY

☐ 10 Hr.　　☐ 12 Hr.　　☐ 24 Hr.　　☐ 26 Hr.

Patient's Name: _____

Patient's Address: _____

_____

Age: _____ Sex: _____ Phone: _____

Date of Birth: _____ Soc. Sec. #: _____

Medication: _____

Doctor: _____ Phone: _____

Hospital: _____ Room: _____

Date of Recording: _____ Started: _____ AM PM

Serial Numbers
　Recorder: _____

　Battery: _____

Connected by: _____

_____

Procedure 12-3: Spirometry

Practice the procedure for performing a spirometry test, and document the procedure in the chart provided.

Procedure 12-4: Peak Flow Rate Measurement

Practice the procedure for measuring peak flow rate, and document the procedure in the chart provided.

CHART	
Date	

Procedure 12-1: Running a 12-Lead, Three-Channel Electrocardiogram

Name: _____ Date: _____

Evaluated by: _____ Score: _____

Performance Objective

Outcome:	Record a 12-lead electrocardiogram.
Conditions:	Using a three-channel electrocardiograph.
Standards:	Given ECG paper and disposable electrodes.
	Time: 15 minutes. Student completed procedure in _____ minutes.
	Accuracy: Satisfactory score on the Performance Evaluation Checklist.

Performance Evaluation Checklist

Trial 1	Trial 2	Point Value	Performance Standards
		•	Worked in a quiet atmosphere away from sources of electrical interference.
		•	Sanitized hands.
		•	Checked the expiration date of the electrodes.
		▷	Explained what may occur if the electrodes are outdated.
		•	Greeted the patient and introduced yourself.
		•	Identified the patient and explained the procedure.
		•	Instructed the patient that he or she will need to lie still, breathe normally, and not talk during the procedure.
		▷	Explained why the patient should lie still and not talk.
		•	Asked the patient to remove appropriate clothing.
		•	Assisted the patient into a supine position on the table.
		•	Made sure that the patient's arms and legs were adequately supported on the table.
		•	Draped the patient properly.
		•	Positioned the electrocardiograph with the power cord pointing away from the patient and not passing under the table.
		•	Worked on the left side of the patient.
		•	Prepared the patient's skin for application of the disposable electrodes.
		▷	Explained why the patient's skin must be prepared properly.
		•	Applied the limb electrodes.
		•	Properly located each chest position and applied the chest electrodes.
		▷	Explained why the tabs of the electrodes should be positioned correctly.
		•	Connected the lead wires to the electrodes.

Trial 1	Trial 2	Point Value	Performance Standards
		•	Arranged the lead wires to follow body contour.
		▷	Explained why the lead wires should follow body contour.
		•	Plugged the patient's cable into the machine and properly supported the cable.
		•	Turned on the electrocardiograph.
		•	Entered the patient's data using the soft-touch keypad.
		▷	Stated the purpose of entering the patient's data.
		•	Reminded the patient to lie still, and pressed the AUTO button to run the recording.
		•	Checked to make sure the standardization mark is 10 mm high.
		•	Checked to make sure the R wave has a positive deflection.
		▷	Stated what would cause the R wave to have a negative deflection.
		•	Observed the recording for artifacts and corrected the problem if they occurred.
		•	Informed the patient that he or she can move and talk.
		•	Turned off the electrocardiograph.
		•	Disconnected the lead wires.
		•	Removed and discarded the disposable electrodes.
		•	Assisted the patient from the table.
		•	Sanitized hands.
		•	Documented the procedure correctly.
		•	Placed the recording in the appropriate place to be reviewed by the provider.
		•	Returned equipment to proper place.
		■	Demonstrated critical thinking skills.
		■	Reassured patients.
		■	Demonstrated empathy for patients' concerns.
		★	Completed the procedure within 15 minutes.
			Totals

CHART

Date	

Evaluation of Student Performance

EVALUATION CRITERIA			COMMENTS
Symbol	**Category**	**Point Value**	
★	Critical Step	16 points	
•	Essential Step	6 points	
■	Affective Competency	6 points	
▷	Theory Question	2 points	

Score calculation: 100 points

    −   points missed

       Score

Satisfactory score: 85 or above

CAAHEP Competencies Achieved

Psychomotor (Skills)
- ☑ I. 2. a. Perform the following procedures: a. electrocardiography.
- ☑ I. 8. Instruct and prepare a patient for a procedure or a treatment.
- ☑ V. 2. Correctly use and pronounce medical terminology in health care interactions.

Affective (Behavior)
- ☑ A. 1. Demonstrate critical thinking skills.
- ☑ A. 2. Reassure patients.
- ☑ A. 3. Demonstrate empathy for patients' concerns.

ABHES Competencies Achieved

- ☑ 2. c. Identify diagnostic and treatment modalities as they relate to each body system.
- ☑ 7. g. Display professionalism through written and verbal communication.
- ☑ 8. e. Perform specialty procedures including but not limited to pediatric care, minor surgery, cardiac, respiratory, OB-GYN, neurological, and gastroenterology.

Procedure 12-2: Applying a Holter Monitor

Name: _____   Date: _____

Evaluated by: _____   Score: _____

Performance Objective

Outcome:	Apply a Holter monitor.
Conditions:	Using a Holter monitor with an internal memory card.
Standards:	Given the following: battery, disposable pouch and lanyard or a belt clip, disposable electrodes, razor, antiseptic wipes, gauze pads, abrasive pad, nonallergenic tape, and a patient diary.
	Time: 20 minutes.　　　　Student completed procedure in _____ minutes.
	Accuracy: Satisfactory score on the Performance Evaluation Checklist.

Performance Evaluation Checklist

Trial 1	Trial 2	Point Value	Performance Standards
		•	Assembled equipment.
		•	Installed a new battery.
		•	Checked the expiration date of the electrodes.
		•	Connected the Holter monitor to the computer.
		•	Entered the patient's demographic data into the computer and downloaded this information to the monitor.
		•	Sanitized hands.
		•	Greeted the patient and introduced yourself.
		•	Identified the patient and explained the procedure.
		•	Instructed the patient in the guidelines for wearing a Holter monitor.
		•	Asked the patient to remove clothing from the waist up.
		•	Positioned the patient in a sitting position.
		•	Located the chest electrode placement sites.
		•	Shaved the patient's chest at each electrode site, if needed.
		•	Rubbed the patient's skin with an alcohol wipe and allowed it to dry.
		•	Slightly abraded the skin.
		▷	Explained why the skin should be abraded.
		•	Attached a lead wire to the snap of each electrode.
		•	Properly applied the electrodes with an attached lead wire.
		▷	Explained why the electrodes should be firmly attached.
		•	Plugged the patient cable into the monitor and turned on the monitor.
		•	Checked the ECG signal quality.

583

Trial 1	Trial 2	Point Value	Performance Standards
		▷	Stated why the signal quality should be clear and strong.
		•	Placed tape over each electrode.
		•	Checked to make sure the date and time displayed on the monitor are accurate.
		•	Started the monitor.
		•	Placed the pouch around the patient's neck and inserted the monitor in the pouch.
		•	Instructed the patient to get dressed.
		•	Completed the patient information section of the diary.
		•	Documented the starting time in the patient diary.
		•	Provided the patient with instructions on completing the diary.
		•	Instructed the patient when to return for removal of the monitor.
		•	Sanitized hands.
		•	Documented the procedure correctly.
		■	Demonstrated critical thinking skills.
		■	Reassured patients.
		■	Demonstrated empathy for patients' concerns.
		★	Completed the procedure within 20 minutes.
			Totals

CHART

Date	

Evaluation of Student Performance

EVALUATION CRITERIA			COMMENTS
Symbol	**Category**	**Point Value**	
★	Critical Step	16 points	
•	Essential Step	6 points	
■	Affective Competency	6 points	
▷	Theory Question	2 points	

Score calculation: 100 points

       −   points missed

         ___ Score

Satisfactory score: 85 or above

CAAHEP Competencies Achieved

Psychomotor (Skills)
- ☑ I. 2. a. Perform the following procedures: a. electrocardiography.
- ☑ I. 8. Instruct and prepare a patient for a procedure or a treatment.
- ☑ V. 2. Correctly use and pronounce medical terminology in health care interactions.

Affective (Behavior)
- ☑ A. 1. Demonstrate critical thinking skills.
- ☑ A. 2. Reassure patients.
- ☑ A. 3. Demonstrate empathy for patients' concerns.

ABHES Competencies Achieved

- ☑ 2. c. Identify diagnostic and treatment modalities as they relate to each body system.
- ☑ 7. g. Display professionalism through written and verbal communication.
- ☑ 8. e. Perform specialty procedures including but not limited to pediatric care, minor surgery, cardiac, respiratory, OB-GYN, neurological, and gastroenterology.

Procedure 12-3: Spirometry Testing

Name: _____   Date: _____

Evaluated by: _____   Score: _____

Performance Objective

Outcome:	Perform a spirometry test.
Conditions:	Using a spirometer.
Standards:	Given the following: disposable tubing, disposable mouthpiece, disposable nose clips, and waste container.
	Time: 20 minutes. Student completed procedure in _____ minutes.
	Accuracy: Satisfactory score on the Performance Evaluation Checklist.

Performance Evaluation Checklist

Trial 1	Trial 2	Point Value	Performance Standards
		•	Sanitized hands.
		•	Assembled and prepared equipment.
		•	Calibrated the spirometer.
		▷	Stated the reason for calibrating the spirometer.
		•	Applied a disposable mouthpiece to the mouthpiece holder.
		•	Greeted the patient and introduced yourself.
		•	Identified the patient and explained the procedure.
		•	Asked the patient if he or she had prepared properly.
		•	Asked the patient to remove heavy or restrictive clothing, to loosen tight clothing, and to discard gum.
		▷	Explained why tight clothing should be loosened.
		•	Measured the patient's weight and height.
		▷	Explained the reason for measuring weight and height.
		•	Asked the patient to sit near the machine.
		•	Entered the patient's data into the computer database of the spirometer.
			Described and demonstrated the breathing maneuver:
		•	Relax and take the deepest breath possible.
		•	Place the mouthpiece in your mouth and seal your lips tightly around it.
		•	Blow out as hard as you can for as long as possible.
		•	Do not block the opening of the mouthpiece with your tongue.
		•	Remove the mouthpiece from your mouth.

587

Trial 1	Trial 2	Point Value	Performance Standards
		▷	Explained why the lips should be tightly sealed around the mouthpiece.
		•	Told the patient the instructions would be repeated during the test.
		•	Encouraged the patient to remain calm.
		•	Gently applied the nose clips.
		▷	Stated the purpose of the nose clips.
		•	Handed the mouthpiece to the patient.
		•	Began the test and actively coached the patient.
		•	Informed the patient of modifications needed if the breathing maneuver was not performed correctly.
		•	Continued the test until three acceptable efforts were obtained.
		•	Gently removed the nose clips from the patient's nose.
		•	Removed the mouthpiece from its holder.
		•	Disposed of the nose clips and mouthpiece in a waste container.
		•	Allowed the patient to remain seated for a few minutes.
		•	Sanitized your hands.
		•	Printed the report and labeled it.
		•	Documented the procedure correctly.
		•	Placed the spirometry report in an appropriate location for review by the provider.
		•	Cleaned the spirometer according to the manufacturer's instructions.
		■	Demonstrated critical thinking skills.
		■	Reassured patients.
		■	Demonstrated empathy for patients' concerns.
		★	Completed the procedure within 20 minutes.
			Totals

CHART

Date	

Evaluation of Student Performance

EVALUATION CRITERIA			COMMENTS
Symbol	**Category**	**Point Value**	
★	Critical Step	16 points	
•	Essential Step	6 points	
■	Affective Competency	6 points	
▷	Theory Question	2 points	

Score calculation: 100 points

−＿＿＿＿ points missed

＿＿＿Score

Satisfactory score: 85 or above

CAAHEP Competencies Achieved

Psychomotor (Skills)
- ☑ I. 2. d. Perform the following procedures: d. pulmonary function testing.
- ☑ I. 8. Instruct and prepare a patient for a procedure or a treatment.
- ☑ I. 10. Perform a quality control measure.
- ☑ 2. Correctly use and pronounce medical terminology in health care interactions.

Affective (Behavior)
- ☑ A. 1. Demonstrate critical thinking skills.
- ☑ B. Reassure patients.
- ☑ A. 3. Demonstrate empathy for patients' concerns.

ABHES Competencies Achieved

- ☑ 2. c. Identify diagnostic and treatment modalities as they relate to each body system.
- ☑ 7. g. Display professionalism through written and verbal communication.
- ☑ 8. e. Perform specialty procedures including but not limited to pediatric care, minor surgery, cardiac, respiratory, OB-GYN, neurological, and gastroenterology.
- ☑ 9. a. Practice quality control

Notes

EVALUATION OF COMPETENCY

Procedure 12-4: Measuring Peak Flow Rate

Name: _____   Date: _____

Evaluated by: _____   Score: _____

Performance Objective

Outcome:	Measure a patient's peak flow rate.
Conditions:	Using a spirometer.
Standards:	Given the following: disposable mouthpiece, waste container.
	Time: 15 minutes. Student completed procedure in _____ minutes.
	Accuracy: Satisfactory score on the Performance Evaluation Checklist.

Performance Evaluation Checklist

Trial 1	Trial 2	Point Value	Performance Standards
		•	Sanitized hands.
		•	Assembled and prepared equipment.
		•	Moved the sliding indicator to the bottom of the scale.
		▷	Stated why the indicator must be moved to the bottom of the scale.
		•	Applied a disposable mouthpiece to the mouthpiece holder.
		▷	Stated the purpose of the disposable mouthpiece.
		•	Greeted the patient and introduced yourself.
		•	Identified the patient and explained the procedure.
		•	Asked the patient to remove heavy or restrictive clothing, to loosen tight clothing, and to discard any gum.
			Described and demonstrated the breathing maneuver:
		•	Relax and take the deepest breath possible.
		•	Place the mouthpiece in your mouth and seal your lips tightly around it.
		•	Blow out as hard and fast as you can.
		•	Try to move the marker as high as you can on the scale.
		•	Do not block the opening of the mouthpiece with your tongue.
		•	Remove the mouthpiece from your mouth.
		•	Told the patient the instructions would be repeated during the test.
		•	Encouraged the patient to remain calm during the procedure.
		▷	Explained why the patient should remain calm.
		•	Placed a new disposable mouthpiece on the peak flow meter.
		•	Slid the marker to the bottom of the numbered scale.

591

Trial 1	Trial 2	Point Value	Performance Standards
		•	Handed the peak flow meter to the patient.
		•	Instructed the patient to stand up straight and look straight ahead.
		•	Began the test and actively coached the patient.
		•	Noted the number where the indicator stopped on the scale and jotted it down on a piece of paper.
		•	Informed the patient of modifications needed if the breathing maneuver was not performed correctly.
		•	Continued the test until three acceptable efforts were obtained.
		▷	Explained why three acceptable efforts must be obtained.
		•	The numbers from the three tests were about the same.
		▷	Stated the significance of the three numbers being about the same.
		•	Took the peak flow meter from the patient.
		•	Removed the mouthpiece from its holder and discarded it in a waste container.
		•	Sanitized your hands.
		•	Noted the highest of the three peak flow measurements.
		•	Documented the procedure correctly.
		•	Cleaned the peak flow meter.
		▷	Explained how to clean the peak flow meter.
		■	Demonstrated critical thinking skills.
		■	Reassured patients.
		■	Demonstrated empathy for patients' concerns.
		★	Completed the procedure within 15 minutes.
			Totals

CHART

Date	

Evaluation of Student Performance

EVALUATION CRITERIA			COMMENTS
Symbol	**Category**	**Point Value**	
★	Critical Step	16 points	
•	Essential Step	6 points	
■	Affective Competency	6 points	
▷	Theory Question	2 points	

Score calculation: 100 points

− _____ points missed

_____ Score

Satisfactory score: 85 or above

CAAHEP Competencies Achieved

Psychomotor (Skills)
- ☑ I. 2. d. Perform the following procedures: d. pulmonary function testing.
- ☑ I. 8. Instruct and prepare a patient for a procedure or a treatment.
- ☑ 2. Correctly use and pronounce medical terminology in health care interactions.

Affective (Behavior)
- ☑ A. 1. Demonstrate critical thinking skills.
- ☑ A. 2. Reassure patients.
- ☑ A. 3. Demonstrate empathy for patients' concerns.

ABHES Competencies Achieved

- ☑ 2. c. Identify diagnostic and treatment modalities as they relate to each body system.
- ☑ 7. g. Display professionalism through written and verbal communications.
- ☑ 8. e. Perform specialty procedures including but not limited to pediatric care, minor surgery, cardiac, respiratory, OB-GYN, neurological, and gastrocntcrology.

13 Colorectal and Male Reproductive Tests and Procedures

√ After Completing	Date Due	Study Guide Pages	STUDY GUIDE ASSIGNMENTS (CTA = Critical Thinking Activity)	Possible Points	Points You Earned
		599	Pretest	10	
		600	Term Key Term Assessment A. Definitions B. Word Parts (Add 1 point for each key term)	11 10	
		601-605	Evaluation of Learning questions	43	
		605	CTA A: gFOBT Patient Preparation	10	
		605-606	CTA B: Capsule Endoscopy (Each question is worth 5 points each)	25	
		606	CTA C: Cologuard Specimen Collection	10	
		607	CTA D: Colorectal Screening (Each space is worth 2 points each)	16	
		608	CTA E: Dear Gabby	10	
		609-610	CTA F: Crossword Puzzle	24	
			Evolve: Apply Your Knowledge questions	12	
			Evolve: Video Evaluation	18	
		599	Posttest	10	
			ADDITIONAL ASSIGNMENTS		
			Total points		

Notes

√ When Assigned by Your Instructor	Study Guide Pages	Practices Required	LABORATORY ASSIGNMENTS (Procedure Number and Name)	Score*
	611-612	5	**Practice for Competency** 13-1 and 13-2: Fecal Occult Blood Testing: Guaiac Slide Test Method and Developing the Hemoccult Slide Test	
	613-616		**Evaluation of Competency** 13-1 and 13-2: Fecal Occult Blood Testing: Guaiac Slide Test Method and Developing the Hemoccult Slide Test	*
	611-612	5	**Practice for Competency** 13-A: Testicular Self-Examination Instructions	
	617-618		**Evaluation of Competency** 13-A: Testicular Self-Examination Instructions	*
			ADDITIONAL ASSIGNMENTS	

Notes

Name: _____   Date: _____

True or False

_____ 1. Hemorrhoids can cause visible red blood to appear on the outside of the stool.

_____ 2. Nonvisible blood in the stool is called occult blood.

_____ 3. Colorectal cancer is a common form of cancer in individuals older than 50 years.

_____ 4. A blue color appearing on a Hemoccult test result is interpreted as a negative result.

_____ 5. If a Hemoccult test result is positive, the provider may order a colonoscopy.

_____ 6. The patient is placed in the prone position for a colonoscopy.

_____ 7. The function of the prostate gland is to produce sperm.

_____ 8. Most prostate cancers are slow growing.

_____ 9. A normal prostate gland feels firm and hard.

_____10. The most common sign of testicular cancer is a small, hard, painless lump on the testicle.

⌕ POSTTEST

True or False

_____ 1. Colorectal cancer usually starts from small precancerous polyps in the colon or rectum.

_____ 2. Consuming red meat may cause a false-positive result on a guaiac fecal occult blood test.

_____ 3. Ibuprofen should be avoided for 7 days before beginning a guaiac fecal occult blood test.

_____ 4. The Hemoccult test should be stored at room temperature after applying a stool specimen to it.

_____ 5. Patient preparation for a sigmoidoscopy includes partial bowel preparation.

_____ 6. After use, a sigmoidoscope must be autoclaved for 20 minutes.

_____ 7. Colonoscopy is performed for the early detection of colorectal cancer.

_____ 8. There are often no symptoms in the early stages of prostate cancer.

_____ 9. A prostate-specific antigen (PSA) level of 20 ng/mL is within normal range.

_____10. Testicular cancer occurs most commonly between the ages of 15 and 34 years.

A. Definitions

Directions: Match each key term with its definition.

_____ 1. Biopsy

_____ 2. Colonoscope

_____ 3. Colonoscopy

_____ 4. Endoscope

_____ 5. Insufflate

_____ 6. Occult blood

_____ 7. Peroxidase

_____ 8. Polyp

_____ 9. Screening

_____10. Sigmoidoscope

_____11. Sigmoidoscopy

A. The visualization of the rectum and the entire colon using a colono-scope

B. Blood occurring in such a small amount that it is not visually detect-able by the unaided eye

C. The surgical removal and examination of tissue from the living body

D. The visual examination of the rectum and sigmoid colon using a sig-moidoscope

E. An abnormal noncancerous growth that protrudes from the mucous membrane of the large intestine.

F. An instrument that consists of a tube and an optical system that is used for direct visual inspection of organs or cavities

G. A substance that is able to transfer oxygen from hydrogen peroxide to oxidize guaiac, causing the guaiac to turn blue

H. An endoscope that is specially designed for passage through the anus to permit visualization of the rectum and sigmoid colon

I. To blow a powder, vapor, or gas (such as air) into a body cavity

J. An endoscope that is specially designed for passage through the anus to permit visualization of the rectum and the entire length of the colon

K. The process of testing to detect disease in an individual who is not yet experiencing symptoms.

B. Word Parts

Directions: Indicate the meaning of each word part in the space provided. List as many medical terms as possible that incorporate the word part in the space provided.

Word Part	Meaning of Word Part	Medical Terms That Incorporate Word Part
1. bi/o		
2. -opsy		
3. colon/o		
4. -scopy		
5. -scope		
6. endo-		
7. -oxia		
8. -ase		
9. ox/I		
10. sigmoid/o		

Directions: Fill in each blank with the correct answer.

1. What conditions can be detected through colorectal tests and procedures?

   _____

   _____

2. List and describe the three parts of the large intestine.

   _____

   _____

   _____

3. What are the functions of the large intestine?

   _____

   _____

4. What is the function of the mucus secreted by the large intestine?

   _____

   _____

5. What is the reason for removing colorectal polyps?

   _____

6. What are the symptoms of colorectal cancer?

   _____

   _____

   _____

7. How does age affect the risk of developing colorectal cancer?

   _____

   _____

8. What are the American Cancer Society's age recommendations for colorectal cancer screening?

   _____

   _____

9. What conditions can cause a false-positive test result on a stool-based colorectal screening test?

   _____

   _____

10. What does it mean if a stool-based colorectal screening test is positive?

   _____

   _____

Chapter **13 Colorectal and Male Reproductive Tests and Procedures**

11. Why must three stool specimens be obtained for a gFOBT?

_____

12. Why is a patient placed on a high-fiber diet for a gFOBT?

_____

_____

13. What medications and vitamin supplements must be discontinued before a gFOBT?

_____

_____

14. What diagnostic tests may be performed if a stool-based colorectal screening test result is positive?

_____

15. Why is it important to perform quality-control methods when developing a gFOBT?

_____

16. How should a gFOBT be stored?

_____

_____

17. What factors can cause a failure of the expected control results to occur on a gFOBT?

_____

_____

18. How does a FIT detect blood in the stool?

_____

_____

19. What are the advantages of a FIT as compared to a gFOBT?

_____

_____

_____

20. What does a FIT-DNA test detect?

_____

_____

21. What is the purpose of performing a sigmoidoscopy?

_____

_____

_____

22. What patient preparation is required for a sigmoidoscopy during the following time parameters?

a. The day before the procedure and continuing until the examination is completed:

_____

_____

b. The evening before the procedure:

_____

_____

c. The day of the procedure:

_____

_____

23. What is the purpose of performing a digital rectal examination (DRE) before a sigmoidoscopy?

_____

_____

_____

24. What is the purpose of insufflating air into the colon during a sigmoidoscopy?

_____

_____

25. What is the purpose of suctioning during sigmoidoscopy?

_____

_____

26. What is the recommended position of the patient during flexible fiberoptic sigmoidoscopy?

_____

27. What parts of the colon are viewed during a colonoscopy?

_____

_____

28. When might a colonoscopy be performed?

_____

_____

29. What is the purpose of a full bowel preparation before a colonoscopy?

_____

_____

30. What does the provider do if the following are discovered during a colonoscopy?

a. Abnormal lesion: _____

b. Polyp: _____

603

31. What is the reason for removing a precancerous polyp during a colonoscopy?

_____

32. Where is the prostate gland located?

_____

_____

33. What are the symptoms of prostate cancer?

_____

_____

_____

34. How is the digital rectal examination used for the early detection of prostate cancer?

_____

_____

35. What do the following PSA levels mean?
   a. Below 4 ng/mL: _____
   b. 4 to 10 ng/mL: _____
   c. Above 10 ng/mL: _____

36. What conditions can cause an elevated PSA level?

_____

37. What patient preparation is required for a PSA test?

_____

_____

38. What tests may be ordered by the provider if the patient has positive prostate screening results?

_____

_____

39. What are the American Cancer Society recommendations for the PSA test and the DRE?

_____

_____

_____

40. When does testicular cancer most commonly occur?

_____

41. What are the risk factors for testicular cancer?

_____

_____

42. When is the best time for a male to perform a testicular self-examination (TSE) and why?

_____

_____

43. What is the most common sign of testicular cancer?

_____

CRITICAL THINKING ACTIVITIES

A. gFOBT Patient Preparation

1. Plan a dinner meal that should be consumed by a patient undergoing a gFOBT. Next to each food item, explain why you included it in the meal.

2. Plan a dinner meal for a patient undergoing a gFOBT that should **NOT** be consumed by a patient undergoing a gFOBT. Next to each food item, explain why the patient should not consume the food item before a gFOBT.

Dinner 1: _____

_____

_____

Dinner 2: _____

_____

_____

B. Capsule Endoscopy

Perform an Internet search for capsule endoscopy. Search for textual information and videos of this procedure. Based on your research, answer the following questions regarding this procedure.

1. What is capsule endoscopy?

_____

_____

_____

_____

_____

2. What conditions can be diagnosed using capsule endoscopy?

_____

_____

_____

3. What patient preparation is required for this procedure?

_____

_____

_____

4. What are the advantages of capsule endoscopy?

_____

_____

_____

5. What are the disadvantages of capsule endoscopy?

_____

_____

_____

_____

C. Cologuard Specimen Collection

For each of the following situations involving the collection of a specimen for a Cologuard test, write **C** if the technique is correct and **I** if it is incorrect.

_____ 1. The Cologuard kit is past its expiration date so the patient contacts the Cologuard laboratory and requests another one.

_____ 2. A patient receives the Cologuard kit and stores it in the refrigerator.

_____ 3. A patient has diarrhea and therefore does not collect the stool specimen until it is gone.

_____ 4. A patient collects the stool specimen during her menstrual period.

_____ 5. A patient accidentally voids some urine into the collection container.

_____ 6. A patient collects an entire bowel movement in the large container included in the kit.

_____ 7. A patient accidentally spills some of the preservative onto her arm and wipes it off with a tissue.

_____ 8. A patient collects a small sample from the bowel movement by scraping the surface of the stool with the probe.

_____ 9. A patient forgets to pour the preservative over the stool specimen before mailing it back the Cologuard laboratory.

_____10. A patient mails the specimen to the Cologuard laboratory 3 days following collection.

606

D. Colorectal Screening

There are advantages and disadvantages to each type of colorectal screening method. Using your textbook and Internet reference sites, indicate these advantages and disadvantages in the chart provided.

Colorectal Screening Method	Advantages	Disadvantages
gFOBT		
FIT		
FIT-DNA test (Cologuard)		
Colonoscopy		

E. Dear Gabby

Gabby broke her wrist while ice skating and wants you to fill in for her. In the space provided, respond to the following letter using the knowledge you have acquired in this chapter.

Dear Gabby:

I am 15 years old, and my mom just took me to a new doctor for a sports physical examination. I am going to play football this fall at my high school. Before this, I had always gone to the doctor I had since I was little, but I had to switch because I am getting older. After the doctor did my physical, he told me that I needed to examine my testicles every month and that the medical assistant would be in to explain how this is done.

Gabby, I was totally shocked, and you can bet I got out of that office before she had a chance to do that. I am too embarrassed to ask my parents about this. Gabby, what is going on? I am only 15 years old. Are my parents taking me to a quack, and should I report this to someone?

Signed,
Don't Know What to Do

_____

_____

_____

_____

_____

_____

_____

608

Directions: Complete the crossword puzzle using the clues provided.

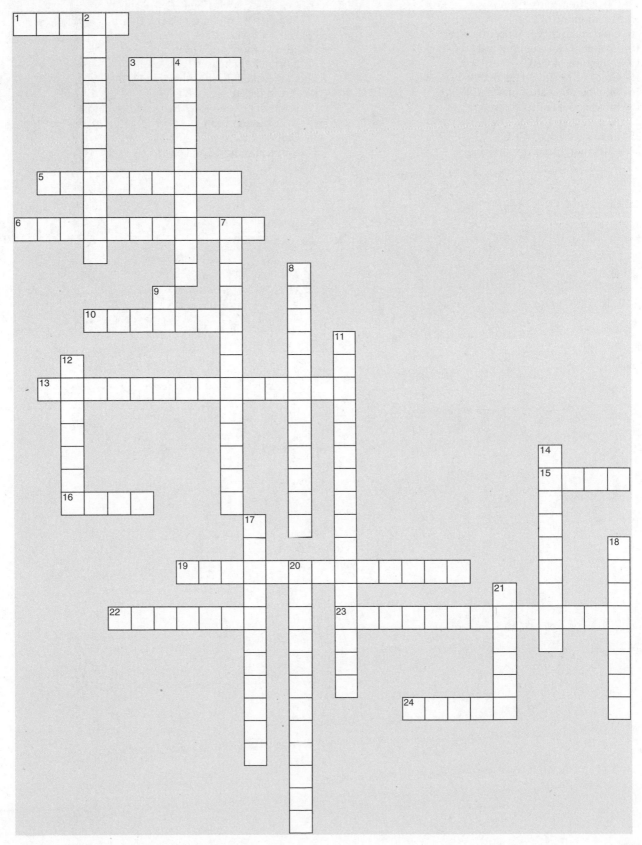

609

Across

1 Majority of large intestine
3 CRC often starts from this
5 Brand name of FIT-DNA test
6 Gold standard for detecting CRC
10 Prostate CA screening test
13 Symptom of CRC
15 Color of positive Hemoccult
16 May be done after elevated PSA
19 Flushes out entire colon
22 Age to start TSE
23 Increases risk of CRC
24 CRC increases after this age

Down

2 Hidden blood
4 Leading cause of male CA deaths
7 Secretes fluid that transports sperm
8 Has an S-shape
9 How to store a gFOBT
11 Normally increases PSA level
12 Can cause false-positive on gFOBT
14 Avoid before a gFOBT
17 Endoscope used to visualize entire colon
18 Attaches to cecum
20 Cause of an invalid gFOBT
21 Surgical removal and exam of tissue

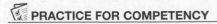 **PRACTICE FOR COMPETENCY**

Procedures 13-1 and 13-2: Fecal Occult Blood Testing: Guaiac Slide Test Method

1. Patient instructions. Instruct the patient in the specimen collection procedure for a fecal occult blood test (e.g., Hemoccult). Document these instructions in the chart provided.
2. Developing the test. Develop a fecal occult blood test, and document the results in the chart provided.

Procedure 13-A: Testicular Self-Examination

Instruct an individual in the procedure for performing a testicular self-examination, and document the procedure in the chart provided.

CHART	
Date	

611

CHART	
Date	

Chapter **13** **Colorectal and Male Reproductive Tests and Procedures**

Procedures 13-1 and 13-2: Fecal Occult Blood Testing: Guaiac Slide Test Method and Developing the Fecal Occult Blood Test

Name: _____   Date: _____

Evaluated by: _____   Score: _____

Performance Objective

Outcome:	Instruct an individual in the specimen collection procedure for a Hemoccult slide test and develop the test.
Conditions:	Given the following: Hemoccult kit, disposable gloves, developing solution, and a waste container.
Standards:	Time: 15 minutes. Student completed procedures in _____ minutes.
	Accuracy: Satisfactory score on the Performance Evaluation Checklist.

Performance Evaluation Checklist

Trial 1	Trial 2	Point Value	Performance Standards
			Instructions for the Hemoccult slide test
		•	Obtained the Hemoccult slide testing kit.
		•	Checked the expiration date on the slides.
		▷	Described what may occur if the slides are outdated.
		•	Greeted the patient and introduced yourself.
		•	Identified the patient and explained the purpose of the test.
		•	Informed the patient when the test should not be performed.
		•	Instructed the patient in the proper preparation required for the test.
		•	Encouraged the patient to adhere to the diet modifications.
		▷	Explained why the patient should follow the diet modifications.
		•	Provided the patient with the Hemoccult slide test kit.
		•	Instructed the patient in completion of the information on the front flap of each card.
		•	Provided instructions on the proper care and storage of the slides.
		▷	Explained why the slides must be stored properly.
			Instructed the patient in the initiation of the test
		•	Began the diet modifications.
		•	Collected a stool specimen from the first bowel movement after the 3-day preparatory period.
			Instructed the patient in the collection of the stool specimen
		•	Filled in the collection date on the front flap.
		•	Used a clean, dry container to collect the stool specimen.

613

Trial 1	Trial 2	Point Value	Performance Standards
		•	Collected the stool sample before it came in contact with toilet bowl water.
		•	Used the wooden applicator to obtain a specimen from one part of the stool.
		•	Opened the front flap of the first cardboard slide.
		•	Spread a thin smear of the specimen over the filter paper in the square labeled A.
		•	Obtained another specimen from a different area of the stool by using the other end of the applicator.
		•	Spread a thin smear of the specimen over the filter paper in the square labeled B.
		•	Closed the front flap of the cardboard slide and filled in the date.
		•	Discarded the applicator in a waste container.
		▷	Explained why a sample is collected from two different parts of the stool.
		•	Instructed the patient to place the slides in a regular envelope to air-dry overnight.
		•	Instructed the patient to continue the testing period on 3 different days until all three specimens have been obtained.
		•	Instructed the patient to place the cardboard slides in the foil envelope and return them to the medical office.
		•	Provided the patient with an opportunity to ask questions.
		•	Made sure the patient understood the instructions.
		•	Documented the procedure correctly.
			Developing the Hemoccult slide test
		•	Assembled equipment.
		•	Checked the expiration date on the developing solution bottle.
		▷	Explained how the solution should be stored.
		•	Sanitized hands and applied gloves.
		•	Opened the back flap of the cardboard slides.
		•	Applied 2 drops of the developing solution to the guaiac test paper underlying the back of each smear.
		•	Did not allow the developing solution to come in contact with skin or eyes.
		•	Read results within 60 seconds.
		★	The results were identical to the evaluator's results.
		▷	Explained why the slides should be read within 60 seconds.
		•	Performed the quality control procedure on each slide.
		•	Read the quality control results after 10 seconds.
		★	The results were identical to the evaluator's results.
		▷	Described what is observed during a normal positive and negative control reaction.

Trial 1	Trial 2	Point Value	Performance Standards
		▷	Stated the purpose of the quality control procedure.
		•	Properly disposed of the slides in a regular waste container.
		•	Removed gloves and sanitized hands.
		•	Documented the results correctly.
		■	Demonstrated critical thinking skills.
		■	Reassured patients.
		■	Demonstrated tactfulness.
		★	Completed the procedure within 15 minutes.
			Totals

CHART

Date	

Evaluation of Student Performance

EVALUATION CRITERIA			COMMENTS
Symbol	**Category**	**Point Value**	
★	Critical Step	16 points	
•	Essential Step	6 points	
■	Affective Competency	6 points	
▷	Theory Question	2 points	

Score calculation: 100 points

− _____ points missed

_____ Score

Satisfactory score: 85 or above

CAAHEP Competencies Achieved

Psychomotor (Skills)
- ☑ I. 10. Perform a quality control measure.
- ☑ II. 2. Record laboratory test results into the patient's record.
- ☑ IV. 1. Instruct a patient regarding a dietary change related to a patient's special dietary needs.
- ☑ V. 3. Coach patients regarding a. office policies b. medical encounters.

Affective (Behavior)
- ☑ A. 1. Demonstrate critical thinking skills.
- ☑ A. 2. Reassure patients.
- ☑ A. 7. Demonstrate tactfulness.

ABHES Competencies Achieved

- ☑ 7. g. Display professionalism through written and verbal communications.
- ☑ 8. e. Perform specialty procedures including but not limited to pediatric care, minor surgery, cardiac, respiratory, OB-GYN, neurological, and gastroenterology.
- ☑ 9. a. Practice quality control.
- ☑ 9. e. (2). Instruct patients in the collection of fecal specimen.

EVALUATION OF COMPETENCY

Procedure 13-A: Testicular Self-Examination Instructions

Name: _____ Date: _____

Evaluated by: _____ Score: _____

Performance Objective

Outcome:	Instruct an individual in the procedure for performing a testicular self-examination (TSE).
Conditions:	None.
Standards:	Time: 10 minutes. Student completed procedure in _____ minutes.
	Accuracy: Satisfactory score on the Performance Evaluation Checklist.

Performance Evaluation Checklist

Trial 1	Trial 2	Point Value	Performance Standards
		•	Greeted the patient and introduced yourself.
		•	Identified the patient and explained that you will be instructing the patient in a TSE.
		•	Explained the purpose of the examination and when to perform it.
			Instructed the patient as follows:
		•	Take a warm bath or shower.
		•	Stand in front of a mirror.
		•	Inspect for any swelling of the skin of the scrotum.
		•	Place the index and middle fingers of both hands on the underside of one testicle and the thumbs on top of the testicle.
		•	Apply a small amount of pressure, and gently roll the testicle between the thumbs and fingers of both hands.
		•	Palpate for lumps, swelling, or any change in the size, shape, or consistency of the testicle.
		▷	Stated the normal characteristics of a testicle.
		•	Locate the epididymis so that you do not confuse it with a lump.
		▷	Stated the characteristics and function of the epididymis.
		•	Repeat the examination on the other testicle.
		•	Report any abnormalities to the provider.
		▷	Stated examples of abnormalities that should be reported.
		•	Documented the procedure correctly.

Chapter **13** Colorectal and Male Reproductive Tests and Procedures

Trial 1	Trial 2	Point Value	Performance Standards
		■	Demonstrated critical thinking skills.
		■	Demonstrated empathy for patients' concerns.
		■	Demonstrated tactfulness.
		★	Completed the procedure within 10 minutes.
			Totals

CHART

Date	

Evaluation of Student Performance

EVALUATION CRITERIA			COMMENTS
Symbol	**Category**	**Point Value**	
★	Critical Step	16 points	
•	Essential Step	6 points	
■	Affective Competency	6 points	
▷	Theory Question	2 points	

Score calculation: 100 points

  − _____ points missed

  _____ Score

Satisfactory score: 85 or above

CAAHEP Competencies Achieved

Psychomotor (Skills)
☑ V. 4. Coach patients regarding a. office policies b. medical encounters.

Affective (Behavior)
☑ A. 1. Demonstrate critical thinking skills.
☑ A. 3. Demonstrate empathy for patients' concerns.
☑ A. 7. Demonstrate tactfulness.

ABHES Competencies Achieved

☑ 7. g. Display professionalism through written and verbal communications.
☑ 8. h. Teach self-examination, disease management and health promotion.

Radiology and Diagnostic Imaging

CHAPTER ASSIGNMENTS

√ After Completing	Date Due	Study Guide Pages	STUDY GUIDE ASSIGNMENTS (CTA = Critical Thinking Activity)	Possible Points	Points You Earned
		623	? Pretest	10	
		624	Term Key Term Assessment A. Definitions B. Word Parts	13 15	
		625–629	Evaluation of Learning questions	46	
		629	CTA A: Instructions for a Lower GI Radiograph	5	
		630	CTA B: Intravenous Pyelogram	5	
		630	CTA C: Magnetic Resonance Imaging	6	
		631	CTA D: Crossword Puzzle	29	
			Evolve: Apply Your Knowledge questions	10	
		623	? Posttest	10	
			ADDITIONAL ASSIGNMENTS		
			Total points		

√ When Assigned by Your Instructor	Study Guide Pages	Practices Required	LABORATORY ASSIGNMENTS (Procedure Number and Name)	Score*
	632-633	3	**Practice for Competency** 14-A: Radiographic Examination Guidelines	
	634-635		**Evaluation of Competency** 14-A: Radiographic Examination Guidelines	*
	632-633	3	**Practice for Competency** 14-B: Diagnostic Imaging Guidelines	
	636-637		**Evaluation of Competency** 14-B: Diagnostic Imaging Guidelines	*
			ADDITIONAL ASSIGNMENTS	

Notes

Name: _____   Date: _____

True or False

_____ 1. A radiologist is a medical doctor specializing in the diagnosis and treatment of disease using radiation and other imaging techniques.

_____ 2. The permanent record of the picture produced on x-ray film is a sonogram.

_____ 3. The purpose of a contrast medium is to make a structure visible on a radiograph.

_____ 4. The patient should be instructed not to wear lotions, powders, or deodorants when having a mammogram.

_____ 5. Mammography can be used to detect breast calcifications.

_____ 6. An upper gastrointestinal (GI) examination assists in diagnosing kidney stones.

_____ 7. An IVP is a radiograph of the kidneys, ureters, and bladder.

_____ 8. Ultrasonography allows for continuous viewing of a structure.

_____ 9. Obstetric ultrasound can be used to determine the gestational age of a fetus.

_____10. A patient must remove all metal before undergoing MRI.

?≡ POSTTEST _____

True or False

_____ 1. Wilhelm Roentgen discovered x-rays in 1895.

_____ 2. Bone is an example of a radiolucent structure.

_____ 3. An instrument used to view internal organs directly in real time is a fluoroscope.

_____ 4. The patient should be instructed not to move during a radiographic examination to prevent blurring of the images on the radiograph.

_____ 5. The breasts must be compressed during mammography to obtain a clear radiograph.

_____ 6. After an upper GI study is performed, the barium causes the stool to have a whitish color for 2 to 3 weeks.

_____ 7. Gas must be removed from the colon before a lower GI study to prevent confusing shadows on the radiograph.

_____ 8. Before performing an IVP, the patient must be asked whether he or she is allergic to penicillin.

_____ 9. Computed tomography produces a series of cross-sectional images.

_____10. A radioactive material is introduced into the body before a nuclear medicine imaging procedure is performed.

A. Definitions

Directions: Match each key term with its definition.

_____ 1. Contrast medium	A. The permanent image produced by x-rays on a radiosensitive receptor device such as a digital detector or radiographic film.
_____ 2. Echocardiogram	B. A provider who specializes in the diagnosis and treatment of disease using radiation and other imaging techniques.
_____ 3. Enema	C. A substance used to make a particular structure visible on a radiograph
_____ 4. Fluoroscope	D. The record obtained with ultrasonography.
_____ 5. Fluoroscopy	E. An injection of fluid into the rectum to aid in the elimination of feces from the colon.
_____ 6. Radiograph	F. The branch of medicine that deals with the use of radiation and other imaging techniques to diagnose and treat disease.
_____ 7. Radiography	G. An instrument used to view internal organs and structures directly in real time.
_____ 8. Radiologist	H. Describing a structure that obstructs the passage of x-rays.
_____ 9. Radiology	I. The taking of permanent records of internal body organs and structures by passing x-rays through the body to act on a radiosensitive receptor device.
_____10. Radiolucent	J. Describing a structure that permits the passage of x-rays.
_____11. Radiopaque	K. An x-ray procedure for viewing internal organs and structures directly in real time.
_____12. Sonogram	L. An ultrasound examination of the heart.
_____13. Ultrasonography	M. The use of high-frequency sound waves to produce an image of an organ or tissue.

B. Word Parts

Directions: Indicate the meaning of each word part in the space provided. List as many medical terms as possible that incorporate the word part in the space provided.

Word Part	Meaning of Word Part	Medical Terms That Incorporate Word Part
1. ech/o		
2. cardi/o		
3. -gram		
4. fluor/o		
5. -scope		
6. -scopy		
7. radi/o		
8. -graph		
9. -graphy		
10. -ologist		
11. -ology		
12. -lucent		
13. -opaque		
14. son/o		
15. ultra-		

Directions: Fill in each blank with the correct answer.

1. Who discovered x-rays?

   _____

2. What is the function of x-rays?

   _____

   _____

3. Why is it important for a patient to prepare properly for a radiographic examination?

   _____

   _____

4. What are the two ways in which radiographs can be taken?

   _____

5. What are the advantages of digital radiography?

   _____

   _____

6. What is the function of a radiopaque contrast medium?

   _____

   _____

7. What are the various ways in which a contrast medium can be administered to a patient?

   _____

   _____

8. Why is barium sulfate frequently used as a contrast medium for examination of the GI tract?

   _____

9. Why should a patient not move during a radiographic examination?

   _____

10. What is the purpose of mammography?

   _____

   _____

11. Why should the patient be instructed not to wear lotions, powders, or deodorants when having a mammogram?

   _____

   _____

625

12. Why must the breasts be compressed during mammography?

_____

_____

13. What is the purpose of a bone density scan?

_____

_____

14. What is osteoporosis?

_____

_____

15. Who is at particular risk for osteoporosis?

_____

16. What information is provided by DXA bone density measurements?

_____

_____

_____

17. What patient preparation is required for a bone density scan?

_____

_____

18. What areas are typically scanned during a DXA scan, and why are these areas scanned?

_____

_____

19. What is the purpose of an upper GI radiographic examination?

_____

_____

20. Why must the GI tract be free of food and fluid before an upper GI radiographic examination is performed?

_____

_____

21. How can the patient prevent constipation after an upper GI examination?

_____

_____

22. What conditions can be diagnosed through a lower GI radiographic examination?

_____

_____

23. Why is it important to remove gas and fecal material from the colon before a lower GI radiographic examination?

_____

_____

24. What is the advantage of the air used with a double-contrast study of the lower GI tract?

_____

_____

25. What is an intravenous pyelogram (IVP)?

_____

_____

26. What conditions can be diagnosed with an IVP?

_____

_____

27. What may the patient experience during an IVP when the iodine enters the bloodstream?

_____

_____

28. Describe the following radiographic examinations:

a. Angiocardiogram: _____

_____

_____

b. Bronchogram: _____

_____

_____

c. Cerebral angiogram: _____

_____

_____

d. Chest radiograph: _____

_____

e. Coronary angiogram: _____

_____

_____

f. Cystogram: _____

_____

_____

Chapter **14** **Radiology and Diagnostic Imaging**

29. What conditions can be detected using ultrasound?

_____

_____

30. What can be determined with an echocardiogram?

_____

_____

31. What are the advantages of ultrasonography?

_____

_____

32. What is the purpose of the gel used with ultrasonography?

_____

_____

33. What is the purpose for performing an obstetric ultrasound?

_____

_____

_____

34. Doppler ultrasound assists in the diagnosis of what conditions?

_____

_____

35. What type of image is produced by computed tomography?

_____

36. What are the primary uses of computed tomography?

_____

_____

37. What type of patient preparation is required for computed tomography?

_____

_____

38. What are the primary uses of magnetic resonance imaging (MRI)?

_____

_____

39. What items must the patient remove before having an MRI scan?

_____

_____

40. What material is used with a nuclear medicine diagnostic imaging procedure?

_____

41. What is the function of a gamma camera used in nuclear medicine?

_____

_____

42. What is the purpose of performing a bone scan?

_____

_____

43. What is a "hot spot" on a bone scan?

_____

_____

44. What is a nuclear cardiac stress test?

_____

_____

45. Describe the two phases of a nuclear cardiac stress test.

_____

_____

46. What can be diagnosed with a PET scan?

_____

CRITICAL THINKING ACTIVITIES

A. Instructions for a Lower GI Radiograph

Trent Douglas has been having pain in his lower abdomen and occult blood in his stool. Dr. Hartman tells you to schedule him for a lower GI radiographic examination at Grant Hospital. In the space provided, explain how you would instruct Mr. Douglas to prepare for this examination. Include the patient preparation and the reason for each of the measures. (Note: The procedure does not require enemas.)

_____

_____

_____

_____

_____

_____

B. Intravenous Pyelogram

Dr. Tristen instructs you to schedule Ellie Ray for an intravenous pyelogram (IVP) at Grant Hospital. After you have explained to Ms. Ray the instructions for preparing for the examination, she asks you the following questions. Respond to them in the space provided.

1. What body structures will be "x-rayed" during the examination?

   _____

2. Why must I perform an enema before the exam?

   _____

   _____

3. Why will iodine be injected into my veins?

   _____

4. Will I feel anything when the iodine is injected?

   _____

   _____

5. What is done if an individual is allergic to iodine?

   _____

   _____

C. Magnetic Resonance Imaging

Jason Zindra, a college baseball player, has been experiencing pain in his left shoulder joint. Dr. Baker schedules him for magnetic resonance imaging (MRI) of the left shoulder. Jason asks you the following questions regarding this procedure. Respond to them in the space provided.

1. Will there be any pain involved with this procedure?

   _____

2. Will I be exposed to x-rays?

   _____

   _____

3. May I wear my eyeglasses during the procedure?

   _____

4. Does the MRI machine make any noise?

   _____

5. Will I be able to move during the procedure?

   _____

   _____

6. Will the technician be in the room with me?

   _____

   _____

D. Crossword Puzzle: Radiology and Diagnostic Imaging

Directions: Complete the crossword puzzle using the clues provided.

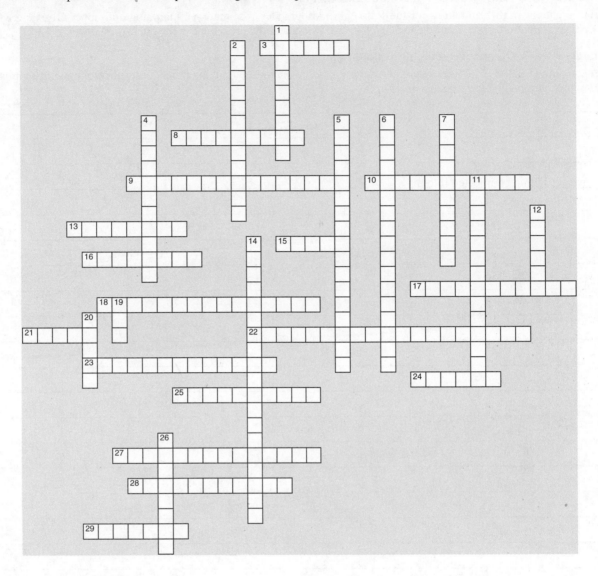

Across

3 Contrast medium example
8 Urinary bladder radiograph
9 Detects osteoporosis
10 View internal organs directly
13 Discovered x-rays
15 Eliminates feces from colon
16 Detects stress fractures
17 Permits passage of x-rays
18 Converts x-rays to electronic signals
21 Remove during an MRI
22 Can tell if it's twins
23 Bile ducts radiograph
24 Produces cross-sectional images
25 Obstructs x-rays
27 US of heart
28 Lung radiograph
29 Diagnoses brain cancer and heart disease

Down

1 Breast radiograph
2 Loss of bone calcium
4 X-ray doctor
5 Coronary artery radiograph
6 Diagnoses blood flow blockages
7 X-ray image
11 May occur during MRI
12 IVP contrast medium
14 Uterus and fallopian tubes radiograph
19 Diagnoses kidney stones
20 Color of radiolucent structure
26 US recording

631

Procedure 14-A: Radiographic Examination Guidelines

Instruct a patient in the guidelines for the following radiographic examinations: mammogram, upper GI examination, lower GI examination, and an intravenous pyelogram. Document the procedure in the chart provided.

Procedure 14-B: Diagnostic Imaging Guidelines

Instruct a patient in the guidelines required for the following diagnostic imaging procedures: ultrasonography, computed tomography, and magnetic resonance imaging.

CHART	
Date	

CHART	
Date	

Procedure 14-A: Radiographic Examinations Guidelines

Name: _____ Date: _____

Evaluated by: _____ Score: _____

Performance Objective

Outcome:	Instruct a patient in the guidelines required for the following radiographic examinations: mammogram, upper GI examination, lower GI examination, and an intravenous pyelogram.
Conditions:	Given the following: a patient instruction sheet for each radiographic examination.
Standards:	Time: 15 minutes. Student completed procedure in _____ minutes.
	Accuracy: Satisfactory score in the Performance Evaluation Checklist.

Performance Evaluation Checklist

Trial 1	Trial 2	Point Value	Performance Standards
		•	Greeted and identified the patient.
		•	Introduced yourself.
			Instructed the patient in the proper preparation for each of the following radiographic examinations:
		•	Mammogram
		•	Upper GI examination
		•	Lower GI examination
		•	Intravenous pyelogram
		•	Documented the procedure correctly.
		■	Reassured patients.
		■	Demonstrated empathy for patients' concerns.
		★	Completed the procedure within 15 minutes.
			Totals

CHART	
Date	

Evaluation of Student Performance

EVALUATION CRITERIA			COMMENTS
Symbol	**Category**	**Point Value**	
★	Critical Step	16 points	
•	Essential Step	6 points	
■	Affective Competency	6 points	
▷	Theory Question	2 points	

Score calculation: 100 points

      − _____ points missed

      _____ Score

Satisfactory score: 85 or above

CAAHEP Competencies Achieved

Psychomotor (Skills)
☑ I. 8. Instruct and prepare a patient for a procedure or a treatment.
☑ IV. 1. Instruct a patient regarding a dietary change related to a patient's special dietary needs.
☑ V. 2. Correctly use and pronounce medical terminology in health care interactions.

Affective (Behavior)
☑ A. 2. Reassure patients.
☑ A. 3. Demonstrate empathy for patients' concerns.

ABHES Competencies Achieved

☑ 2. c. Identify diagnostic and treatment modalities as they relate to each body system.
☑ 7. g. Display professionalism through written and verbal communication.

Procedure 14-B: Diagnostic Imaging Guidelines

Name: _____   Date: _____

Evaluated by: _____   Score: _____

Performance Objective

Outcome:	Instruct a patient in the guidelines required the following diagnostic imaging procedures: ultrasonography, computed tomography, and magnetic resonance imaging.
Conditions:	Given the following: a patient instruction sheet for each diagnostic imaging procedure.
Standards:	Time: 15 minutes. Student completed procedure in _____ minutes
	Accuracy: Satisfactory score in the Performance Evaluation Checklist.

Performance Evaluation Checklist

Trial 1	Trial 2	Point Value	Performance Standards
		•	Greeted and identified the patient.
		•	Introduced yourself.
			Instructed patient in the proper preparation for each of the following diagnostic imaging procedures:
		•	Ultrasonography
		•	Computed tomography
		•	Magnetic resonance imaging
		•	Nuclear medicine
		•	Documented the procedure correctly.
		■	Reassured patients.
		■	Demonstrated empathy for patients' concern.
		★	Completed the procedure within 15 minutes.
			Totals

CHART	
Date	

Evaluation of Student Performance

EVALUATION CRITERIA			COMMENTS
Symbol	**Category**	**Point Value**	
★	Critical Step	16 points	
•	Essential Step	6 points	
■	Affective Competency	6 points	
▷	Theory Question	2 points	

Score calculation: 100 points

−＿＿＿ points missed

＿＿＿Score

Satisfactory score: 85 or above

CAAHEP Competencies Achieved

Psychomotor (Skills)
☑ I. 8. Instruct and prepare a patient for a procedure or a treatment.
☑ IV. 1. Instruct a patient regarding a dietary change related to a patient's special dietary needs.
☑ V. 2. Correctly use and pronounce medical terminology in health care interactions.

Affective (Behavior)
☑ A. 2. Reassure patients.
☑ A. 3. Demonstrate empathy for patients' concerns.

ABHES Competencies Achieved

☑ 2. c. Identify diagnostic and treatment modalities as they relate to each body system.
☑ 7. g. Display professionalism through written and verbal communication.

CHAPTER ASSIGNMENTS

√ After Completing	Date Due	Study Guide Pages	STUDY GUIDE ASSIGNMENTS (CTA = Critical Thinking Activity)	Possible Points	Points You Earned
		643	Pretest	10	
		644	Term Key Term Assessment	23	
		645-651	Evaluation of Learning questions	60	
		651-652	CTA A: Triglycerides Test Requirements	10	
		653	CTA B: Laboratory Test Directory	20	
		653	CTA C: Identifying Abnormal Values	10	
		653	CTA D: Laboratory Report	14	
		654	CTA E: Patient Test Information	14	
		655	CTA F: Test Kit Package Insert (3 points for each section)	42	
		656-657	CTA G: Crossword Puzzle	32	
			Evolve: Road to Recovery: Laboratory Test Categories (Record points earned)		
			Evolve: Apply Your Knowledge questions	10	
		643	Posttest	10	
			ADDITIONAL ASSIGNMENTS		
			Total points		

√ When Assigned by Your Instructor	Study Guide Pages	Practices Required	LABORATORY ASSIGNMENTS (Procedure Number and Name)	Score*
	658	2	**Practice for Competency** 15-1: Operate an Emergency Eyewash Station	
	662-664		☑ **Evaluation of Competency** 15-1: Operate an Emergency Eyewash Station	*
	659-661	3	**Practice for Competency** 15-A: Collecting a Specimen for Transport to an Outside Laboratory	
	665-666		☑ **Evaluation of Competency** 15-A: Collecting a Specimen for Transport to an Outside Laboratory	*

Notes

Name: _____   Date: _____

True or False

_____ 1. When the body is in homeostasis, an imbalance exists in the body.

_____ 2. A screening test is performed on healthy individuals to assist in the early detection of disease.

_____ 3. A laboratory request form provides the outside laboratory with information needed for accurate testing and reporting of results.

_____ 4. The clinical diagnosis is indicated on a laboratory request to correlate laboratory data with the needs of the provider.

_____ 5. The purpose of a laboratory report is to indicate the patient's diagnosis.

_____ 6. A patient who is fasting in preparation for a laboratory test is permitted to drink diet soda.

_____ 7. A specimen is a small sample taken from the body to represent the nature of the whole.

_____ 8. A laboratory report marked QNS indicates the patient did not prepare properly.

_____ 9. Fecal occult blood testing is an example of a CLIA-waived test.

_____10. The purpose of quality control is to prevent accidents in the laboratory.

?⃞ **POSTTEST**

True or False

_____ 1. Laboratory test results are most frequently used to assist in the diagnosis of a patient's condition.

_____ 2. The test menu of a laboratory directory is an alphabetical listing of all the tests performed by the outside laboratory.

_____ 3. A panel consists of a combination of laboratory tests.

_____ 4. A lipid panel includes a glucose test.

_____ 5. The purpose of patient preparation for a laboratory test is to ensure that the test results fall within the reference range.

_____ 6. A comprehensive metabolic panel requires that the patient undergoes fasting.

_____ 7. Antibiotics taken by the patient before the collection of a throat specimen for a culture may produce a false-positive test result.

_____ 8. The purpose of CLIA is to prevent exposure of employees to bloodborne pathogens.

_____ 9. A laboratory performing nonwaived tests must be certified by CLIA and adhere to the CLIA regulations.

_____10. A qualitative test result indicates the exact amount of an analyte present in the body.

Chapter **15** **Introduction to the Clinical Laboratory**

Directions: Match each key term with its definition.

_____ 1. Analyte

_____ 2. Calibration

_____ 3. CLIA nonwaived test

_____ 4. CLIA waived test

_____ 5. Clinical diagnosis

_____ 6. Clinical laboratory

_____ 7. Control

_____ 8. Critical value

_____ 9. Fasting

_____ 10. Homeostasis

_____ 11. Laboratory test

_____ 12. Package insert

_____ 13. Panel

_____ 14. Qualitative test

_____ 15. Quality control

_____ 16. Quantitative test

_____ 17. Reagent

_____ 18. Reference range

_____ 19 Screening test

_____ 20. Serum

_____ 21. Specimen

_____ 22. Test system

_____ 23. Unique identifier

A. A facility in which tests are performed on biologic specimens to obtain information regarding the health of a patient.

B. The state in which body systems are functioning normally and the internal environment of the body is in equilibrium; the body is in a healthy state.

C. A combination of laboratory tests that have been determined to be the most sensitive and specific means of identifying a disease state or evaluating a particular organ or organ system.

D. A printed document developed by a test manufacturer that provides detailed information on the use of the test and how to perform the test.

E. A solution that is used to monitor a test system to ensure reliable and accurate test results.

F. A test that indicates whether or not a particular analyte is present in a specimen and may also provide an approximate indication of the amount of the analyte present.

G. The application of methods and means to ensure that test results are reliable and valid and that errors are detected and eliminated.

H. A patient test result that is dangerously abnormal and is life-threatening requiring immediate attention.

I. A test that indicates the exact amount of an analyte that is present in a specimen with the results being reported in measurable units.

J. A body substance that is being identified or measured in a laboratory test.

K. A chemical that reacts with a specimen to allow measurement of an analyte.

L. A certain established and acceptable range within which the laboratory test results of a healthy individual are expected to fall.

M. A tentative diagnosis of a patient's condition obtained through an evaluation of the health history and the physical examination, without the benefit of laboratory or diagnostic tests.

N. Abstaining from food or fluids (except water) for a specified amount of time before the collection of a specimen.

O. A laboratory test that meets the criteria for being a simple procedure that is easy to perform and has a low risk of erroneous test results.

P. A laboratory test performed routinely on apparently healthy individuals to assist in the early detection of disease.

Q. The clear, straw-colored part of the blood that remains after the solid elements and the clotting factor fibrinogen have been separated out of it.

R. A mechanism to check the precision and accuracy of an automated analyzer to determine, if it is providing accurate test results.

S. A small sample taken from the body to represent the nature of the whole.

T. The clinical analysis and study of a body substance to obtain objective data for the diagnosis, treatment, and management of a patient's condition.

U. A setup that includes all of the test components required to perform a laboratory test, such as test devices, controls, and test reagents.

V. A complex laboratory test that does not meet the criteria for waiver and is subject to the CLIA regulations.

W. Information directly associated with an individual that reliably identifies the individual as the person for whom the service or treatment is intended.

Directions: Fill in each blank with the correct answer.

1. What is the purpose of a laboratory test results?

   _____

   _____

2. What changes may occur in the body when a pathological condition is present?

   _____

   _____

3. What are the advantages of performing laboratory tests in a POL?

   _____

   _____

4. What is CLIA and what is its purpose?

   _____

   _____

5. What is a CLIA-waived test?

   _____

   _____

6. Where are CLIA nonwaived tests usually performed?

   _____

7. What may occur if a POL is not maintained at room temperature?

   _____

   _____

8. What guidelines should be followed regarding the refrigerator in a POL?

   _____

   _____

   _____

9. What is an emergency eyewash station?

   _____

   _____

10. How long should the eyes be flushed following exposure to a hazardous substance and why?

   _____

   _____

645

11. What may occur if there is a delay in treatment following exposure of the eyes to a hazardous substance?

_____

12. What are two examples of outside laboratories?

_____

13. What general information is included for each test in a laboratory test directory?

_____

_____

14. List five examples of specimens collected from the body for laboratory analysis.

_____

_____

15. Identify the purpose of each of the following categories of laboratory tests:

a. Hematology: _____

_____

b. Clinical chemistry: _____

_____

c. Immunology and blood banking: _____

_____

d. Urinalysis: _____

_____

e. Microbiology: _____

_____

f. Parasitology: _____

_____

g. Cytology: _____

h. Histology: _____

16. Why must laboratory test results be compared with the reference ranges supplied by the laboratory performing the test?

_____

_____

17. What is a specific panel?

_____

_____

18. What tests are included in the following panels?

    a. Comprehensive metabolic panel: _____

    _____

    b. Hepatic panel: _____

    _____

    c. Prenatal panel: _____

    _____

    d. Thyroid panel: _____

    _____

19. What is the purpose of the following panels?

    a. Hepatic panel: _____

    b. Lipid panel: _____

    c. Prenatal panel: _____

    d. Thyroid panel: _____

20. List five uses of laboratory test results.

_____

_____

_____

21. When is a laboratory test ordered to assist in a differential diagnosis?

_____

22. List three examples of laboratory screening tests.

_____

23. What is the purpose of a laboratory request?

_____

_____

Chapter **15** **Introduction to the Clinical Laboratory**

24. What is the reason for indicating the following on a laboratory request form?

    a. Patient's date of birth and gender: _____

    _____

    b. Date of collection of the specimen: _____

    _____

    c. Source of a microbiologic specimen: _____

    _____

    d. Clinical diagnosis: _____

    _____

    e. Medications the patient is taking: _____

    _____

25. How is an electronic laboratory request transmitted to an outside laboratory?

    _____

    _____

26. Why is a critical value reported immediately to the provider by an outside laboratory?

    _____

27. What are the two most common unique identifiers used to label specimens?

    _____

28. What two methods can be used to label a specimen?

    _____

29. What should the MA do if the patient needs to collect a specimen at home?

    _____

    _____

30. List examples of factors that may affect the test results of laboratory tests.

    _____

    _____

31. Why is it important for the MA to explain the reason for the advance preparation to the patient?

    _____

32. What is the purpose of fasting for 8 to 12 hours?

    _____

    _____

33. What may occur if a specimen for transport to an outside laboratory is collected or handled improperly?

    _____

    _____

34. What would cause a specimen to be rejected by an outside laboratory due to a labeling problem?

_____

_____

35. Why is it important to properly identify a patient?

_____

_____

36. Why must the appropriate container be used to collect a specimen?

_____

_____

37. What occurs if an insufficient amount of a specimen is submitted to an outside laboratory for testing?

_____

_____

38. What is the purpose of a biohazard specimen bag?

_____

_____

39. What is a laboratory lockbox?

_____

40. What are the guidelines for POLs that hold a certificate of waiver?

_____

_____

41. What regulations must be followed by laboratories performing nonwaived tests?

_____

_____

_____

_____

42. List examples of CLIA-waived blood chemistry and immunologic tests.

_____

_____

_____

43. What is included in a laboratory test system?

_____

_____

649

44. What is the purpose of a test kit package insert?

_____

_____

45. What is a unitized test device?

_____

_____

46. What is a procedure reference card and what is its purpose?

_____

_____

47. Describe a CLIA-waived automated analyzer.

_____

_____

48. What is the purpose of quality control?

_____

_____

49. What are the storage requirements for most test components?

_____

_____

50. What should be written on the label of a control that is stable only for a certain period of time after opening it?

_____

_____

51. What is the purpose of calibrating an automated analyzer?

_____

_____

52. What checks are performed by an internal control?

_____

_____

53. What is the purpose of an external control?

_____

_____

54. What types of results are produced by the following external controls?

a. Low-level control:

_____

_____

b. High-level control:

_____

_____

55. What may cause an external control procedure to fail to produce expected results?

_____

_____

_____

56. What should be done if the external control procedure does not perform as expected?

_____

_____

57. What is the difference between a qualitative test and a quantitative test?

_____

_____

_____

58. How should a qualitative test result be documented?

_____

_____

59. How should a quantitative test result be documented?

_____

_____

60. List five laboratory safety guidelines that should be followed for specimen collection and testing in the POL.

_____

_____

_____

_____

_____

_____

CRITICAL THINKING ACTIVITIES

A. Triglycerides Test Requirements

Your provider has ordered a triglycerides test on a patient that will be analyzed at an outside laboratory. You are required to collect the specimen and prepare it for transport to the outside laboratory. Using Figure 15-3 in your textbook as a reference, respond to the following questions in the space provided.

1. What is the amount and type of specimen required for this test?

_____

2. What type of container should be used to collect the specimen?

_____

3. What patient preparation is required for this test?

_____

_____

4. What should be done with the specimen once it is collected?

_____

_____

_____

5. How should you store the specimen while awaiting pickup by the laboratory courier?

_____

6. What would cause the laboratory to reject the specimen?

_____

_____

7. What are the uses of a triglycerides test?

_____

_____

8. What are the limitations of this test?

_____

_____

9. When would be the best time to collect this specimen (AM or PM)? Explain the reason for your answer.

_____

_____

_____

10. When the laboratory report is returned, the triglycerides test result is 250 mg/dL. How is this value interpreted?

_____

B. Laboratory Test Directory

Access the test menu for an online laboratory test directory and complete the information for each test in the chart presented below. Test menus can be accessed at the following websites:

https://www.labcorp.com/test-menu/search

https://dlolab.com/virtual-test-guide

Name of Test	Specimen Type and Amount (volume)	Collection Container	Collection and Processing Requirements	Causes for Rejection
CBC with differential				
PT/INR				
Lipid Panel				
ABO Blood Grouping				
Urinalysis with Microscopic Examination				

C. Identifying Abnormal Values

Refer to the laboratory report in your textbook (see Figure 15-6), and circle the abnormal values.

D. Laboratory Report

Refer to the computer-generated laboratory report in your textbook (Figure 15-6). Using the reference range values listed in this report; determine whether the following tests fall within their normal reference range or whether they are high or low. Mark each test according to the following: N = normal, H = high, L = low.

1. Glucose: 140 mg/dL: _____

2. BUN: 15 mg/dL: _____

3. Creatinine: 1.7 mg/dL: _____

4. Calcium: 10.2 mg/dL: _____

5. Sodium: 156 mmol/L: _____

6. Potassium: 5.5 mmol/L: _____

7. Chloride: 84 mmol/L: _____

8. Carbon dioxide: 18 mEq/L: _____

9. Total protein: 4.0 g/dL: _____

10. Albumin: 3.5 g/dL: _____

11. Total bilirubin: 0.8 mg/dL: _____

653

12. ALP: 80 U/L: _____

13. AST: 24 U/L: _____

14. ALT: 44 U/L: _____

E. Patient Test Information

Your provider has ordered an oral glucose tolerance test for Elise Van den Berg at a hospital laboratory. Using the OGTT information sheet in your textbook (Figure 15-10), answer the following questions.

1. What conditions can be diagnosed (or screened) with an OGTT?

   _____

   _____

2. Would it be a good idea for Mrs. Van den Berg to bring her toddler to the testing facility? Explain the reason for your answer.

   _____

   _____

3. Mrs. Van den Berg asks you the following questions. Answer the questions and, when possible, explain the reason for your answer.

   a. Would spaghetti be a good meal to have in the 3 days prior to the test?

   _____

   b. Can I schedule the test in the afternoon? _____

   c. How long do I need to fast? _____

   d. Can I drink water during the fasting period? _____

   e. Can I have a low-calorie protein shake the morning of the test? _____

   f. How long will I be at the testing facility? _____

   g. How long will I have to drink the glucose solution? _____

   h. Can I knit during the collection period? _____

   i. Can I go outside to smoke during the collection period? _____

   j. Can I practice my back flips during the collection period? _____

   k. Can I drink anything during the collection period?

   _____

   _____

   l. Are there any side effects that might occur during the collection period?

   _____

   _____

F. Test Kit Product Insert

Obtain a package insert from a CLIA-waived test kit. The package insert can be obtained from an actual test kit or by using a search engine on the Internet such as Google (e.g., Hemoccult package insert). Provide a brief description of the information included in each section of the package insert in the space provided. Examples of brand names of CLIA-waived test kits include the following:

Hemoccult fecal occult blood test	QuickVue hCG pregnancy test
ColoScreen fecal occult blood test	OSOM hCG urine pregnancy test
QuickVue iFOB test	OraQuick Advance HIV-1/2 test
Chemstrip urine test strips	QuickVue In-Line Strep A test
Multistix 10 SG	OSOM Ultra Strep A test
OSOM Mono test	ICON DS Strep A test
Clearview Mono test	QuickVue Influenza a + b test

Name of Test Kit: _____

Section	Information
Intended use	
Summary and explanation	
Principles of the procedure	
Precautions and warnings	
Reagents and materials provided	
Materials not provided	
Storage and stability	
Specimen collection and handling	
Test procedure	
Interpretation and reading results	
Quality control	
Limitations of the procedure	
Expected values	
Performance characteristics	

Chapter **15 Introduction to the Clinical Laboratory**

Directions: Complete the crossword puzzle using the clues provided.

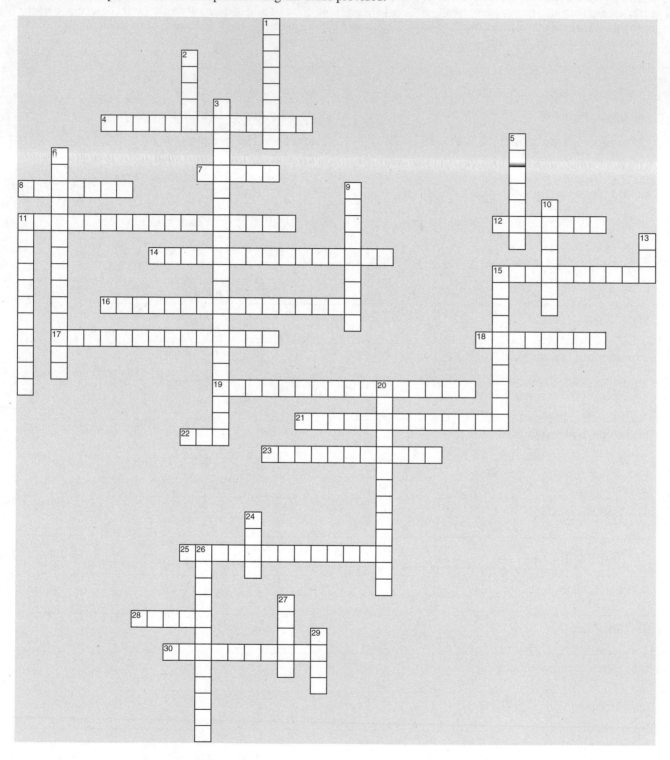

Across

4 Provides info on performing lab test
7 Specimen collected with a SST
8 A substance being identified
11 Tentative diagnosis
12 Cause of specimen rejection
14 Approximate amount of analyte present
15 Determines CAD risk
16 Is that you?
17 Where healthy test results fall
18 Alphabetic listing of tests
19 Cause of failed control results
21 Detects disease early
22 Not enough specimen?
23 Healthy body
25 Dangerously low test result
28 Common type of specimen
30 Has a low risk of erroneous test results

Down

1 Sample of the body
2 For documenting control results
3 Which disease is it?
5 Stores specimens awaiting pickup
6 Accurate and reliable test results
9 What are the results?
10 No food or fluid (except water)
11 Test system working OK?
13 In-house laboratory
15 Order a laboratory test
20 Complex CLIA lab test
24 To improve quality of lab testing
26 Example of CLIA-waived test
27 More than one lab test
29 As soon as possible

Chapter **15** **Introduction to the Clinical Laboratory**

Procedure 15-1: Operate and Inspect an Emergency Eyewash Station

Operate and inspect an emergency eyewash station. Document the inspection on the eyewash inspection tag presented below.

EMERGENCY EYEWASH STATION INSPECTION

INSPECT UNIT CAREFULLY BEFORE SIGNING

DATE	BY	DATE	BY

DO NOT REMOVE THIS TAG

Procedure 15-A: Collecting Specimen for Transport to an Outside Laboratory

1. Laboratory requisition. Complete the Laboratory Request form on page 633 using a classmate as a patient. The tests that have been ordered by the provider include the following: basic metabolic panel, lipid panel, CBC (with differential), and rheumatoid arthritis factor.
2. Specimen collection. Practice the procedure for collecting a specimen for transport to an outside laboratory, and document the procedure in the chart provided.

CHART	
Date	

CHART	
Date	

Chapter **15** **Introduction to the Clinical Laboratory**

LABORATORY REQUEST
Biomedical Laboratories, Inc.
100 Main Street
Athens, Georgia 45760

Patient's Name (Last)	(First)	(MI)	Sex	Date of Birth MO DAY YEAR	Collection Time : AM PM	Fasting YES NO	Collection Date MO DAY YEAR

NPI/UPIN	Physician's ID #	Patient's SS #	Patient's ID #	Urine hrs/vol hrs____ vol____

PATIENT

Physician's Name (Last, First)	Physician's Signature	Patient's Address	Phone
Medicare # (Include prefix/suffix)	☐ Primary ☐ Secondary	City	State ZIP
Medicaid # State	Physician's Provider #	Name of Responsible Party (if different from patient)	
Diagnosis/Signs/Symptoms in ICD-10 Format (Highest Specificity) REQUIRED		Address of Responsible Party (if different from patient) APT #	
		City State ZIP	

RESP. PARTY

INSURANCE

Patient's Relationship to Responsible Party	■ 1–Self	☐ 2–Spouse	☐ 3–Child	☐ 4–Other

Performance Lab ☐	Carrier	Group #	Employee #	Mem

Insurance Company Name	Plan	Carrier Code
Subscriber/Member #	Location	Group #
Insurance Address	Physician's Provider #	
City	State	ZIP
Employer's Name or Number	Insured SS # (If not patient)	Worker's Comp ☐ Yes ☐ No

I hereby authorize the release of medical information related to the service subscribed herein and authorize payment directed to LabCorp.

X _____
Patient's Signature   Date

MEDICARE ADVANCE BENEFICIARY NOTICE

I have read the ABN on the reverse. If Medicare denies payment, I agree to pay for the identified test(s).

X _____
Patient's Signature   Date

NOTE: WHEN ORDERING TESTS FOR WHICH MEDICARE OR MEDICAID REIMBURSEMENT WILL BE SOUGHT, PHYSICIANS SHOULD ONLY ORDER TESTS THAT ARE MEDICALLY NECESSARY FOR THE DIAGNOSIS OR TREATMENT OF THE PATIENT. COMPONENTS OF THE ORGAN OR DISEASE PANELS/COMBINATIONS PRINTED BELOW ARE SHOWN ON THE REVERSE SIDE AND MAY ALSO BE ORDERED INDIVIDUALLY BELOW. COMPONENTS MAY BE BILLED SEPARATELY PER CARRIER POLICY.

PANELS (See reverse for components)

80049	Basic Metabolic Panel	(SST)
80054	Comp Metabolic Panel	(SST)
80051	Electrolyte Panel	(SST)
80058	Hepatic Panel	(SST)
80059	Hepatitis Panel	(SST)
80061	Lipid Panel	(SST)
80091	Thyroid Panel	(SST)
80055	Prenatal Panel	(RED)(LAV)
80072	Rheumatoid Panel	(SST)

HEMATOLOGY

85025	CBC w Diff	(LAV)
85027	CBC w/o Diff	(LAV)
85014	Hematocrit	(LAV)
85018	Hemoglobin	(LAV)
85595	Platelet Count	(LAV)
85041	RBC Count	(LAV)
85048	WBC Count	(LAV)
85007	WBC Differential	(LAV)
89190	Nasal Smear, Eosin	(Nasal Smear)
85060	Pathologist Consult–Peripheral Smear	(LAV)

ALPHABETICAL/COMBINATION TESTS

86900 86901	ABO and Rh	(LAV)
82040	Albumin	(SST)
84075	Alkaline Phosphatase	(SST)
84460	ALT (SGPT)	(SST)
82150	Amylase, Serum	(SST)
86038	Antinuclear Antibodies	(SST)
84450	AST (SGOT)	(SST)
82607 82746	B₁₂ and Folate	(SST)
82250	Bilirubin, Total	(SST)

ALPHABETICAL TESTS CON'T

84520	BUN	(SST)
82310	Calcium	(SST)
80156	Carbamazepine (Tegretol®)	(SER)
82378	CEA	(SST)
82465	Cholesterol, Total	(SST)
82565	Creatinine	(SST)
80162	Digoxin	(SER)
82670	Estradiol	(SST)
82728	Ferritin, Serum	(SST)
82985	Fructosamine	(SST)
83001	FSH	(SST)
83001 83002	FSH and LH	(SST)
82977	GGT	(SST)
82947	Glucose, Plasma	(GRY)
82947	Glucose, Serum	(SST)
82950	Glucose, 2-hr. PP	(SST)
83036	Glycohemoglobin, Total	(LAV)
84703	hCG, Beta Subunit, Qual	(SST)
84702	hCG, Beta Subunit, Quant	(SST)
83718	HDL Cholesterol	(SST)
86677	*Helicobacter pylori*, IgG	(SST)
86706	Hep B Surface Antibody	(SST)
87340	Hep B Surface Antigen	(SST)
86803	Hep C Antibody	(SST)
83036	Hemoglobin A₁C	(LAV)
86701	HIV Antibodies	(SST)
83540	Iron, Total	(SST)
83540 83550	Iron and IBC	(SST)
83615	LDH	(SST)

ALPHABETICAL TESTS CON'T

83002	LH	(SST)
83690	Lipase	(SER)
80178	Lithium (Eskalith®)	(SER)
83735	Magnesium, Serum	(SST)
80184	Phenobarbital (Luminal®)	(SER)
80185	Phenytoin (Dilantin®)	(SER)
84132	Potassium	(SST)
84146	Prolactin, Serum	(SST)
84153	Prostate-Specific Antigen	(SST)
84066	Prostatic Acid Phos	(SST)
84155	Protein, Total	(SST)
85610	Prothrombin Time (PT)	(BLU)
85610 85730	PT and PTT Activated	(BLU)
85730	PTT Activated	(BLU)
86431	Rheumatoid Arthritis Factor	(SST)
86592	RPR	(SST)
86762	Rubella Antibodies, IgG	(SST)
85651	Sed Rate	(LAV)
84295	Sodium	(SST)
84403	Testosterone	(SST)
80198	Theophylline	(SER)
84436	Thyroxine (T₄)	(SST)
84478	Triglycerides	(SST)
84480	Triiodothyronine (T₃)	(SST)
84443	TSH, High Sensitivity	(SST)
84550	Uric Acid	(SST)
81003	Urinalysis Microscopic on Positives	(URN)
81001	Urinalysis with Microscopic	(URN)
80164	Valproic Acid (Depakene®)	(SER)

MICROBIOLOGY See Reverse Side

■ENDOCERVICAL ■THROAT ■URINE
■STOOL ■URETHRAL INDICATE SOURCE

87070	Aerobic Bacterial Culture	(Bact Trnspt)
87490 87590	*Chlamydia*/GC DNA Probe w/ Confirmation on Positives	(Probe Trnspt)
87490 87590	*Chlamydia*/GC DNA Probe Without Confirmation	(Probe Trnspt)
87490	*Chlamydia* DNA Probe	(Probe Trnspt)
87081	Genital, Beta-Hemolytic Strep Cult, Group B	(Bact Trnspt)
87070	Genital Culture, Routine	(Bact Trnspt)
87070	Lower Respiratory Culture	(Steril Trnspt)
87590	*N. gonorrhoeae* DNA Probe	(Probe Trnspt)
87015 87211	Ova and Parasites	(O & P Kit)
87081 X2 87045	Stool Culture	(Fecal Trnspt)
87081	Throat, Beta-Hemolytic Strep Cult, Group A	(Bact Trnspt)
87060	Upper Respiratory Culture, Routine	(Bact Trnspt)
87086	Urine Culture, Routine	(Urn Cul Trnspt)

Clinical Information/Medications

OTHER TESTS/INDIVIDUAL COMPONENTS
TEST #   TEST NAMES

LAB USE ONLY	STAT ☐ 998074	VENIPUNCTURE ☐ 998085	TRAVEL ☐ 998096	NON LABCORP ☐ 998239	VERBAL ORDER ☐ 998250	CHART ORDER ☐ 998261	HANDWRITTEN ☐ 998272	24 HR TUV ☐ 998283	PST/PSC #

CONTAINERS RECEIVED	SST SPUN	USST UNSPUN	SER SERUM TRNSPT	FRZ FRZ TRNS	RED RED	LAV LAVENDER	SLD SLIDE	BLU LT. BLUE	GRY GREY	GRN GREEN	RYB RYL BLU	YEL ACD	PLS PLASMA	URN URINE	24U 24 HR URINE	TA-U TART. ACID	FL FLUID	OT OTHER	BACT TRANSP	O & P KIT	PROBE TRNSP	URN CULT TRNSP	STERIL TRNSP	FECAL TRNSP	VIRAL TRNSP

300-0384

661

Procedure 15-1: Operating an Emergency Eyewash Station

Name: _____   Date: _____

Evaluated by: _____   Score: _____

Performance Objective

Outcome:	Operate and inspect an emergency eyewash station.
Conditions:	Using an emergency eyewash station.
	Given a disinfectant.
Standards:	Time: 5 minutes. Student completed procedure in _____ minutes.
	Accuracy: Satisfactory score on the Performance Evaluation Checklist.

Performance Evaluation Checklist

Trial 1	Trial 2	Point Value	Performance Standards
			Operate the Emergency Eyewash Station
		•	Immediately proceeded to the emergency eyewash station after the eye(s) came in contact with a hazardous substance.
		•	Asked for assistance, if needed.
		•	Activated the eyewash station using the activation lever.
		•	Held both eyelids apart with your thumbs and forefingers.
		▷	Stated why the eyelids must be held apart.
		•	Lowered your eyes into the stream of water and flushed both eyes simultaneously.
		•	If necessary, removed contact lenses.
		▷	Stated why contact lenses should be removed.
		•	Continued to hold the eyelids apart and gently rolled your eyeballs from left to right and up and down.
		▷	Stated why the eyeballs should be gently rolled.
		•	Continued to flush the eyes for a full 15 minutes.
		▷	Explained why the eyes should be flushed for a minimum of 15 minutes.
		•	Returned the activation lever to its resting position.
		•	Sought medical attention immediately to determine whether further treatment was required.
		•	Cleaned, disinfected, rinsed, and completely dried the eyewash device.
			Inspect the Emergency Eyewash Station
		•	Made sure the access route to the eyewash station is well lit and free of obstructions.
		▷	Stated what may occur if there is a delay in reaching the eyewash station.
		•	Made sure the eyewash station is well-lit and the area around the eyewash station is free of clutter.

Trial 1	Trial 2	Point Value	Performance Standards
		▷	Stated why the area around the station should be free of clutter.
		•	Made sure the nozzle covers are in place and in good condition.
		▷	Stated the purpose of the nozzle covers.
		•	Made sure the eyewash bowl is clean and free of debris.
		•	Activated the eyewash device using the activation lever.
		•	Made sure the water flow from the nozzles occurred in one second or less following activation of the eyewash.
		•	Made sure the nozzle covers come off automatically when the eyewash device is activated.
		•	Activated the eyewash station for approximately three minutes.
		▷	Stated the purpose of flushing the eyewash station.
		•	Made sure that water flows continuously without the use of the hands.
		•	Made sure the nozzle heads are not clogged and that water flows equally from both nozzle heads.
		•	Returned the activation lever to its resting position.
		•	Cleaned, disinfected, rinsed, and completely dried the eyewash device.
		•	Replaced the nozzle covers on the nozzle heads.
		•	Reported any problems to the appropriate personnel.
		•	Documented the inspection date and signed your initials on the eyewash inspection tag.
		▷	Stated how often the eyewash station should be inspected.
		■	Demonstrated critical thinking skills.
		■	Demonstrated self-awareness.
		★	Completed the procedure within 20 minutes.
		Totals	

Evaluation of Student Performance

EVALUATION CRITERIA			COMMENTS
Symbol	**Category**	**Point Value**	
★	Critical Step	16 points	
•	Essential Step	6 points	
■	Affective Competency	6 points	
▷	Theory Question	2 points	

Score calculation: 100 points

− _____ points missed

_____ Score

Satisfactory score: 85 or above

663

CAAHEP Competencies Achieved

Psychomotor (Skills)

- ☑ III. 1. Participate in bloodborne pathogen training.
- ☑ XII. 1. Comply with safety practices.
- ☑ XII. 2. Demonstrate proper use of a. eyewash.

Affective (Behavior)

- ☑ A. 1. Demonstrate critical thinking skills.
- ☑ A. 8. Demonstrate self-awareness.

ABHES Competencies Achieved

- ☑ 8. a. Practice standard precautions and perform disinfection/sterilization techniques.
- ☑ 8. g. Recognize and respond to medical office emergencies.

EVALUATION OF COMPETENCY

Procedure 15-A: Collecting a Specimen for Transport to an Outside Laboratory

Name: _____ Date: _____

Evaluated by: _____ Score: _____

Performance Objective

Outcome:	Collect a specimen for transport to an outside laboratory.
Conditions:	Given the appropriate supplies for the specimen collection and transport (will be based upon the type of specimen collected).
Standards:	Time: 10 minutes. Student completed procedure in _____ minutes.
	Accuracy: Satisfactory score on the Performance Evaluation Checklist.

Performance Evaluation Checklist

Trial 1	Trial 2	Point Value	Performance Standards
		•	Informed the patient of any advance preparation or special instructions.
		•	Notified the patient of the time to report to the medical office for the specimen collection.
		•	Reviewed the collection and handling requirements in the laboratory directory for the test(s) ordered by the provider.
		•	Greeted the patient and introduced yourself. Identified the patient and explained the procedure.
		•	Determined whether the patient prepared properly for the test.
		•	Sanitized hands and assembled equipment and supplies.
		•	Completed a laboratory request form.
		•	Labeled each specimen container.
		▷	Explained the importance of properly labeling specimen containers.
			Collected the specimen incorporating the following guidelines:
		•	Followed the OSHA Standard.
		•	Collected the specimen according to the requirements specified in the laboratory directory.
		•	Collected the proper type and amount of specimen required for the test.
		•	Securely tightened the lids on specimen containers.
		•	Discarded used collection materials in a biohazard waste container.
		•	Processed the specimen according to the requirements specified in the laboratory directory.
			Prepared the specimen for transport:
		•	Placed the specimen in a biohazard specimen bag.
		•	Transmitted the laboratory request electronically and/or place the request in the outside pocket of the specimen bag.

665

Trial 1	Trial 2	Point Value	Performance Standards
		•	Properly stored the specimen awaiting pickup following the storage requirements in the laboratory directory.
		•	Documented the procedure correctly.
		■	Reassured patients.
		★	Completed the procedure within 10 minutes.
			Totals

CHART	
Date	

Evaluation of Student Performance

EVALUATION CRITERIA			COMMENTS
Symbol	**Category**	**Point Value**	
★	Critical Step	16 points	
•	Essential Step	6 points	
■	Affective Competency	6 points	
▷	Theory Question	2 points	

Score calculation: 100 points

    −   points missed

       ___ Score

Satisfactory score: 85 or above

CAAHEP Competencies Achieved

Psychomotor (Skills)
☑ III. 2. Select appropriate barrier/personal protective equipment (PPE).

Affective (Behavior)
☑ A. 2. Reassure patients.

ABHES Competencies Achieved

☑ 9. d. Collect, label, and process specimens.

16 Urinalysis

CHAPTER ASSIGNMENTS

√ After Completing	Date Due	Study Guide Pages	STUDY GUIDE ASSIGNMENTS (CTA = Critical Thinking Activity)	Possible Points	Points You Earned
		671	Pretest	10	
			Key Term Assessment		
		672	A. Definitions	22	
		673	B. Word Parts (Add 1 point for each key term)	16	
		673-678	Evaluation of Learning questions	55	
		678	CTA A: First-Voided Specimen	3	
		678-679	CTA B: Clean-Catch Specimen	4	
		679	CTA C: Urine Reagent Strip Test Package Insert	6	
			Evolve: Chemical Testing of Urine (Record points earned)		
		680-681	CTA D: Crossword Puzzle	26	
			Evolve: Road to Recovery: Urinalysis Terminology (Record points earned)		
			Evolve: Apply Your Knowledge questions	10	
			Evolve: Video Evaluation	24	
		671	Posttest	10	
			ADDITIONAL ASSIGNMENTS		
			Total points		

√ When Assigned By Your Instructor	Study Guide Pages	Practices Required	LABORATORY ASSIGNMENTS (Procedure Number and Name)	Score*
	683-684	3	**Practice for Competency** 16-1: Collection of a Clean-Catch Midstream Urine Specimen	
	689-691		**Evaluation of Competency** 16-1: Collection of a Clean-Catch Midstream Urine Specimen	*
	683-684		**Practice for Competency** 16-2: Collection of a 24-Hour Urine Specimen	
	693-695		**Evaluation of Competency** 16-2: Collection of a 24-Hour Urine Specimen	
	683-684	5	**Practice for Competency** 16-A: Assessing Color and Appearance of a Urine Specimen	
	697-698		**Evaluation of Competency** 16-A: Assessing Color and Appearance of a Urine Specimen	*
	683-687	5	**Practice for Competency** 16-3: Chemical Assessment of a Urine Specimen Using a Reagent Strip	
	699-702		**Evaluation of Competency** 16-3: Chemical Assessment of a Urine Specimen Using a Reagent Strip	*
	683-684	2	**Practice for Competency** 16-4: Prepare a Urine Specimen for Microscopic Examination	
	703-705		**Evaluation of Competency** 16-4: Prepare a Urine Specimen for Microscopic Examination	*
	683-684	2	**Practice for Competency** 16-5: Perform a CLIA-Waived Urine Pregnancy Test	
	707-708		**Evaluation of Competency** 16-5: Perform a CLIA-Waived Urine Pregnancy Test	*
			ADDITIONAL ASSIGNMENTS	

Notes

Name _____   Date _____

? PRETEST

True or False

_____ 1. Approximately 95% of urine consists of water.

_____ 2. Frequency is the condition of having to urinate often.

_____ 3. An excessive increase in urine output is called *polyuria*.

_____ 4. A clean-catch midstream urine specimen is required, if the urine is being cultured and examined for bacteria.

_____ 5. Urinalysis consists of a physical, chemical, and microscopic examination of urine.

_____ 6. A urine specimen that is light yellow indicates that bacteria are present in the specimen.

_____ 7. The pH of most urine specimens is neutral.

_____ 8. Blood may normally be present in the urine due to menstruation.

_____ 9. Hematuria refers to the presence of blood in the urine.

_____10. HCG is a hormone that is present in the urine and blood of a pregnant woman.

? POSTTEST

True or False

_____ 1. Urea is a waste product derived from the breakdown of protein.

_____ 2. A normal adult excretes approximately 250 mL of urine each day.

_____ 3. Vomiting can result in oliguria.

_____ 4. The distal urethra normally contains microorganisms.

_____ 5. A 24-hour urine specimen may be collected to assist in the diagnosis of a UTI.

_____ 6. If a urine specimen is allowed to stand for more than 1 hour at room temperature, the pH becomes more acidic.

_____ 7. If a freshly voided specimen is cloudy, the patient may have a UTI.

_____ 8. The normal specific gravity of urine ranges from 1.005 to 1.030.

_____ 9. Dysuria is the inability to control urination at night.

_____10. Casts are formed in the urinary bladder.

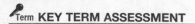
A. Definitions

Directions: Match each key term with its definition.

_____ 1. Anuria

_____ 2. Bilirubinuria

_____ 3. Dysuria

_____ 4. Frequency

_____ 5. Glycosuria

_____ 6. Hematuria

_____ 7. Ketonuria

_____ 8. Ketosis

_____ 9. Micturition

_____ 10. Nephron

_____ 11. Nocturia

_____ 12. Nocturnal enuresis

_____ 13. Oliguria

_____ 14. pH

_____ 15. Polyuria

_____ 16. Proteinuria

_____ 17. Pyuria

_____ 18. Retention

_____ 19. Specific gravity

_____ 20. Urgency

_____ 21. Urinalysis

_____ 22. Urinary incontinence

A. Decreased or scanty output of urine
B. The presence of protein in the urine
C. Inability of an individual to control urination at night during sleep (bedwetting)
D. The presence of bilirubin in the urine
E. Increased output of urine
F. The presence of pus in the urine
G. The presence of glucose in the urine
H. The physical, chemical, and microscopic analysis of urine
I. The presence of ketone bodies in the urine
J. The act of voiding urine
K. An accumulation of large amounts of ketone bodies in the tissues and body fluids
L. The measurement of the amount of dissolved substances present in the urine compared with the same amount of distilled water
M. The unit that describes the acidity or alkalinity of a solution
N. The functional unit of the kidney that filters waste substances from the blood and dilutes them with water to produce urine
O. The inability to empty the bladder; urine is being produced normally but is not being voided
P. The immediate need to urinate
Q. Failure of the kidneys to produce urine
R. Difficult or painful urination
S. The condition of having to urinate often
T. Blood present in the urine
U. Excessive (voluntary) urination during the night
V. The inability to retain urine

B. Word Parts

Directions: Indicate the meaning of each word part in the space provided. List as many medical terms as possible that incorporate the word part in the space provided.

Word Part	Meaning of Word Part	Medical Terms That Incorporate Word Part
1. an-		
2. ur/o		
3. -ia		
4. bilirubino/o		
5. dys-		
6. glyc/o		
7. hemato/o		
8. keton/o		
9. -osis		
10. noct/i		
11. olig/o		
12. poly		
13. py/o		
14. supra		
15. pub/o		
16. -ic		

☑ EVALUATION OF LEARNING

Directions: Fill in each blank with the correct answer.

1. List two functions of the urinary system.

   _____

2. What is the function of the urinary bladder?

   _____

3. What is the function of the ureters?

   _____

4. How does the function of the urethra differ in the male and female?

   _____

   _____

5. What is the urinary meatus?

_____

6. Most of the urine (95%) is composed of what substance?

_____

7. How much urine does the normal adult excrete each day and what causes this amount to vary?

_____

_____

8. What are four conditions that cause polyuria?

_____

_____

9. What are four conditions that cause oliguria?

_____

_____

10. What type of urine specimen is required for the detection of a UTI?

_____

11. Why is a first-voided morning specimen often preferred for urine testing?

_____

_____

12. What is the purpose of performing the clean-catch midstream urine collection procedure?

_____

_____

13. What type of test is performed on a first-catch urine specimen?

_____

14. Why must these guidelines be followed for the collection of a first-catch urine specimen?

   a. Not cleansing the genital area before collection of the specimen:

_____

   b. Collection of only 15 to 30 mL of the initial stream of urine:

_____

15. What is the purpose of a 24-hour urine specimen?

_____

_____

16. Why should a patient not void directly into a 24-hour urine specimen container that contains a preservative?

_____

17. List three changes that may take place in a urine specimen, if it is allowed to stand at room temperature for more than 1 hour.

_____

_____

_____

18. Why does concentrated urine tend to be a darker yellow?

_____

_____

19. What can cause a freshly voided urine specimen to be cloudy?

_____

_____

20. What is the odor of a urine specimen that has been allowed to stand at room temperature for a long period of time?

_____

21. What is the purpose of testing the specific gravity of urine?

_____

22. What are four conditions that cause an increase in the specific gravity of urine?

_____

_____

23. What is the normal range for the specific gravity of urine?

_____

24. Why does concentrated urine have a higher specific gravity?

_____

25. What conditions can be evaluated and diagnosed through the chemical examination of urine?

_____

_____

26. What is the normal range for the pH of urine?

_____

27. What may cause an increase in the pH of urine?

_____

28. Why does urine become more alkaline if it is not preserved?

_____

_____

29. What may cause glycosuria?

_____

_____

30. What conditions may cause proteinuria?

_____

_____

31. What may cause ketonuria?

_____

_____

32. How is bilirubin normally eliminated from the body?

_____

_____

33. What conditions may cause bilirubin to appear in the urine?

_____

34. What may cause blood to appear in the urine?

_____

_____

35. Why should a nitrite test be performed on a first-voided morning specimen?

_____

_____

36. Why should a nitrite test not be performed on a urine specimen that has been left standing at room temperature?

_____

_____

37. What conditions cause leukocyturia?

_____

_____

38. What should be done if a urine specimen is unable to be tested within 1 hour of voiding?

_____

_____

39. How should urine reagent strips be stored?

_____

_____

676

40. How does a quality control test ensure the reliability of reagent strip urine testing?

_____

_____

41. What problems may cause a urine strip quality control test to fail to produce expected results?

_____

_____

42. When should a urine reagent strip quality control test be performed?

_____

_____

43. What is the purpose of performing a microscopic examination of the urine?

_____

_____

44. What is urine sediment?

_____

45. Why is a first-voided urine specimen recommended for a microscopic examination of the urine?

_____

_____

46. What effect does concentrated and dilute urine have on red blood cells?

_____

Concentrated urine: _____

_____

Dilute urine: _____

_____

47. What condition may be indicated by an elevated number of white blood cells in the urine sediment?

_____

48. What are urinary casts?

_____

_____

49. What is the name of the vaginal infection caused by yeast?

_____

50. List three reasons for performing a pregnancy test.

_____

_____

51. What is the name of the hormone that is present in the urine and blood only of a pregnant woman?

_____

52. What is the preferred specimen for a urine pregnancy test?

_____

53. What may occur is the specific gravity of a urine specimen is less than 1.007?

_____

54. What is the purpose of an internal control built into a urine pregnancy test?

_____

_____

55. What conditions (other than a normal pregnancy) can result in a positive urine pregnancy test?

_____

CRITICAL THINKING ACTIVITIES

A. First-Voided Specimen

You have instructed Jim Pratt to collect a first-voided morning urine specimen, which is to be brought to the medical office for testing. Mr. Pratt asks the following questions. Respond to them in the spaces provided.

1. Why is a first-voided specimen needed for the testing?

_____

_____

2. Can I collect the specimen in an empty peanut butter jar?

_____

_____

3. Why must the specimen be preserved until it is brought to the medical office?

_____

_____

B. Clean-Catch Specimen

You have just instructed Ann Berger to obtain a clean-catch midstream urine specimen at the medical office. Mrs. Berger asks the following questions. Respond to them in the spaces provided.

1. What is the purpose of cleansing the urinary meatus?

_____

_____

2. Why must a front-to-back motion be used to clean the urinary meatus?

_____

_____

Chapter **16** **Urinalysis**

3. Why must a small amount of urine first be voided into the toilet?

_____

_____

4. Why should the inside of the specimen container not be touched?

_____

_____

C. Urine Reagent Strip Test Package Insert

Obtain the package insert for a CLIA-waived reagent strip test for the chemical testing of urine (e.g., Multistix 10 SG). Using the package insert, answer the following questions in the spaces provided. (*Note:* A package insert for Multistix 10 SG can be obtained on the Internet by performing a search for *Multistix 10 SG package insert*).

1. What is the brand name of the test?

_____

2. This test assists in the diagnosis of what conditions?

_____

_____

_____

3. What type of urine specimen is recommended for this test?

_____

4. What substances can be detected by this test?

_____

_____

_____

_____

5. Explain the proper storage and handling of this test.

_____

_____

6. List any substances or techniques that may interfere with obtaining an accurate reading (e.g., not reading the test at the prescribed time).

_____

_____

_____

D. Crossword Puzzle: Urinalysis

Directions: Complete the crossword puzzle using the clues provided.

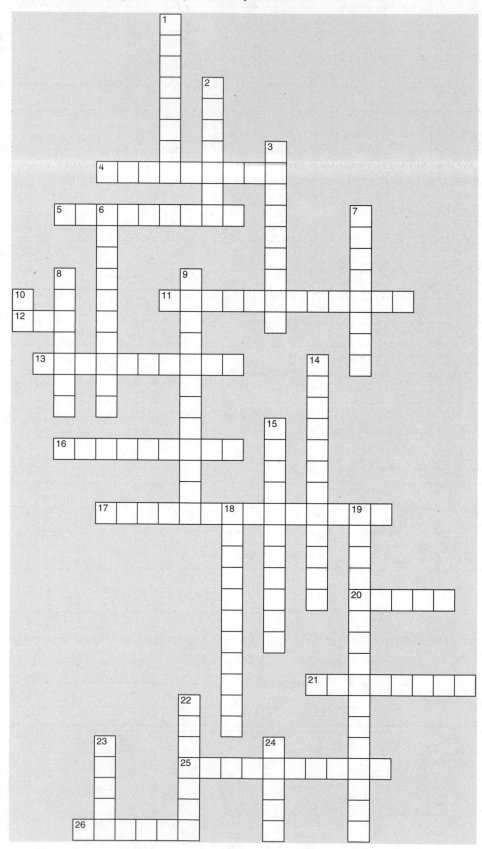

Across

4 Yellow urine pigment
5 Promotes dryness
11 Lives 120 days
12 Makes preg test +
13 Tx for UTI
16 Cause of bilirubinuria
17 Security for urine drug testing
20 UTI bacteria
21 Cause of oliguria
25 Physical, chemical, and microscopic
26 No urine produced

Down

1 This drug causes polyuria
2 Kidney unit
3 Cannot empty bladder
6 Cause of ketonuria
7 Cause of cloudy urine
8 Sym of UTI
9 Normal cause of hematuria
10 Acid or alkaline?
14 WBCs in the urine
15 Act of voiding urine
18 Spec for preg test
19 Cause of glycosuria
22 Difficult or painful urination
23 Neutral pH
24 Most of urine

Notes

Procedure 16-1: Collection of a Clean-Catch Midstream Urine Specimen. Instruct an individual in the procedure for collecting a clean-catch midstream urine specimen and document the procedure in the chart provided.

Procedure 16-2: Collection of a 24-Hour Urine Specimen: Instruct an individual in the procedure for collecting a 24-hour urine specimen and document the procedure in the chart provided.

Procedure 16-A: Color and Appearance of a Urine Specimen. Assess the color and appearance of a urine specimen and document the results in the chart provided.

Procedure 16-3: Chemical Assessment of a Urine Specimen Using a Reagent Strip.
a. Perform a Multistix 10 SG quality control test, and document results on the quality control log on the next page.
b. Perform a chemical assessment of a urine specimen using a Multistix 10 SG reagent strip. Document the results on the laboratory report form provided. Circle any abnormal results.

Procedure 16-4: Prepare a Urine Specimen for Microscopic Examination. Prepare a urine specimen for microscopic analysis examination by the provider using the Kova Method. Examine the specimen to observe the microscopic structures and indicate those that you were able to identify in the space below.

_____

_____

_____

Procedure 16-5: Perform a CLIA-Waived Urine Pregnancy Test. Perform a CLIA-waived urine pregnancy test, and document results in the chart provided.

CHART	
Date	

683

CHART	
Date	

684

URINALYSIS QUALITY CONTROL LOG		
Name of Test: _____ Date: _____	Name of Control: _____ Lot #: _____ Exp. Date: _____	Technician: _____
TEST	EXPECTED RESULT (specified in package insert accompanying the control)	CONTROL RESULT
Glucose		
Bilirubin		
Ketone		
Specific gravity		
Blood		
pH		
Protein		
Urobilinogen		
Nitrite		
Leukocytes		

Multistix® 10 SG Reagent Strips for Urinalysis

PATIENT

DATE   TIME

Test						
LEUKOCYTES	NEGATIVE ☐		TRACE ☐	SMALL + ☐	MODERATE ++ ☐	LARGE +++ ☐
NITRITE	NEGATIVE ☐		POSITIVE ☐	POSITIVE ☐	(Any degree of uniform pink color is found)	
UROBILINOGEN	NORMAL 0.2 ☐	NORMAL 1 ☐	mg/dL 2 ☐	4 ☐	8 ☐ (1mg = approx. 1 BU)	
PROTEIN	NEGATIVE ☐	TRACE ☐	mg/dL 30 * ☐	100 ++ ☐	300 +++ ☐	2000 OR MORE ☐
pH	5.0 ☐	6.0 ☐	6.5 ☐	7.0 ☐	7.5 ☐	8.0 ☐ · · · 8.5 ■
BLOOD	NEGATIVE ☐	NON-HEMOLYZED TRACE ☐	NON-HEMOLYZED MODERATE ☐	HEMOLYZED TRACE ☐	SMALL + ☐	MODERATE ++ ☐ · · · LARGE +++ ☐
SPECIFIC GRAVITY	1.000 ☐	1.006 ☐	1.010 ☐	1.015 ☐	1.020 ☐	1.025 ☐ · · · 1.030 ☐
KETONE	NEGATIVE ☐	mg/dL	TRACE 5 ☐	SMALL 15 ☐	MODERATE 40 ☐	LARGE 80 ☐ · · · LARGE 160 ☐
BILIRUBIN	NEGATIVE ☐		SMALL + ☐	MODERATE ++ ☐	LARGE +++ ☐	
GLUCOSE	NEGATIVE ☐	g/L (%) mg/dL	1/10 (tr.) 100 ☐	1/6 250 ☐	1/2 500 ☐	1 1000 ☐ · · · 2 or more 2000 or more ☐

(Modified and printed with permission of Siemens Medical Solutions Diagnostic, Tarrytown, NY 10591.)

Multistix® 10 SG Reagent Strips for Urinalysis

PATIENT

DATE   TIME

Test						
LEUKOCYTES	NEGATIVE ☐		TRACE ☐	SMALL + ☐	MODERATE ++ ☐	LARGE +++ ☐
NITRITE	NEGATIVE ☐		POSITIVE ☐	POSITIVE ☐	(Any degree of uniform pink color is found)	
UROBILINOGEN	NORMAL 0.2 ☐	NORMAL 1 ☐	mg/dL 2 ☐	4 ☐	8 ☐ (1mg = approx. 1 BU)	
PROTEIN	NEGATIVE ☐	TRACE ☐	mg/dL 30 * ☐	100 ++ ☐	300 +++ ☐	2000 OR MORE ☐
pH	5.0 ☐	6.0 ☐	6.5 ☐	7.0 ☐	7.5 ☐	8.0 ☐ · · · 8.5 ☐
BLOOD	NEGATIVE ☐	NON-HEMOLYZED TRACE ☐	NON-HEMOLYZED MODERATE ☐	HEMOLYZED TRACE ☐	SMALL + ☐	MODERATE ++ ☐ · · · LARGE +++ ☐
SPECIFIC GRAVITY	1.000 ☐	1.006 ☐	1.010 ☐	1.015 ☐	1.020 ☐	1.025 ☐ · · · 1.030 ☐
KETONE	NEGATIVE ☐	mg/dL	TRACE 5 ☐	SMALL 15 ☐	MODERATE 40 ☐	LARGE 80 ☐ · · · LARGE 160 ☐
BILIRUBIN	NEGATIVE ☐		SMALL + ☐	MODERATE ++ ☐	LARGE +++ ☐	
GLUCOSE	NEGATIVE ☐	g/L (%) mg/dL	1/10 (tr.) 100 ☐	1/6 250 ☐	1/2 500 ☐	1 1000 ☐ · · · 2 or more 2000 or more ☐

(Modified and printed with permission of Siemens Medical Solutions Diagnostic, Tarrytown, NY 10591.)

Multistix® 10 SG Reagent Strips for Urinalysis

PATIENT

DATE   TIME

LEUKOCYTES	NEGATIVE ☐		TRACE ☐	SMALL + ☐	MODERATE ++ ☐	LARGE +++ ☐
NITRITE	NEGATIVE ☐		POSITIVE ☐	POSITIVE ☐	(Any degree of uniform pink color is found)	
UROBILINOGEN	NORMAL 0.2 ☐	NORMAL 1 ☐	mg/dL 2 ☐	4 ☐	8 ☐ (1mg = approx. 1 BU)	
PROTEIN	NEGATIVE ☐	TRACE ☐	mg/dL 30 ☐ *	100 ++ ☐	300 +++ ☐	2000 OR MORE ☐
pH	5.0 ☐	6.0 ☐	6.5 ☐	7.0 ☐	7.5 ☐	8.0 ☐	8.5 ☐
BLOOD	NEGATIVE ☐	NON-HEMOLYZED TRACE ☐	NON-HEMOLYZED MODERATE ☐	HEMOLYZED TRACE ☐	SMALL + ☐	MODERATE ++ ☐	LARGE +++ ☐
SPECIFIC GRAVITY	1.000 ☐	1.006 ☐	1.010 ☐	1.015 ☐	1.020 ☐	1.025 ☐	1.030 ☐
KETONE	NEGATIVE ☐	mg/dL	TRACE 5 ☐	SMALL 15 ☐	MODERATE 40 ☐	LARGE 80 ☐	LARGE 160 ☐
BILIRUBIN	NEGATIVE ☐		SMALL + ☐	MODERATE ++ ☐	LARGE +++ ☐	
GLUCOSE	NEGATIVE ☐	g/L (%) mg/dL	1/10 (tr.) 100 ☐	1/6 250 ☐	1/2 500 ☐	1 1000 ☐	2 or more 2000 or more ☐

(Modified and printed with permission of Siemens Medical Solutions Diagnostic, Tarrytown, NY 10591.)

Multistix® 10 SG Reagent Strips for Urinalysis

PATIENT

DATE   TIME

LEUKOCYTES	NEGATIVE ☐		TRACE ☐	SMALL + ☐	MODERATE ++ ☐	LARGE +++ ☐
NITRITE	NEGATIVE ☐		POSITIVE ☐	POSITIVE ☐	(Any degree of uniform pink color is found)	
UROBILINOGEN	NORMAL 0.2 ☐	NORMAL 1 ☐	mg/dL 2 ☐	4 ☐	8 ☐ (1mg = approx. 1 BU)	
PROTEIN	NEGATIVE ☐	TRACE ☐	mg/dL 30 ☐ *	100 ++ ☐	300 +++ ☐	2000 OR MORE ☐
pH	5.0 ☐	6.0 ☐	6.5 ☐	7.0 ☐	7.5 ☐	8.0 ☐	8.5 ☐
BLOOD	NEGATIVE ☐	NON-HEMOLYZED TRACE ☐	NON-HEMOLYZED MODERATE ☐	HEMOLYZED TRACE ☐	SMALL + ☐	MODERATE ++ ☐	LARGE +++ ☐
SPECIFIC GRAVITY	1.000 ☐	1.006 ☐	1.010 ☐	1.015 ☐	1.020 ☐	1.025 ☐	1.030 ☐
KETONE	NEGATIVE ☐	mg/dL	TRACE 5 ☐	SMALL 15 ☐	MODERATE 40 ☐	LARGE 80 ☐	LARGE 160 ☐
BILIRUBIN	NEGATIVE ☐		SMALL + ☐	MODERATE ++ ☐	LARGE +++ ☐	
GLUCOSE	NEGATIVE ☐	g/L (%) mg/dL	1/10 (tr.) 100 ☐	1/6 250 ☐	1/2 500 ☐	1 1000 ☐	2 or more 2000 or more ☐

(Modified and printed with permission of Siemens Medical Solutions Diagnostic, Tarrytown, NY 10591.)

Chapter **16** **Urinalysis**

Notes

Procedure 16-1: Collection of a Clean-Catch Midstream Urine Specimen

Name: _____ Date: _____

Evaluated by: _____ Score: _____

Performance Objective

Outcome:	Instruct a patient in the procedure for collecting a clean-catch midstream urine specimen.
Conditions:	Given the following: sterile specimen container and label, personal antiseptic towelettes, and tissues.
Standards:	Time: 10 minutes. Student completed procedure in _____ minutes.
	Accuracy: Satisfactory score on the Performance Evaluation Checklist.

Performance Evaluation Checklist

Trial 1	Trial 2	Point Value	Performance Standards
		•	Sanitized hands.
		•	Greeted the patient and introduced yourself.
		•	Identified the patient and explained the procedure.
		•	Assembled equipment.
		•	Labeled specimen container.
			Instructed the female patient by telling her to
		•	Wash hands and open antiseptic towelettes.
		•	Remove lid from specimen container without touching inside of container or lid.
		•	Place the lid on a paper towel with the opening facing upward.
		•	Pull down undergarments and sit on the toilet.
		•	Expose the urinary meatus by spreading the labia apart with one hand.
		•	Cleanse each side of the urinary meatus with a front-to-back motion using a separate towelette on each side of the meatus.
		▷	Explained why a front-to-back motion should be used.
		•	After use, discard each towelette into toilet.
		•	Cleanse directly across the meatus using a third towelette and discard it.
		•	Void a small amount of urine into the toilet, while continuing to hold the labia apart.
		▷	Explained the purpose of voiding into the toilet.
		•	Without stopping the urine flow, collect the next amount of urine by voiding into the sterile container.
		•	Fill container approximately half full with urine without touching the inside of the container.
		▷	Stated why the inside of the container should not be touched.

689

Trial 1	Trial 2	Point Value	Performance Standards
		•	Void the last amount of urine into the toilet.
		•	Replace specimen container lid.
		•	Wipe area dry with a tissue, flush the toilet, and wash hands.
			Instructed the male patient by telling him to
		•	Wash hands and open antiseptic towelettes, and remove lid from specimen container.
		•	Pull down undergarments and stand in front of toilet.
		•	Retract the foreskin of the penis if uncircumcised.
		•	Cleanse area around the meatus and the urethral opening by wiping each side of the meatus with a separate antiseptic towelette.
		•	Cleanse directly across the meatus using a third antiseptic towelette.
		•	Discard each towelette into the toilet after use.
		•	Void a small amount of urine into the toilet.
		•	Collect the next amount of urine by voiding into the sterile container without touching the inside of the container.
		•	Fill container approximately half full with urine.
		•	Void the last amount of urine into the toilet.
		•	Replace lid on specimen container.
		•	Wipe area dry with a tissue, flush the toilet, and wash hands.
			Performed the following:
		•	Provided patient with instructions on what to do with specimen.
		•	Tested specimen or prepared it for transport to an outside laboratory.
		•	Documented the procedure correctly.
		■	Reassured patients.
		★	Completed the procedure within 10 minutes.
			Totals

CHART	
Date	

Evaluation of Student Performance

EVALUATION CRITERIA			COMMENTS
Symbol	**Category**	**Point Value**	
★	Critical Step	16 points	
•	Essential Step	6 points	
■	Affective Competency	6 points	
▷	Theory Question	2 points	

Score calculation: 100 points

− _____ points missed

_____ Score

Satisfactory score: 85 or above

CAAHEP Competencies Achieved

Psychomotor (Skills)

☑ I. 8. Instruct and prepare a patient for a procedure or treatment.

Affective (Behavior)

☑ A. 2. Reassure patients.

ABHES Competencies Achieved

☑ 7. g. Display professionalism through written and verbal communications.
☑ 9. e. (1). Instruct patient in the collection of urine specimens.

Notes

Chapter **16** **Urinalysis**

Procedure 16-2: Collection of a 24-Hour Urine Specimen

Name: _____ Date: _____

Evaluated by: _____ Score: _____

Performance Objective

Outcome:	Instruct a patient in the procedure for collecting a 24-hour urine specimen.
Conditions:	Given a large urine specimen container and label, written instructions, and a laboratory requisition.
Standards:	Time: 10 minutes. Student completed procedure in _____ minutes.
	Accuracy: Satisfactory score on the Performance Evaluation Checklist.

Performance Evaluation Checklist

Trial 1	Trial 2	Point Value	Performance Standards
		•	Sanitized hands.
		•	Greeted and introduced yourself.
		•	Identified the patient and explained the procedure.
		•	Assembled equipment.
		•	Labeled the specimen container.
			Instructed the patient in the collection of the specimen:
		•	Empty your bladder when you get up in the morning as usual.
		•	Write the date and start time on the container label.
		•	The next time you need to urinate, void into the collecting container.
		•	Pour the urine into the large specimen container.
		•	Tightly screw the lid onto the container.
		•	Store the container in the refrigerator or in an ice chest.
		•	Repeat these steps each time you urinate.
		•	Collect all of your urine in a 24-hour period, and store it in the designated container.
		•	Urinate in the collection container before having a bowel movement.
		▷	Stated when the patient must start the collection process again from the beginning.
		•	On the following morning, get up at the same time.
		•	Void into the collection container for the last time, and pour the urine into the large specimen container.
		•	Put the lid on the container tightly.
		•	Write the date and time the test ended on the container label.
		•	Return the urine specimen container to the office the same morning as completing the test.

Trial 1	Trial 2	Point Value	Performance Standards
			Performed the following:
		•	Provided the patient with the 24-hour specimen container, a collecting container, and written instructions.
		•	Provided the patient with a Material Safety Data Sheet (MSDS), if the specimen container contains a preservative.
		▷	Stated the purpose of the MSDS.
		•	Documented instructions given to the patient in his or her medical record
			Processed the specimen:
		•	Asked the patient whether there were any problems when he or she returned the specimen container.
		▷	Explained what should be done if the specimen was undercollected or overcollected.
		•	Prepared the specimen for transport to the laboratory.
		•	Completed a laboratory request form.
		•	Documented the procedure correctly.
		■	Reassured patients.
		★	Completed the procedure within 5 minutes.
			Totals

CHART

Date	

Evaluation of Student Performance

EVALUATION CRITERIA			COMMENTS
Symbol	**Category**	**Point Value**	
★	Critical Step	16 points	
•	Essential Step	6 points	
■	Affective Competency	6 points	
▷	Theory Question	2 points	

Score calculation: 100 points

       –   points missed

          ___Score

Satisfactory score: 85 or above

CAAHEP Competencies Achieved

Psychomotor (Skills)
☑   I. 8. Instruct and prepare a patient for a procedure.

Affective (Behavior)
☑   A. 2. Reassure patients.

ABHES Competencies Achieved

☑   7. g. Display professionalism through written and verbal communications.
☑   9. e. 1) Instruct patients in the collection of urine specimens.

Notes

Procedure 16-A: Assessing Color and Appearance of a Urine Specimen

Name: _____   Date: _____

Evaluated by: _____   Score: _____

Performance Objective

Outcome:	Assess the color and appearance of a urine specimen.
Conditions:	Given a transparent container and a urine specimen.
Standards:	Time: 5 minutes. Student completed procedure in _____ minutes.
	Accuracy: Satisfactory score on the Performance Evaluation Checklist.

Performance Evaluation Checklist

Trial 1	Trial 2	Point Value	Performance Standards
			Color
		•	Sanitized hands and applied gloves.
		•	Transferred urine specimen to a transparent container.
		•	Assessed the color of the urine specimen.
		★	The assessment was identical to the evaluator's assessment.
			Appearance
		•	Assessed the appearance of the urine specimen in the transparent container.
		★	The assessment was identical to the evaluator's assessment.
		•	Documented the results correctly.
		•	Properly disposed of urine specimen.
		•	Sanitized hands and removed gloves.
		■	Demonstrated critical thinking skills.
		■	Reassured patients.
		★	Completed the procedure within 5 minutes.
			TOTALS

CHART	
Date	

Evaluation of Student Performance

<table>
<tr><th colspan="3">EVALUATION CRITERIA</th><th>COMMENTS</th></tr>
<tr><th>Symbol</th><th>Category</th><th>Point Value</th><td rowspan="9"></td></tr>
<tr><td>★</td><td>Critical Step</td><td>16 points</td></tr>
<tr><td>•</td><td>Essential Step</td><td>6 points</td></tr>
<tr><td>■</td><td>Affective Competency</td><td>6 points</td></tr>
<tr><td>▷</td><td>Theory Question</td><td>2 points</td></tr>
<tr><td colspan="3">Score calculation: 100 points</td></tr>
<tr><td colspan="3">−   points missed</td></tr>
<tr><td colspan="3">___Score</td></tr>
<tr><td colspan="3">Satisfactory score: 85 or above</td></tr>
</table>

CAAHEP Competencies Achieved

Psychomotor (Skills)

☑ I. 11. c. Collect specimens and perform CLIA waived urinalysis.
☑ II. 2. Record laboratory test results into the patient's record.

Affective (Behavior)

☑ A. 1. Demonstrate critical thinking skills.
☑ A. 2. Reassure patients.

ABHES Competencies Achieved

☑ 9. b. (1). Perform selected CLIA-waived tests that assist with diagnosis and treatment: urinalysis.

Procedure 16-3: Chemical Assessment of a Urine Specimen Using a Reagent Strip

Name: _____ Date: _____

Evaluated by: _____ Score: _____

Performance Objective

Outcome:	Perform a chemical assessment of a urine specimen using a reagent strip.
Conditions:	Given the following: disposable gloves, Multistix 10 SG reagent strips, urine container, timer, and a laboratory report form.
Standards:	Time: 5 minutes. Student completed procedure in _____ minutes.
	Accuracy: Satisfactory score on the performance evaluation checklist.

Performance Evaluation Checklist

Trial 1	Trial 2	Point Value	Performance Standards
		•	If necessary, performed a quality control procedure.
		▷	Stated when a quality control procedure should be performed.
		•	Obtained a freshly voided urine specimen from patient.
		▷	Explained why the container used to collect the specimen should be clean.
		•	Sanitized hands.
		•	Assembled equipment.
		•	Checked the expiration date of the reagent strips.
		▷	Stated why expiration date should be checked.
		•	Applied gloves.
		•	Removed a reagent strip from container and recapped immediately.
		▷	Explained why container should be recapped immediately.
		•	Did not touch the test areas with fingers or lay the strip on the table.
		▷	Explained why the test areas should not be touched with fingers or table surface.
		•	Mixed the urine specimen thoroughly.
		•	Removed the lid and completely immersed the reagent strip in urine specimen.
		•	Removed the strip immediately and ran the edge against the rim of the urine container. Started the timer.
		▷	Explained why excess urine should be removed from the strip.
		•	Held the reagent strip in a horizontal position and placed it as close as possible to the corresponding color blocks on color chart.

Trial 1	Trial 2	Point Value	Performance Standards
		▷	Explained why the strip should be held in a horizontal position.
		•	Did not lay the strip directly on the color chart.
		•	Read the results at the exact reading times specified on the color chart.
		▷	Explained why the results must be read at specified times.
		★	The results were identical to the evaluator's results.
		•	Disposed of the strip in a regular waste container
		•	Removed gloves and sanitized hands.
		•	Documented the results correctly.
		■	Demonstrated critical thinking skills.
		■	Reassured patients.
		★	Completed the procedure within 5 minutes.
			TOTALS

CHART

Date	

Evaluation of Student Performance

EVALUATION CRITERIA			COMMENTS
Symbol	Category	Point Value	
★	Critical Step	16 points	
•	Essential Step	6 points	
■	Affective Competency	6 points	
▷	Theory Question	2 points	

Score calculation: 100 points

    −   points missed
          ___Score

Satisfactory score: 85 or above

CAAHEP Competencies Achieved

Psychomotor (Skills)

☑   I. 10. Perform a quality control measure.
☑   I. 11. c. Collect specimens and perform CLIA waived urinalysis.
☑   II. 2. Record laboratory test results into the patient's record.

Affective (Behavior)

☑   A. 1. Demonstrate critical thinking skills.
☑   A. 2. Reassure patients.

ABHES Competencies Achieved

☑   9. a. Practice quality control.
☑   9. b. (1) Perform selected CLIA-waived tests that assist with diagnosis and treatment: urinalysis.

Multistix® 10 SG Reagent Strips for Urinalysis

PATIENT

DATE   TIME

LEUKOCYTES	NEGATIVE ☐		TRACE ☐	SMALL + ☐	MODERATE ++ ☐	LARGE +++ ☐
NITRITE	NEGATIVE ☐		POSITIVE ☐	POSITIVE ☐	(Any degree of uniform pink color is found)	
UROBILINOGEN	NORMAL 0.2 ☐	NORMAL 1 ☐	mg/dL 2 ☐	4 ☐	8 ☐	(1mg = approx. 1 BU)
PROTEIN	NEGATIVE ☐	TRACE ☐	mg/dL 30 ☐ *	100 ++ ☐	300 +++ ☐	2000 OR MORE ☐
pH	5.0 ☐	6.0 ☐	6.5 ☐	7.0 ☐	7.5 ☐	8.0 ☐	8.5 ☐
BLOOD	NEGATIVE ☐	NON-HEMOLYZED TRACE ☐	NON-HEMOLYZED MODERATE ☐	HEMOLYZED TRACE ☐	SMALL + ☐	MODERATE ++ ☐	LARGE +++ ☐
SPECIFIC GRAVITY	1.000 ☐	1.006 ☐	1.010 ☐	1.015 ☐	1.020 ☐	1.025 ☐	1.030 ☐
KETONE	NEGATIVE ☐	mg/dL	TRACE 5 ☐	SMALL 15 ☐	MODERATE 40 ☐	LARGE 80 ☐	LARGE 160 ☐
BILIRUBIN	NEGATIVE ☐		SMALL + ☐	MODERATE ++ ☐	LARGE +++ ☐	
GLUCOSE	NEGATIVE ☐	g/L (%) mg/dL	1/10 (tr.) 100 ☐	1/6 250 ☐	1/2 500 ☐	1 1000 ☐	2 or more 2000 or more ☐

(Modified and printed with permission of Siemens Medical Solutions Diagnostic, Tarrytown, NY 10591.)

Multistix® 10 SG Reagent Strips for Urinalysis

PATIENT

DATE   TIME

LEUKOCYTES	NEGATIVE ☐		TRACE ☐	SMALL + ☐	MODERATE ++ ☐	LARGE +++ ☐
NITRITE	NEGATIVE ☐		POSITIVE ☐	POSITIVE ☐	(Any degree of uniform pink color is found)	
UROBILINOGEN	NORMAL 0.2 ☐	NORMAL 1 ☐	mg/dL 2 ☐	4 ☐	8 ☐	(1mg = approx. 1 BU)
PROTEIN	NEGATIVE ☐	TRACE ☐	mg/dL 30 ☐ *	100 ++ ☐	300 +++ ☐	2000 OR MORE ☐
pH	5.0 ☐	6.0 ☐	6.5 ☐	7.0 ☐	7.5 ☐	8.0 ☐	8.5 ☐
BLOOD	NEGATIVE ☐	NON-HEMOLYZED TRACE ☐	NON-HEMOLYZED MODERATE ☐	HEMOLYZED TRACE ☐	SMALL + ☐	MODERATE ++ ☐	LARGE +++ ☐
SPECIFIC GRAVITY	1.000 ☐	1.006 ☐	1.010 ☐	1.015 ☐	1.020 ☐	1.025 ☐	1.030 ☐
KETONE	NEGATIVE ☐	mg/dL	TRACE 5 ☐	SMALL 15 ☐	MODERATE 40 ☐	LARGE 80 ☐	LARGE 160 ☐
BILIRUBIN	NEGATIVE ☐		SMALL + ☐	MODERATE ++ ☐	LARGE +++ ☐	
GLUCOSE	NEGATIVE ☐	g/L (%) mg/dL	1/10 (tr.) 100 ☐	1/6 250 ☐	1/2 500 ☐	1 1000 ☐	2 or more 2000 or more ☐

(Modified and printed with permission of Siemens Medical Solutions Diagnostic, Tarrytown, NY 10591.)

EVALUATION OF COMPETENCY

Procedure 16-4: Prepare a Urine Specimen for Microscopic Examination: Kova Method

Name: _____   Date: _____

Evaluated by: _____   Score: _____

Performance Objective

Outcome:	Prepare a urine specimen for microscopic analysis by the provider.
Conditions:	Given the following: disposable gloves; first-voided morning urine specimen; Kova urine centrifuge tube, cap, pipet, slide, and stain; test tube rack; urine centrifuge; and mechanical stage microscope.
Standards:	Time: 15 minutes. Student completed procedure in _____ minutes.
	Accuracy: Satisfactory score on the Performance Evaluation Checklist.

Performance Evaluation Checklist

Trial 1	Trial 2	Point Value	Performance Standards
		•	Sanitized hands.
		•	Assembled equipment.
		•	Applied gloves.
		•	Mixed urine specimen with pipet.
		▷	Stated the purpose of mixing the specimen.
		•	Poured urine specimen into urine centrifuge tube to the 12-mL mark.
		•	Capped the tube.
		•	Centrifuged specimen for 5 minutes.
		▷	Stated the purpose of centrifuging the specimen.
		•	Removed the tube from the centrifuge without disturbing the sediment.
		•	Removed the cap.
		•	Inserted Kova pipet into the urine tube and seated it firmly.
		•	Inverted the tube and poured off the supernatant.
		•	Removed pipet from the tube.
		•	Added one drop of Kova stain to the tube.
		▷	Stated the purpose of the stain.
		•	Placed pipet back in tube and mixed specimen thoroughly.
		•	Placed urine tube in test tube rack.
		•	Transferred a sample of the specimen to the Kova slide.
		•	Did not overfill or underfill the well of the Kova slide.
		•	Placed pipet in the urine tube.

Trial 1	Trial 2	Point Value	Performance Standards
		•	Allowed specimen to sit for 1 minute.
		▷	Explained the purpose of allowing the specimen to sit 1 minute.
		•	Placed the slide on the stage of the microscope.
		•	Properly focused the specimen under low power.
		•	Placed the slide on the stage of the microscope.
		•	Properly focused the specimen for the provider.
		•	Removed the slide from the stage when the provider is finished examining the specimen.
		•	Disposed of the slide and pipet in a regular waste container.
		•	Rinsed the remaining urine down the sink.
		•	Capped the empty urine tube and disposed of it in a regular waste container.
		•	Removed gloves and sanitized hands.
		■	Demonstrated critical thinking skills.
		★	Completed the procedure within 15 minutes.
			Totals

CHART

Date	

Evaluation of Student Performance

EVALUATION CRITERIA			COMMENTS
Symbol	**Category**	**Point Value**	
★	Critical Step	16 points	
•	Essential Step	6 points	
■	Affective Competency	6 points	
▷	Theory Question	2 points	

Score calculation: 100 points

     −   points missed

         ___ Score

Satisfactory score: 85 or above

CAAHEP Competencies Achieved

Psychomotor (Skills)

☑ I. 9. Assist provider with a patient exam.

Affective (Behavior)

☑ A. 1. Demonstrate critical thinking skills.

ABHES Competencies Achieved

☑ 8. c. Assist provider with general/physical examination.

Notes

Procedure 16-5: Perform a CLIA-Waived Urine Pregnancy Test

Name: _____   Date: _____

Evaluated by: _____   Score: _____

Performance Objective

Outcome:	Perform a CLIA-waived urine pregnancy test.
Conditions:	Given the following: disposable gloves, urine pregnancy test kit, first-voided morning urine specimen, waste container.
Standards:	Time: 5 minutes. Student completed procedure in _____ minutes.
	Accuracy: Satisfactory score on the Performance Evaluation Checklist.

Performance Evaluation Checklist

Trial 1	Trial 2	Point Value	Performance Standards
		•	Sanitized hands.
		•	Assembled equipment.
		•	Checked the expiration date on the pregnancy test kit.
		▷	Explained why the expiration date should be checked.
		•	If necessary, ran controls on the pregnancy test and documented results in the quality control log.
		▷	Stated when controls should be run.
		•	Applied gloves.
		•	Rotated the specimen container to mix the urine specimen.
		•	Inspected the foil pouch to make sure it is not torn or punctured.
		•	Removed the test cassette from its pouch and placed it on a clean, dry, level surface.
		•	Added 3 drops of urine to the well on the test cassette.
		•	Did not handle or move the cassette again until the test is ready for interpretation.
		•	Disposed of the pipet in a regular waste container.
		•	Waited 3 minutes and read the results.
		•	Interpreted the test results.
		★	The results were identical to the evaluator's results.
		▷	Described the appearance of a positive and a negative test result.
		▷	Explained what should be done if a blue internal control line does not appear within 3 minutes.
		•	Disposed of the test cassette in a regular waste container.
		•	Removed gloves and sanitized hands.
		•	Documented the results correctly.

Trial 1	Trial 2	Point Value	Performance Standards
		■	Demonstrated critical thinking skills.
		■	Reassured patients.
		★	Completed the procedure within 5 minutes.
			TOTALS

CHART

Date	

Evaluation of Student Performance

EVALUATION CRITERIA			COMMENTS
Symbol	**Category**	**Point Value**	
★	Critical Step	16 points	
•	Essential Step	6 points	
■	Affective Competency	6 points	
▷	Theory Question	2 points	

Score calculation: 100 points

− _____ points missed

_____ Score

Satisfactory score: 85 or above

CAAHEP Competencies Achieved

Psychomotor (Skills)

☑ I. 10. Perform a quality control measure.
☑ I. 11. c. Collect specimens and perform CLIA waived urinalysis.
☑ II. 2. Record laboratory test results into the patient's record.

Affective (Behavior)

☑ A. 1. Demonstrate critical thinking skills.
☑ A. 2. Reassure patients.

ABHES Competencies Achieved

☑ 9. a. Practice quality control.
☑ 9. b. (1) Perform selected CLIA-waived tests that assist with diagnosis and treatment: urinalysis.

17 Phlebotomy

CHAPTER ASSIGNMENTS

√ After Completing	Date Due	Study Guide Pages	STUDY GUIDE ASSIGNMENTS (CTA = Critical Thinking Activity)	Possible Points	Points You Earned
		713	? Pretest	10	
		714	Term Key Term Assessment		
			A. Definitions	16	
		714	B. Word Parts	13	
			(Add 1 point for each key term)		
		715-719	Evaluation of Learning questions	50	
		720	CTA A: Antecubital Veins	5	
			Evolve: Got Blood? (Record points earned)		
		720-721	CTA B: Venipuncture-Vacutainer Method	15	
		721-722	CTA C: Venipuncture Situations	7	
		722	CTA D: Vasovagal Warning Signals	20	
		723	CTA E: Skin Puncture	8	
		724	CTA F: Crossword Puzzle	29	
			Evolve: Apply Your Knowledge questions	10	
			Evolve: Video Evaluation	42	
		713	? Posttest	10	
			ADDITIONAL ASSIGNMENTS		
			Total points		

√ When Assigned By Your Instructor	Study Guide Pages	Practices Required	LABORATORY ASSIGNMENTS (Procedure Number and Name)	Score*
	725	5	**Practice for Competency** 17-1: Venipuncture—Vacutainer Method	
	727-730		**Evaluation of Competency** 17-1: Venipuncture—Vacutainer Method	*
	725-726	5	**Practice for Competency** 17-2: Venipuncture—Butterfly Method	
	731-734		**Evaluation of Competency** 17-2: Venipuncture—Butterfly Method	*
	725	2	**Practice for Competency** 17-3: Separating Serum From a Blood Specimen	
	735-737		**Evaluation of Competency** 17-3: Separating Serum From a Blood Specimen	*
	725-726	3	**Practice for Competency** 17-4: Skin Puncture—Disposable Lancet	
	739-741		**Evaluation of Competency** 17-4: Skin Puncture—Disposable Lancet	*
			ADDITIONAL ASSIGNMENTS	

Notes

Name:_____ Date:_____

_____

True or False

_____ 1. An individual who collects blood specimens is known as a vampire.

_____ 2. The purpose of applying a tourniquet when performing venipuncture is to make the patient's veins stand out.

_____ 3. The tourniquet should be left on the patient's arm for at least 2 minutes before performing a venipuncture.

_____ 4. Serum is obtained from whole blood that has been centrifuged.

_____ 5. A 25-gauge needle is recommended for performing venipuncture with the Vacutainer method.

_____ 6. The size of the collection tube used to obtain a venous blood specimen depends on the size of the patient's veins.

_____ 7. The correct order of draw evacuated blood collection tubes is red, lavender, gray, and green.

_____ 8. Veins are most likely to collapse in patients with large veins and thick walls.

_____ 9. Hemolysis of a blood specimen results in inaccurate test results.

_____10. When obtaining a capillary specimen, the first drop of blood should be used for the test.

📄 **POSTTEST**
_____

True or False

_____ 1. Venous reflux can be prevented by filling the collection tube to the exhaustion of the vacuum.

_____ 2. If the tourniquet is applied too tightly, inaccurate test results may occur.

_____ 3. The median cubital vein is the best vein to use for venipuncture.

_____ 4. On standing, a blood specimen to which an anticoagulant has been added separates into plasma, buffy coat, and red blood cells.

_____ 5. Whole blood is obtained by using a tube containing an anticoagulant.

_____ 6. An evacuated blood collection tube with a lavender stopper contains EDTA.

_____ 7. A red-stoppered tube is used to collect a blood specimen for most blood chemistry tests.

_____ 8. Not filling a tube to the exhaustion of the vacuum can result in hemolysis of the blood specimen.

_____ 9. If the needle is removed from the arm before removing the tourniquet, internal and external bleeding will occur around the puncture site.

_____10. If a fibrin clot forms in the serum layer of a blood specimen, it will lead to inaccurate test results.

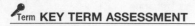 **KEY TERM ASSESSMENT**

A. Definitions

Directions: Match each key term with its definition.

_____ 1. Antecubital space

_____ 2. Anticoagulant

_____ 3. Buffy coat

_____ 4. Evacuated collection tube

_____ 5. Hematoma

_____ 6. Hemoconcentration

_____ 7. Hemolysis

_____ 8. Osteochondritis

_____ 9. Osteomyelitis

_____10. Phlebotomist

_____11. Phlebotomy

_____12. Plasma

_____13. Serum

_____14. Venipuncture

_____15. Venous reflux

_____16. Venous stasis

A. The liquid part of blood, consisting of a clear, straw-colored fluid that makes up approximately 55% of the blood volume

B. A substance that inhibits blood clotting

C. A health professional trained in the collection of blood specimens

D. The breakdown of blood cells

E. A sterile glass or plastic blood collection tube with a color-coded closure that contains a vacuum

F. The temporary cessation or slowing of the venous blood flow

G. A thin, light-colored layer of white blood cells and platelets that lies between a top layer of plasma and a bottom layer of red blood cells when an anticoagulant has been added to a blood specimen

H. The surface of the arm in front of the elbow

I. Inflammation of bone and cartilage

J. An increase in the concentration of the nonfilterable blood components in the blood vessels as a result of a decrease in the fluid content of the blood

K. Plasma from which the clotting factor fibrinogen has been removed

L. Incision of a vein for the removal of blood

M. Inflammation of the bone or bone marrow as a result of bacterial infection

N. A swelling or mass of coagulated blood caused by a break in a blood vessel

O. Puncturing of a vein

P. The backflow of blood (from a collection tube) into the patient's vein

B. Word Parts

Directions: Indicate the meaning of each word part in the space provided. List as many medical terms as possible that incorporate the word part in the space provided.

Word Part	Meaning of Word Part	Medical Terms That Incorporate Word Part
1. ante-		
2. anti-		
3. hemat/o		
4. -oma		
5. hem/o		
6. -lysis		
7. oste/o		
8. myel/o		
9. -itis		
10. phleb/o		
11. -otomy		
12. ven/o		
13. -ous		

714

Chapter **17 Phlebotomy**

EVALUATION OF LEARNING

Directions: Fill in each blank with the correct answer.

1. What is the purpose of phlebotomy?

   _____

2. List the three major areas of blood collection and the type of specimen obtained.

   _____

   _____

   _____

3. What two methods can be used to perform a venipuncture?

   _____

   _____

4. What are the advantages of using the Vacutainer method of venipuncture?

   _____

5. When is the butterfly method used for venipuncture?

   _____

   _____

6. What reference source should be consulted to determine the collection and handling requirements of tests performed at an outside laboratory?

   _____

7. Why should a patient be identified using two unique identifiers?

   _____

   _____

8. What might occur if the wrong collection tube is used to collect a blood specimen?

   _____

9. What occurs if an expired collection tube is used to collect a blood specimen?

   _____

10. What is the purpose of a laboratory request?

    _____

11. How should a barcode label be placed on a blood collection tube and why?

    _____

    _____

12. Why should the patient be notified right before the needle is being inserted?

    _____

    _____

13. Explain how to prevent venous reflux.

_____

_____

14. What is the purpose of the tourniquet?

_____

_____

15. What may occur if the tourniquet is too tight or too loose?

Too tight. _____

Too loose: _____

16. What can occur if the tourniquet is left on the patient's arm for longer than a minute?

_____

_____

17. What occurs if the venipuncture needle is removed before the tourniquet?

_____

_____

18. Why are the antecubital veins preferred for performing a venipuncture?

_____

_____

_____

19. What are the advantages of using the median cubital vein as a venepuncture site?

_____

20. What should be determined through palpation after a suitable vein has been located?

_____

21. List four techniques that can be used to make veins more prominent.

_____

_____

_____

_____

22. Why should the veins of the hand be used only as a last resort for venipuncture?

_____

_____

_____

23. How is a serum specimen obtained?

_____

_____

24. How is a whole blood specimen obtained?

_____

_____

25. List the three layers into which blood separates when it is mixed with an anticoagulant.

_____

_____

26. List the layers into which blood separates when an anticoagulant is not added to it.

_____

_____

27. List six OSHA safety precautions that must be followed when performing a venipuncture and separating serum or plasma from whole blood.

_____

_____

_____

_____

_____

28. What needle gauges are used for the Vacutainer method and when is each used?

_____

_____

29. What is the purpose of the flange on the plastic holder of the Vacutainer system?

_____

_____

30. What additive is present in the following evacuated blood collection tubes?

Red: _____

Gold and marbled red/gray: _____

Lavender: _____

Light blue: _____

Green: _____

Gray: _____

Royal blue: _____

31. What color stopper must be used to collect the blood specimen for each of the tests listed?

CBC: _____

Prothrombin time: _____

Oral glucose tolerance test: _____

Most blood chemistry tests: _____

Blood gas determinations: _____

Lead test: _____

Blood alcohol test: _____

32. Why is it important to use the correct order of draw when performing a venipuncture?

_____

_____

33. Why is it important to mix a tube containing an anticoagulant immediately after drawing it?

_____

_____

34. What are the ranges for the gauge and length of needle used for the butterfly method of venipuncture?

_____

_____

35. What sites should be avoided when performing a venepuncture?

_____

_____

36. How can the cephalic and basilic veins be prevented from rolling during a venipuncture?

_____

_____

37. What is typically observed when performing a venipuncture on a vein that collapses?

_____

38. What are three ways in which a hematoma may occur?

_____

_____

_____

39. List four ways to prevent a blood specimen from becoming hemolyzed.

_____

_____

_____

_____

718

40. What should be done if the patient experiences dizziness or fainting during or after a venepuncture?

_____

_____

41. List examples of substances dissolved in the serum of blood.

_____

_____

42. What is the purpose of performing laboratory tests on serum?

_____

_____

43. List the proper size tube that must be used to obtain the following serum specimens:

2 mL of serum: _____

6 mL of serum: _____

4 mL of serum: _____

44. What is a fibrin clot, and why should it be avoided in a serum specimen?

_____

_____

45. How does a serum separator tube function in the collection of a serum specimen?

_____

_____

_____

46. What is the preferred site for a skin puncture for the following individuals?

a. Adult: _____

b. Infant: _____

47. Why is it important not to penetrate the skin too deeply when performing a skin puncture?

_____

_____

48. How is blade length determined for a skin puncture?

_____

_____

49. What are two examples of microcollection devices?

_____

_____

50. Why should a finger puncture not be performed on the index finger?

_____

_____

719

A. Antecubital Veins

Practice palpating the antecubital veins on at least five classmates. Use a tourniquet applied to each person's arm, and ask the individual to clench his or her fist. Document the individual's name and which vein would be considered the best to use on each person when performing venipuncture.

	NAME	SUITABLE VEIN
1.		
2.		
3.		
4.		
5.		

B. Venipuncture—Vacutainer Method

Using the principles outlined in the Vacutainer venipuncture procedure, indicate what may occur under the following circumstances:

1. A collection tube is used that is past its expiration date.

2. The collection tube is not labeled.

3. The tourniquet is not applied tightly enough.

4. The tourniquet is left on for 5 minutes.

5. The area cleansed with an antiseptic is not allowed to dry before the venipuncture is made.

6. The collection tube is inserted past the indentation in the plastic holder before the vein is entered.

7. An angle of less than 15 degrees is used when performing venipuncture.

8. An angle of more than 15 degrees is used when performing venipuncture.

_____

_____

9. The needle is moved after inserting it.

_____

_____

10. Venous reflux occurs when using an EDTA collection tube.

_____

_____

11. The collection tube is removed before it has filled to the exhaustion of the vacuum.

_____

_____

12. The needle is removed from the arm before the tourniquet is removed.

_____

_____

13. A gauze pad is not placed slightly above the puncture site before removing the needle.

_____

_____

14. The patient bends the arm at the elbow after the needle is removed.

_____

_____

15. The patient lifts a heavy object after the venipuncture.

_____

_____

C. Venipuncture Situations

You are responsible for performing the venipunctures in your medical office. In the space provided, explain what you would do in each of the following situations:

1. The patient asks you if the venipuncture will hurt.

_____

_____

2. On palpating the patient's vein, you find that it feels stiff and hard.

_____

_____

3. You have attempted one venipuncture in a patient with small veins using the Vacutainer method of venipuncture; however, the vein collapsed, and you were unable to obtain blood.

_____

_____

4. The patient moves during the procedure, causing the needle to come out of his arm.

_____

_____

5. You have inserted the needle in the vein but notice a sudden swelling around the puncture site.

_____

_____

6. You inadvertently puncture the brachial artery after inserting the needle.

_____

_____

7. The patient begins to sweat and tells you that he or she feels warm and light-headed.

_____

_____

D. Vasovagal Syncope Warning Signals

Create a profile of an individual who is exhibiting the warning signals of vasovagal syncope (fainting) following these guidelines:

1. Using a blank piece of paper, colored pencils, crayons, or markers, draw a figure of an individual exhibiting the warning signals of vasovagal syncope. Be as creative as possible.

2. Do not use any text on your drawing other than to label items you have drawn in your picture. (A picture is worth a thousand words!)

3. Try to include as many of the warning signals of vasovagal syncope as possible.

4. In the classroom, find a partner, and trade drawings. Identify the warning signals in your partner's drawing. With your partner, discuss the cause and symptoms of vasovagal syncope and how to treat it. Also discuss prevention methods for vasovagal syncope. List this information in the space provided below.

Cause and Symptoms: _____

_____

_____

Treatment: _____

_____

_____

Prevention Methods: _____

_____

_____

722

E. Skin Puncture

The medical assistant is performing a skin puncture on an adult patient to obtain a capillary blood specimen for a hemoglobin test. For each of the following situations, write C if the technique is correct and I if the technique is incorrect. If the technique is correct, explain the rationale for performing it that way; if incorrect, explain what might happen if the technique were performed in the incorrect manner.

_____ 1. Before making the puncture, the medical assistant asks the patient to rinse her hand in warm water.

_____

_____

_____ 2. The puncture is made with the patient in a standing position.

_____

_____

_____ 3. The site is allowed to dry thoroughly after it is cleansed with an antiseptic wipe.

_____

_____

_____ 4. The specimen is collected from the lateral part of the tip of the ring finger.

_____

_____

_____ 5. The puncture is made perpendicular to the lines of the fingerprint.

_____

_____

_____ 6. The depth of the puncture is 4 mm.

_____

_____

_____ 7. The first drop of blood is wiped away.

_____

_____

_____ 8. The puncture site is squeezed excessively to obtain the blood specimen.

_____

_____

F. Crossword Puzzle: Phlebotomy

Directions: Complete the crossword puzzle using the clues provided.

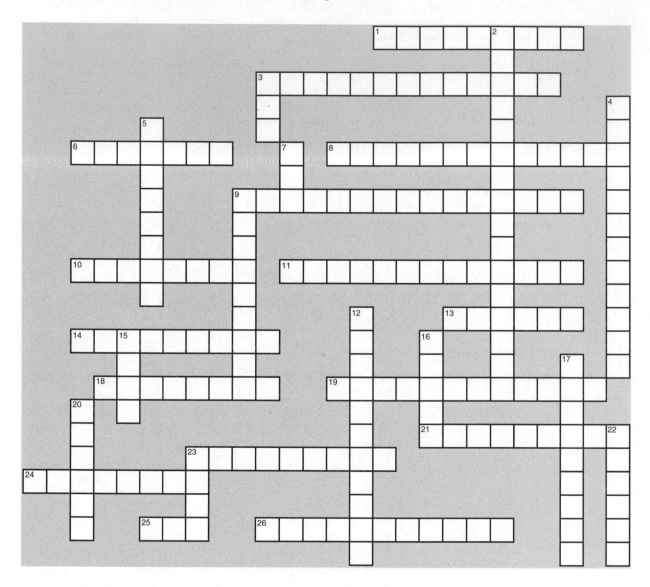

Across
1. What BP does during fainting
3. Makes RBCs clot quicker
6. Rolling vein
8. Best VP vein
9. Inflammation of bone and cartilage
10. Outdated tube problem
11. Inhibits blood clotting
13. Faint position
14. PT tube color
18. EDTA tube color
19. Backflow of blood
21. For small veins
23. Broken RBCs
24. Bad bruise
25. No additive tube
26. Based on size of pt's finger

Down
2. In front of the elbow
3. Select lavender tube for this test
4. Collects blood
5. First drop of capillary blood?
7. Contains a "separating" gel
9. Time limit for tourniquet
12. Do not use for skin puncture
15. Fluoride/oxalate tube color
16. Don't use to palpate vein
17. WBCs and platelets
20. Fainting warning signal
22. Color of serum
23. Last choice veins

724

Procedure 17-1: Venipuncture Vacutainer Method. Practice the procedure for collecting a venous blood specimen using the Vacutainer method. Document the procedure in the chart provided.

Procedure 17-2: Venipuncture Butterfly Method. Practice the procedure for collecting a venous blood specimen using the butterfly method. Document the procedure in the chart provided.

Procedure 17-3: Separating Serum From a Blood Specimen. Practice the procedure for separating serum from a blood specimen.

Procedure 17-4: Skin Puncture: Disposable Lancet. Obtain a capillary blood specimen using a disposable lancet.

CHART	
Date	

725

CHART	
Date	

Procedure 17-1: Venipuncture—Vacutainer Method

Name: _____ Date: _____

Evaluated by: _____ Score: _____

Performance Objective

Outcome:	Perform a venipuncture using the Vacutainer method.
Conditions:	Given the following: disposable gloves, tourniquet, antiseptic wipe, blood collection needle with a safety shield, plastic tube holder, collection tubes with labels, gauze pad, adhesive bandage, biohazard sharps container, biohazard specimen bag, and a laboratory request form.
Standards:	Time: 10 minutes. Student completed procedure in _____ minutes.
	Accuracy: Satisfactory score on the Performance Evaluation Checklist.

Performance Evaluation Checklist

Trial 1	Trial 2	Point Value	Performance Standards
		•	Reviewed requirements for collecting and handling for the tests ordered.
		•	Sanitized hands.
		•	Greeted the patient and introduced yourself.
		•	Identified the patient.
		•	Seated the patient in a phlebotomy chair.
		•	Asked patient if he or she prepared properly.
			Prepared the equipment
		•	Assembled equipment.
		•	Selected the proper collection tubes.
		•	Checked the expiration date on the tubes.
		▷	Stated the purpose of checking the expiration date.
		•	Completed a laboratory request.
		•	Labeled the collection tubes.
		•	Screwed the plastic holder onto the plastic holder and tightened securely.
		•	Opened the gauze packet.
		•	Positioned the collection tubes in the correct order of draw.
		•	Tapped collection tubes with a powdered additive below the stopper.
		▷	Stated the purpose for tapping the tube.
		•	Placed the first tube loosely in the plastic holder.
			Prepared the patient
		•	Explained the procedure to the patient and reassured patient.

727

Trial 1	Trial 2	Point Value	Performance Standards
		•	Performed a preliminary assessment of both arms.
		•	Correctly applied the tourniquet.
		•	Asked patient to clench fist.
		▷	Stated the purpose of the tourniquet and clenched fist.
		•	Assessed the veins of both arms.
		•	Determined the best vein to use.
		•	Positioned the patient's arm correctly.
		•	Thoroughly palpated the selected vein.
		•	Did not leave the tourniquet on for more than 1 minute.
		▷	Explained why the tourniquet should not be left on for more than 1 minute.
		•	Removed tourniquet and cleansed the puncture site.
		•	Allowed puncture site to air dry.
		▷	Explained why the site should be allowed to air dry.
		•	Did not touch the site after cleansing.
		•	Placed supplies within comfortable reach of the nondominant hand.
		•	Reapplied tourniquet and applied gloves.
			Performed the venipuncture
		•	Correctly positioned safety shield and removed cap from the needle.
		•	Properly held the Vacutainer setup (bevel up) with the dominant hand.
		•	Positioned the tube with the label facing downward.
		▷	Explained why the label should face downward.
		•	Grasped the patient's arm and anchored the vein correctly.
		•	Positioned the Vacutainer setup at a 15-degree angle to the arm, with the needle pointing in the same direction as the vein to be entered.
		•	Positioned the needle approximately $1/8$ inch below the place where the vein is to be entered.
		•	Told the patient that a small stick will be felt.
		•	With one continuous motion, entered the skin and then the vein.
		•	Stabilized the Vacutainer setup.
		▷	Stated why the Vacutainer setup should be stabilized.
		•	Pushed the tube forward slowly to the end of the holder using the flange.
		•	Allowed collection tube to fill to the exhaustion of the vacuum.
		▷	Explained why the tube should be allowed to fill to the exhaustion of the vacuum.

Trial 1	Trial 2	Point Value	Performance Standards
		•	Removed the tube from the plastic holder using the flange.
		•	Immediately and gently inverted tube 5 times, if it contained a clot activator and 8 to 10 times if it contained an anticoagulant.
		•	Inserted the next tube into the holder using the flange.
		•	Continued until the last tube was filled.
		★	Removed the tourniquet and asked the patient to unclench fist.
		•	Removed the last tube from the holder.
		▷	Stated why the last tube should be removed.
		•	Placed gauze pad slightly above puncture site and withdrew the needle slowly and at the same angle as that for penetration.
		•	Immediately moved gauze over puncture site and applied pressure.
		•	Activated the safety shield away from yourself.
		•	Immediately disposed of holder and needle in a biohazard sharps container.
		•	Instructed patient to apply pressure with the gauze pad for 1 to 2 minutes.
		▷	Stated why pressure should be applied.
		•	Applied adhesive bandage to puncture site.
		•	Placed tube in an upright position in a test tube rack.
		•	Removed gloves and sanitized hands.
		•	Documented the procedure correctly.
		•	Processed the specimens, if needed.
		•	Prepared the specimen for transport to an outside laboratory.
		■	Demonstrated critical thinking skills.
		■	Reassured patients.
		■	Demonstrated empathy for patient's concerns.
		★	Completed the procedure within 10 minutes.
			Totals

CHART

Date	

Evaluation of Student Performance

EVALUATION CRITERIA			COMMENTS
Symbol	**Category**	**Point Value**	
★	Critical Step	16 points	
•	Essential Step	6 points	
■	Affective Competency	6 points	
▷	Theory Question	2 points	

Score calculation: 100 points

       −   points missed

           ___ Score

Satisfactory score: 85 or above

CAAHEP Competencies Achieved

Psychomotor (Skills)

☑ I. 2. b. Perform the following procedures: venipuncture.
☑ III. 10. Demonstrate proper disposal of biohazardous material a. sharps b. regulated waste.

Affective (Behavior)

☑ A. 1. Demonstrate critical thinking skills.
☑ A. 2. Reassure patients.
☑ A. 3. Demonstrate empathy for patients' concerns.

ABHES Competencies Achieved

☑ 8. a. Practice standard precautions and perform disinfection/sterilization techniques.
☑ 9. c. Dispose of biohazardous materials.
☑ 9. d. (1). Collect, label and process specimens: Perform venipuncture a. Evacuated tube system.

Procedure 17-2: Venipuncture—Butterfly Method

Name: _____   Date: _____

Evaluated by: _____   Score: _____

Performance Objective

Outcome:	Perform a venipuncture using the butterfly method.
Conditions:	Given the following: disposable gloves, tourniquet, antiseptic wipe, winged infusion set, plastic holder, collection tubes with labels, gauze pad, adhesive bandage, biohazard sharps container, biohazard specimen bag, and a laboratory request form.
Standards:	Time: 10 minutes. Student completed procedure in _____ minutes.
	Accuracy: Satisfactory score on the Performance Evaluation Checklist.

Performance Evaluation Checklist

Trial 1	Trial 2	Point Value	Performance Standards
		•	Reviewed requirements for collecting and handling the blood specimen.
		•	Sanitized hands.
		•	Greeted the patient and introduced yourself.
		•	Identified patient.
		▷	Stated why the patient must be correctly identified.
		•	Asked patient if he or she prepared properly.
		▷	Explained why it is important for the patient to prepare properly.
			Prepared the equipment
		•	Assembled equipment.
		•	Selected the proper collection tubes.
		•	Checked the expiration date of the tubes.
		•	Completed a laboratory request.
		•	Labeled the collection tubes.
		•	Removed the winged infusion set from its package.
		•	Extended the tubing to its full length and stretched it.
		▷	Explained why the tubing should be extended and stretched.
		•	Screwed the plastic holder onto the Luer adapter and tightened it securely.
		•	Opened the gauze packet.
		•	Positioned the collection tubes in the correct order of draw.
		•	Tapped collection tubes with a powdered additive below the stopper.
		▷	Stated why tubes with powdered additives must be tapped.

Trial 1	Trial 2	Point Value	Performance Standards
		•	Placed the first tube loosely in the plastic holder with the label facing downward.
		▷	Explained why the label should be facing downward.
			Prepared the patient
		•	Explained the procedure to the patient and reassured patient.
		•	Performed a preliminary assessment of both arms.
		•	Correctly applied the tourniquet and asked patient to clench fist.
		•	Assessed the veins of both arms.
		•	Determined the best vein to use.
		•	Positioned the patient's arm correctly.
		▷	Stated why arm must be positioned correctly.
		•	Thoroughly palpated the selected vein.
		▷	Stated the purpose of palpating the vein.
		•	Did not leave the tourniquet on for more than 1 minute.
		•	Removed tourniquet and cleansed the puncture site.
		•	Allowed puncture site to air dry.
		•	Did not touch the site after cleansing.
		•	Placed supplies within comfortable reach.
		•	Reapplied tourniquet and applied gloves.
			Performed the venipuncture
		•	Grasped the winged infusion set correctly.
		•	Removed the protective sheath from the needle.
		•	Positioned the needle with the bevel up.
		▷	Explained why the bevel should be up.
		•	Grasped patient's arm and anchored the vein correctly.
		•	Positioned the needle at a 15-degree angle to arm, with needle pointing in the same direction as the vein to be entered.
		•	Positioned the needle approximately $1/8$ inch below the place where the vein is to be entered.
		•	Told the patient that a small stick will be felt.
		•	With one continuous motion, entered the skin and then the vein.
		▷	Explained why a continuous motion should be used.
		•	Decreased the angle of the needle to 5 degrees.
		•	Seated the needle.

Trial 1	Trial 2	Point Value	Performance Standards
		▷	Stated the purpose of seating the needle.
		•	Opened the butterfly wings and rested them flat against the skin.
		•	Kept the tube and holder in a downward position.
		•	Slowly pushed the tube forward to the end of the plastic holder.
		•	Allowed collection tube to fill to the exhaustion of the vacuum.
		▷	Explained why the tube should be filled to the exhaustion of the vacuum.
		•	Removed the tube from the plastic holder.
		•	Immediately and gently inverted collection tube 5 times, if it contained a clot activator and 8 to 10 times, if it contained an anticoagulant.
		▷	Explained why a tube with an anticoagulant must be inverted immediately.
		•	Inserted the next tube into the holder.
		•	Continued until the last tube was filled.
		★	Removed the tourniquet and asked the patient to unclench fist.
		▷	Stated why the tourniquet must be removed before the needle.
		•	Removed the last tube from the holder.
		•	Placed gauze pad slightly above puncture site. Grasped the setup just below the wings and withdrew the needle slowly and at the same angle as that for penetration.
		•	Immediately moved gauze over puncture site and applied pressure.
		•	Instructed the patient to apply pressure with the gauze.
		•	Activated the safety shield on the needle.
		•	Properly disposed of the winged infusion set and plastic holder in a biohazard sharps container.
		•	Continued to apply pressure for 1 to 2 minutes.
		•	Applied adhesive bandage.
		•	Placed the tubes in an upright position in a test tube rack.
		•	Removed gloves and sanitized hands.
		•	Documented the procedure correctly.
		•	If needed process that blood specimen.
		•	Prepare the specimen for transport to an outside laboratory.
		■	Demonstrated critical thinking skills.
		■	Reassured patients.
		■	Demonstrated empathy for patient's concerns.
		★	Completed the procedure within 10 minutes.

Trial 1	Trial 2	Point Value	Performance Standards
			Totals

CHART

Date	

Evaluation of Student Performance

EVALUATION CRITERIA			COMMENTS
Symbol	**Category**	**Point Value**	
★	Critical Step	16 points	
•	Essential Step	6 points	
■	Affective Competency	6 points	
▷	Theory Question	2 points	

Score calculation: 100 points

− _____ points missed

_____ Score

Satisfactory score: 85 or above

2015 CAAHEP Competencies Achieved

Psychomotor (Skills)

☑ I. 2. b. Perform the following procedures: venipuncture.
☑ III. 10. Demonstrate proper disposal of biohazardous material a. sharps b. regulated waste.

Affective (Behavior)

☑ A. 1. Demonstrate critical thinking skills.
☑ A. 2. Reassure patients.
☑ A. 3. Demonstrate empathy for patients' concerns.

ABHES Competencies Achieved

☑ 8. a. Practice standard precautions and perform disinfection/sterilization techniques.
☑ 9. c. Dispose of biohazardous materials.
☑ 9. d. (1). Collect, label and process specimens: Perform venipuncture b. Winged infusion set.

Procedure 17-3: Separating Serum from a Blood Specimen

Name: _____   Date: _____

Evaluated by: _____   Score: _____

Performance Objective

Outcome:	Separate serum from a blood specimen.
Conditions:	Given the following: red collection tube setup, test tube rack, disposable pipet, transfer tube and label, disposable gloves, face shield or mask and an eye protection device, centrifuge, and a biohazard sharps container.
Standards:	Time: 20 minutes. Student completed procedure in _____ minutes.
	Accuracy: Satisfactory score on the Performance Evaluation Checklist.

Performance Evaluation Checklist

Trial 1	Trial 2	Point Value	Performance Standards
		•	Collected the blood specimen by performing a venipuncture.
		▷	Stated why a red-closure tube should be used.
		•	Placed the specimen tube in an upright position for 30 to 45 minutes at room temperature while keeping the stopper on the specimen tube.
		▷	Explained why the specimen tube must be placed in an upright position.
		•	Placed the specimen tube in the centrifuge, with the closure end upward.
		▷	Stated why the closure must remain on the specimen tube.
		•	Balanced the specimen with the same type and weight of tube.
		▷	Stated the purpose for balancing the centrifuge.
		•	Centrifuged the specimen for 10 minutes.
		▷	Explained the purpose of centrifugation.
		•	Allowed the centrifuge to come to a complete stop.
		•	Did not open the lid or try to stop the centrifuge with your hand.
		•	Put on a face shield or a mask and an eye protection device and applied gloves.
		▷	Stated the purpose of wearing personal protective equipment.
		•	Removed the specimen tube from the centrifuge without disturbing the contents.
		▷	Explained what must be done if the contents of the tube are disturbed.
		•	Carefully removed the closure from the tube.
		•	Squeezed the bulb of the pipet and placed the tip of the pipet against the side of the tube approximately ¼ inch above the cell layer.
		▷	Explained why the bulb should be squeezed before inserting the pipet into serum.
		•	Released the bulb to suction serum into the pipet.

735

Trial 1	Trial 2	Point Value	Performance Standards
		•	Transferred serum to the transfer tube.
		•	Did not disturb the cell layer.
		•	Continued pipetting until as much serum as possible was removed.
		•	Capped the transfer tube tightly and held it up to the light to examine it for hemolysis.
		▷	Explained what should be done if hemolysis is present in the specimen.
		•	Made sure that the proper amount of serum was obtained.
		•	Properly disposed of equipment.
		•	Removed gloves and sanitized hands.
		•	Prepared the specimen for transport to an outside laboratory.
		•	Documented the procedure correctly.
		■	Demonstrated critical thinking skills.
		■	Demonstrated empathy for patients' concerns.
		★	Completed the procedure within 20 minutes.
			Totals

Evaluation of Student Performance

EVALUATION CRITERIA			COMMENTS
Symbol	**Category**	**Point Value**	
★	Critical Step	16 points	
•	Essential Step	6 points	
■	Affective Competency	6 points	
▷	Theory Question	2 points	

Score calculation: 100 points

      −   points missed

        ___Score

Satisfactory score: 85 or above

CAAHEP Competencies Achieved

Psychomotor (Skills)
- ☑ I. 2. b. Perform the following procedures: venipuncture.
- ☑ III. 10. Demonstrate proper disposal of biohazardous material: (a) sharps, (b) regulated waste.

Affective (Behavior)
- ☑ A. 1 Demonstrated critical thinking skills.
- ☑ A. 3. Demonstrated empathy for patients' concerns.

ABHES Competencies Achieved

- ☑ 8. a. Practice standard precautions and perform disinfection/sterilization techniques.
- ☑ 9. c. Dispose of biohazardous materials.
- ☑ 9. d. (1). Collect, label and process specimens: Perform venipuncture.

737

Notes

Procedure 17-4: Skin Puncture—Disposable Lancet

Name: _____   Date: _____

Evaluated by: _____   Score: _____

Performance Objective

Outcome:	Obtain a capillary blood specimen.
Conditions:	Given the following: disposable gloves, antiseptic wipe, CoaguChek lancet, gauze pad, adhesive bandage, and a biohazard sharps container.
Standards:	Time: 5 minutes. Student completed procedure in _____ minutes.
	Accuracy: Satisfactory score on the Performance Evaluation Checklist.

Performance Evaluation Checklist

Trial 1	Trial 2	Point Value	Performance Standards
		•	Sanitized hands.
		•	Greeted the patient and introduced yourself.
		•	Identified the patient.
		•	Asked patient if he or she prepared properly.
		•	Assembled equipment.
		•	Opened sterile gauze packet.
		•	Explained the procedure to the patient and reassured patient.
		•	Seated patient in chair.
		•	Extended the palmar surface of patient's hand facing up.
		•	Selected a puncture site.
		•	Warmed site if needed.
		▷	Explained why the site should be warmed.
		•	Cleansed puncture site and allowed it to air dry.
		▷	Explained why the site should be allowed to air dry.
		•	Did not touch the site after cleansing.
		•	Applied gloves.
		•	Firmly grasped patient's finger.
		•	Positioned the lancet firmly on the fleshy portion of the fingertip slightly to the side of center.
		•	Told the patient that he or she will feel a small stick.
		▷	Explained why the patient should be alerted to the stick.

739

Trial 1	Trial 2	Point Value	Performance Standards
		•	Depressed the activation button without moving the lancet or finger until an audible click is heard.
		▷	Stated why the lancet and finger should not be moved.
		•	Disposed of lancet in biohazard sharps container.
		•	Waited a few seconds to allow blood flow to begin.
		•	Wiped away the first drop of blood with a gauze pad.
		▷	Stated why the first drop of blood should be wiped away
		•	Allowed a second large, well-rounded drop of blood to form by holding the hand in a downward position and applying gentle continuous pressure.
		•	Did not squeeze finger to obtain blood.
		•	Collected the blood specimen on a test strip or in the appropriate microcollection device.
		•	Instructed patient to hold a gauze pad over puncture site with pressure.
		•	Remained with patient until bleeding stopped.
		•	Applied an adhesive bandage, if needed.
		•	Tested the blood specimen following the manufacturer's instructions.
		•	Removed gloves.
		•	Sanitized hands.
		■	Demonstrated critical thinking skills.
		■	Reassured patients.
		■	Demonstrated empathy for patients' concerns.
		★	Completed the procedure within 5 minutes.
			Totals

Evaluation of Student Performance

EVALUATION CRITERIA			COMMENTS
Symbol	**Category**	**Point Value**	
★	Critical Step	16 points	
•	Essential Step	6 points	
■	Affective Competency	6 points	
▷	Theory Question	2 points	

Score calculation: 100 points

— _____ points missed

_____ Score

Satisfactory score: 85 or above

Psychomotor (Skills)

- ☑ I. 2. c. Perform the following procedures: capillary puncture.
- ☑ III. 10. Demonstrate proper disposal of biohazardous material: a. sharps; b. regulated waste.

Affective (Behavior)

- ☑ A. 1. Demonstrate critical thinking skills.
- ☑ A. 2. Reassure patients.
- ☑ A. 3. Demonstrate empathy for patients' concerns.

ABHES Competencies Achieved

- ☑ 8. a. Practice standard precautions and perform disinfection/sterilization techniques.
- ☑ 9. c. Dispose of biohazardous materials.
- ☑ 9. d. (2). Collect, label, and process specimens: Perform capillary puncture.

18 Hematology

CHAPTER ASSIGNMENTS

√ After Completing	Date Due	Study Guide Pages	STUDY GUIDE ASSIGNMENTS (CTA = Critical Thinking Activity)	Possible Points	Points You Earned
		747	Pretest	10	
			Key Term Assessment		
		748	A. Definitions	26	
		749	B. Word Parts (Add 1 point for each key term)	26	
		750-755	Evaluation of Learning questions	67	
		756	CTA A: CBC Reference Ranges	17	
		756-759	CTA B: Diseases	40	
		760	CTA C: Hematocrit	5	
		760	CTA D: Iron Content of Food	10	
		760-761	CTA E: Iron-Deficiency Anemia	20	
		762	CTA F: PT/INR Test Requirements	9	
		763	CTA G: Dear Gabby	10	
			Evolve: Name That Cell: Identification of Blood Cells (Record points earned)		
		764-765	CTA H: Crossword Puzzle	35	
			Evolve: Time for a Test: Hematologic Tests (Record points earned)		
			Evolve: Apply Your Knowledge questions	10	
			Evolve: Video Evaluation	38	
		747	Posttest	10	

√ After Completing	Date Due	Study Guide Pages	STUDY GUIDE ASSIGNMENTS (CTA = Critical Thinking Activity)	Possible Points	Points You Earned
			ADDITIONAL ASSIGNMENTS		
			Total points		

√ When Assigned by Your Instructor	Study Guide Pages	Practices Required	LABORATORY ASSIGNMENTS (Procedure Number and Name)	Score*
	767-769	3	**Practice for Competency** 18-A: CLIA-Waived Hemoglobin Test	
	771-773		**Evaluation of Competency** 18-A: CLIA-Waived Hemoglobin Test	*
	767-770	3	**Practice for Competency** 18-1: CLIA-Waived Hematocrit Test	
	775-777		**Evaluation of Competency** 18-1: CLIA-Waived Hematocrit Test	*
	767-770	10	**Practice for Competency** 18-2: Preparation of a Blood Smear for a Differential Cell Count	
	779-781		**Evaluation of Competency** 18-2: Preparation of a Blood Smear for a Differential Cell Count	*
	767-770	3	**Practice for Competency** 18-B: CLIA-Waived PT/INR Test	
	783-784		**Evaluation of Competency** 18-B: CLIA-Waived PT/INR Test	*
			ADDITIONAL ASSIGNMENTS	

Notes

Name: _____   Date: _____

True or False

_____ 1. Plasma makes up approximately 55% of the blood volume.

_____ 2. A mature erythrocyte has a biconcave shape and contains a nucleus.

_____ 3. Erythrocytes are responsible for defending the body against infection.

_____ 4. The life span of a red blood cell is 120 days.

_____ 5. The function of hemoglobin is to assist in blood clotting.

_____ 6. Leukocytosis is an abnormal increase in the number of leukocytes.

_____ 7. Another name for a thrombocyte is a platelet.

_____ 8. A low hemoglobin reading occurs with polycythemia.

_____ 9. An increase in neutrophils occurs during an acute infection.

_____10. The PT test measures how long it takes for an individual's blood to form a clot.

? POSTTEST

True or False

_____ 1. The function of the plasma is to transport antibodies, enzymes, and hormones.

_____ 2. The red bone marrow of the sternum produces red blood cells in an adult.

_____ 3. The reference range for a RBC count for an adult female is 4 to 5.5 million/cubic mm of blood.

_____ 4. The reference range for hemoglobin for an adult male is 12 to 16 g/dL.

_____ 5. The reference range for a WBC count is 4500 to 11,000/cubic mm of blood.

_____ 6. Leukocytes do their work in the tissues.

_____ 7. Bilirubin is an orange-colored pigment that is a by-product from the breakdown of hemoglobin.

_____ 8. An immature form of a neutrophil is known as a seg.

_____ 9. The primary function of a neutrophil is to form antibodies.

_____10. The function of warfarin is to inhibit the growth of bacteria in the body.

A. Definitions

Directions: Match each key term with its definition.

_____ 1. Ameboid movement

_____ 2. Anemia

_____ 3. Anisocytosis

_____ 4. Anticoagulant

_____ 5. Bilirubin

_____ 6. Diapedesis

_____ 7. Erythrocyte

_____ 8. Hematology

_____ 9. Hematopoiesis

_____10. Hemoglobin

_____11. Hemolysis

_____12. Hypochromic

_____13. Leukocyte

_____14. Leukocytosis

_____15. Leukopenia

_____16. Macrocytic

_____17. Microcytic

_____18. Morphology

_____19. Normochromic

_____20. Normocytic

_____21. Oxyhemoglobin

_____22. Phagocytosis

_____23. Polycythemia

_____24. Thrombocyte

_____25. Thrombocytopenia

_____26. Thrombocytosis

A. An abnormal decrease in the number of white blood cells (less than 4500/cubic mm of blood)

B. The breakdown of erythrocytes with the release of hemoglobin into the plasma

C. Movement used by leukocytes that permits them to propel themselves from the capillaries into the tissues

D. The ameboid movement of blood cells (especially leukocytes) through the wall of a capillary and out into the tissues

E. A disorder in which there is an increase in the number of RBCs or the amount of hemoglobin

F. A condition in which there is a decrease in the number of erythrocytes or in the amount of hemoglobin in the blood

G. Hemoglobin that has combined with oxygen

H. The study of blood

I. An abnormal increase in the number of white blood cells (greater than 11,000/ cubic mm of blood)

J. An orange-colored bile pigment that is a by-product of heme destruction from the hemoglobin molecule

K. The engulfing and destruction of foreign particles, such as pathogens and damaged cells

L. The protein- and iron-containing pigment of erythrocytes that transports oxygen to the tissues of the body

M. A substance that inhibits blood clotting

N. A red blood cell with a decreased concentration of hemoglobin

O. An abnormally small red blood cell

P. An abnormally large red blood cell

Q. A red blood cell with a normal concentration of hemoglobin

R. A normal-sized red blood cell

S. A variation in the size of red blood cells

T. Platelets

U. White blood cell

V. An abnormal decrease in the number of thrombocytes

W. Red blood cell

X. An abnormal increase in the number of thrombocytes

Y. The study of the size, shape, and structure of a blood cell

Z. The process of blood cell formation

B. Word Parts

Directions: Indicate the meaning of each word part in the space provided. List as many medical terms as possible that incorporate the word part in the space provided.

Word Part	Meaning of Word Part	Medical Terms That Incorporate Word Part
1. anis/o		
2. cyt/o		
3. -ia		
4. -osis		
5. anti-		
6. -coagulant		
7. hemat/o		
8. -ology		
9. -lysis		
10. hypo-		
11. chrom/o		
12. -ic		
13. leuk/o		
14. -penia		
15. micro-		
16. norm/o		
17. phag/o		
18. poly-		
19. erythro-		
20. an-		
21. thrombo-		
22. macr/o		
23. -globin		
24. dia-		
25. bili-		
26. morpho-		

Directions: Fill in each blank with the correct answer.

1. What is included in the study of blood (hematology)?

_____

_____

2. List 5 examples of hematologic tests.

_____

_____

3. How many pints of blood are contained in the human body?

_____

4. What is the function of plasma?

_____

_____

5. What percentage of the total blood volume is made up of formed elements?

_____

6. What cells make up the formed elements of blood?

_____

7. Where are the formed elements produced?

_____

8. What is the function of red blood cells?

_____

9. Where are erythrocytes produced in an adult?

_____

_____

10. What are the advantages of a RBC having a biconcave shape?

_____

_____

11. What gives blood its red color?

_____

12. A hemoblobin molecule can combine with how many oxygen molecules?

_____

13. Describe the appearance of arterial blood and venous blood.

_____

_____

14. What is the average life span of a red blood cell?

_____

15. What happens to the iron and bilirubin that are released from the breakdown of hemoglobin?

Iron: _____

Bilirubin: _____

16. What is the function of leukocytes?

_____

17. Where do leukocytes do their work?

_____

18. Why do the capillaries in an infected area dilate during inflammation?

_____

_____

19. What is the purpose of diapedesis?

_____

20. What is the difference in appearance between granulocytes and agranulocytes?

Granulocytes: _____

Agranulocytes: _____

21. What is the purpose of inflammation?

_____

_____

22. What are the 4 symptoms of inflammation?

_____

23. What is contained in pus?

_____

24. Why are neutrophils also known as "segs"?

_____

25. What are 3 ways in which neutrophils fight infection?

_____

_____

_____

751

26. What causes an increase in eosinophils?

_____

27. What is the function of the following substances released by basophils?

Histamine: _____

Heparin: _____

28. What is the function of lymphocytes?

_____

29. What are 5 viral diseases that cause an increase in lymphocytes?

_____

_____

30. What is the function of macrophages (derived ffrom monocytes)?

_____

_____

31. Describe what happens when each of the following occur during the blood-clotting mechanism in the body:

Lining of a blood vessel breaks: _____

_____

Platelets become stickly: _____

_____

Platelet plug: _____

_____

Fibrin network forms: _____

_____

Blood clot formation: _____

_____

32. What is the purpose of a CBC?

_____

_____

33. What are the CLIA-waived and moderate complexity tests included in a CBC?

CLIA-waived tests: _____

Moderate complexity tests: _____

_____

34. What is the reference range for hemoglobin in an adult?

Adult female: _____

Adult male: _____

35. What conditions cause a decreased hemoglobin level?

_____

_____

36. What type of patients are at risk for developing iron-deficiency anemia?

_____

_____

37. When is a hematocrit performed?

_____

_____

38. What makes up the buffy coat?

_____

39. What is the reference range for a hematocrit in an adult?

Adult female: _____

Adult male: _____

40. What causes a decrease and increase in the RBC count?

Decrease in RBC count: _____

_____

Increase in RBC count: _____

41. What is measured by each of the following red blood cell indices?

MCV: _____

MCH: _____

MCHC: _____

RDW: _____

42. What is the most common cause of microcytic anemia?

_____

43. What are the most common causes of macrocytic anemia?

_____

_____

44. Hypochromia occurs with what type of conditions?

_____

45. What is the reference range for a WBC count for an adult?

_____

753

46. What conditions result in an inrease in the WBC count?

_____

_____

47. What takes place during a WBC differential count?

_____

_____

48. What are the reference ranges for a WBC differential count in an adult?

Neutrophils: _____

Eosinophils: _____

Basophils: _____

Lymphocytes: _____

Monocytes: _____

49. What are the advantages of the following methods for performing a WBC differential count?

Automatic method: _____

Manual method:_____

50. Why must the WBCs be stained when performing a manual WBC differential count?

_____

_____

51. What is the function of platelets?

_____

52. What is the reference range for a platelet count in an adult?

_____

53. What signs and symptoms may warrant the ordering of a platelet count on a patient?

_____

_____

54. What does the PT test measure?

_____

55. What is the reference range for a PT test of an adult?

_____

56. What do the following PT results mean?

a. PT result more than 12 seconds: _____

b. PT result less than 9 seconds: _____

57. What is the purpose of performing an INR on PT test results?

_____

58. What is the reference range for an INR result of a healthy individual with a normal clotting ability?

_____

59. What is the risk of the following INR results?

   a. Low INR: _____

   b. Elevated INR: _____

60. How does warfarin work to prevent blood clotting?

_____

_____

61. What are conditions for which warfarin is prescribed?

_____

_____

62. How can atrial fibrillation cause a stroke?

_____

_____

63. What is the goal of warfarin therapy?

_____

_____

64. How often should a patient on long-term warfarin therapy have a PT/INR test?

_____

65. What color closure of tube should be used to collect a specimen for a PT/INR test?

_____

66 Why is it important to fill the collection tube for a PT/INR test to the exhaustion of the vacuum?

_____

_____

67. What are the advantages of PT/INR home testing?

_____

_____

_____

A. CBC Reference Ranges

Refer to Table 18-1 in your textbook: CBC Purpose and Reference Ranges. Using the reference range values listed in this table, determine whether the following tests fall within their normal reference ranges or whether they are high or low. Mark each test according to the following: N = normal, H = high, L = low.

_____ 1. RBC count (female): $4.8 \times 10^6/mm^3$

_____ 2. RBC count (male): $3.6 \times 10^6/mm^3$

_____ 3. WBC: $13.5 \times 10^3/mm^3$

_____ 4. Hemoglobin (female): 14 g/dL

_____ 5. Hemoglobin (male): 12 g/dL

_____ 6. Hematocrit (female): 50%

_____ 7. Hematocrit (male): 50%

_____ 8. Platelet count: $100 \times 10^3/mm^3$

_____ 9. MCV: 96 f/L

_____ 10. MCH: 36 pg

_____ 11. MCHC: 30 mg/dL

_____ 12. RDW: 12.3%

_____ 13. Neutrophils: 89%

_____ 14. Eosinophils: 0%

_____ 15. Basophils: 8%

_____ 16. Lymphocytes: 14%

_____ 17. Monocytes 6%

B. Diseases

1. You and your classmates work at a large clinic. It is National Disease Awareness Week. The providers at your clinic ask you to develop informative, creative, and colorful brochures for patients about various diseases. Choose a condition from the list, and design a brochure using the blank Frequently Asked Questions (FAQ) brochure provided on the following page. Each student in the class should select a different disease. On a separate sheet of paper, write three true/false questions relating to the information in your brochure.

2. Present your brochure to the class. After all the brochures have been presented, each student should ask three questions to the entire class to see how well the class understands the diseases that were presented. (*Note:* Students can take notes during the presentations and refer to them when answering the questions.)

Conditions

1. Addison's disease

2. Amyotrophic lateral sclerosis

3. Aplastic anemia

4. Bell's palsy

5. Cirrhosis

6. Crohn's disease

7. Cushing's syndrome

8. Cystic fibrosis

9. Degenerative disc disease

10. Epilepsy

11. Hemolytic anemia

12. Hemophilia

13. Hernia

14. Hodgkin's disease

15. Hyperthyroidism

16. Hypothyroidism

17. Leukemia

18. Lupus erythematosus

19. Multiple sclerosis

20. Muscular dystrophy

21. Parkinson's disease

22. Peptic ulcer

23. Pernicious anemia

24. Polycythemia

25. Sickle-cell anemia

26. Ulcerative colitis

FAQ
ON:

Q: A:

Q: A:

Q: A:

Q: A:

Illustration

Q:

A:

Q:

A:

Q:

A:

Q:

A:

C. Hematocrit

Label the layers of this microhematocrit capillary tube that has been centrifuged. Place an arrow at the point where you would take the hematocrit reading.

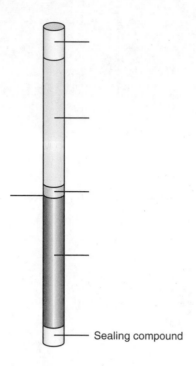

Sealing compound

D. Iron Content of Food

Consuming food that is high in iron helps to prevent iron-deficiency anemia. To become familiar with foods that are high in iron content and foods that contain little or no iron, plan the following two meals. One meal should be as high as possible in iron content, and the other meal should not contain any iron at all.

Meal 1: High in iron

_____

_____

_____

Meal 2: Contains no iron

_____

_____

_____

_____

E. Iron-Deficiency Anemia

Create a profile of an individual who has iron-deficiency anemia following these guidelines:

1. Using colored pencils, crayons, or markers, draw a figure of an individual exhibiting iron-deficiency anemia. Be as creative as possible.

2. Do not use any text on your drawing other than to label items you have drawn in your picture. (A picture is worth a thousand words!)

3. Try to include all of the symptoms of iron-deficiency anemia in your drawing. The Iron-Deficiency Anemia Patient Coaching Box in your textbook can be used as a reference source.

4. In the classroom, find a partner and trade drawings. Identify the symptoms of iron-deficiency anemia in your partner's drawing. With your partner, discuss what treatment is recommended and also what this person could do to prevent iron-deficiency anemia.

IRON-DEFICIENCY ANEMIA

F. PT/INR Test Requirements

Your provider has ordered a PT/INR test on a patient that will be analyzed at an outside laboratory. You are required to collect the specimen and prepare it for transport to the outside laboratory. Using Figure 18-12 in your textbook as a reference, respond to the following questions in the space provided.

1. What is the amount and type of specimen required for this test?

   _____

2. What type of collection container should be used to collect the specimen?

   _____

3. What are the collection and processing requirements for this specimen?

   _____

   _____

   _____

4. How should you store the specimen while awaiting pickup by the laboratory courier?

   _____

5. What should be done if the testing will not take place within 24 hours following collection of the specimen?

   _____

   _____

   _____

6. What would cause the laboratory to reject the specimen?

   _____

   _____

   _____

7. What are the reference ranges for each of the following:

   a. INR for patients with normal clotting ability: _____

   b. INR for patients on moderate intensity warfarin therapy: _____

   c. INR for patients on higher intensity warfarin therapy: _____

   d. PT reference range: _____

8. What are the uses of a PT/INR test?

   _____

   _____

   _____

   _____

9. What are the limitations of this test?

   _____

   _____

G. Dear Gabby

Gabby is attending her high school class reunion and wants you to fill in for her. In the space provided, respond to the following letter. (First research the symptoms of iron poisoning in children and include this information in your response).

Dear Gabby,

I am a stay-at-home mom with two adorable children, ages 2 and 4. I have been feeling run down and tired lately, so I bought some iron pills from the drugstore. They came individually packaged in foil and plastic. They are hard to open, so I cut each package open and transferred the iron pills to a little plastic baggie. When I told my mother about what I thought was a great idea, she became very concerned. She told me that I could possibly be putting my children at danger. She said that iron is poisonous to children and that I should not do that. Gabby, my mom has always been overprotective. Is this just another one of her episodes?

Signed,

Curious in Kansas

_____

_____

_____

_____

_____

_____

_____

_____

H. Crossword Puzzle: Hematology

Directions: Complete the crossword puzzle using the clues provided.

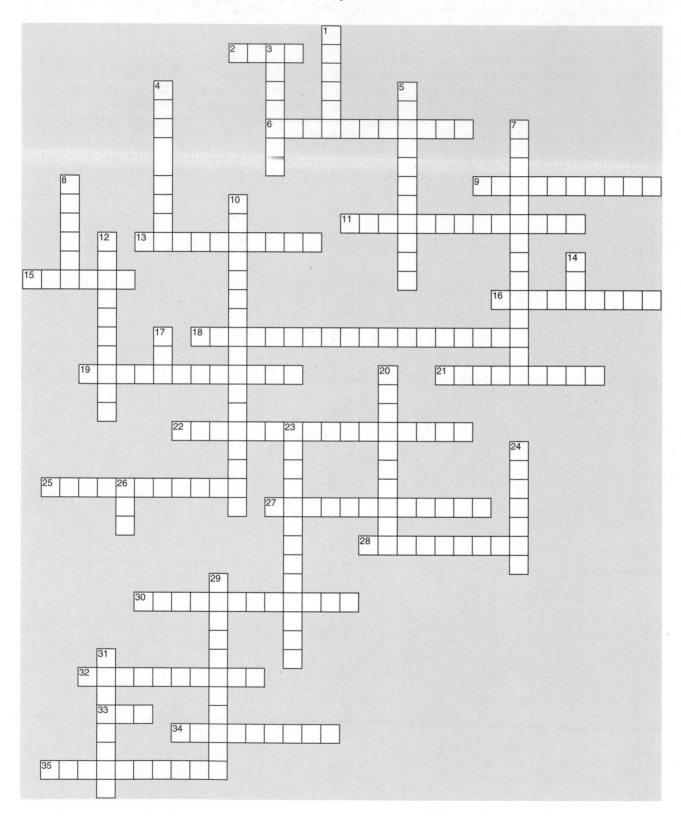

Across

2 Immature neutrophil
6 AKA red blood cell
9 Where blood cells are made
11 Process of blood cell formation
13 Carries oxygen
15 Liquid part of blood
16 Color tube for PT/INR
18 Cause of blood pooling in atrium
19 Too many RBCs
21 Contains platelets and WBCs
22 Less than 150,000 platelets
25 First responders to invaders
27 Above 11,000 WBCs
28 AKA white blood cell
30 Variation in size of RBCs
32 Size, shape, and structure
33 Measurement of average size of RBC
34 Color of arterial blood
35 Help determine cause of anemia

Down

1 Blood clotting test
3 RBC lacks this
4 Small red skin spots
5 Scavengers
7 Common cause of anemia
8 Decrease in RBCs
10 Indication for warfarin
12 Study of blood
14 AKA thrombophlebitis
17 Frequently performed lab test
20 Produces antibodies
23 Hemoglobin and oxygen
24 Where leukocytes work
26 Lives 120 days
29 Increased in allergic reactions
31 Warfarin brand name

Notes

Procedure 18-A: CLIA-Waived Hemoglobin Determination

a. Run controls on a CLIA-waived hemoglobin analyzer, and document results on the quality control log on p. 709.
b. Perform a hemoglobin test on a patient using a CLIA-waived hemoglobin analyzer, and document results in the chart provided. Circle any values that fall outside the normal range.

Procedure 18-1: Perform a CLIA-Waived Hematocrit Test

Perform a CLIA-waived hematocrit test in duplicate, and document results in the chart provided. Circle any values that fall outside the normal range.

Procedure 18-2: Preparation of a Blood Smear for a WBC Differential Count

Prepare a blood smear for a WBC differential count and prepare it for transport to an outside laboratory. Document the procedure in the chart provided. Examine the slides under a microscope to observe the blood cells and indicate blood cells that you were able to identify in the space below:

_____

_____

Procedure 18-B: Perform a CLIA-Waived PT/INR Test

a. Run controls on a CLIA-waived PT/INR analyzer, and document results on the quality control log on p. 710.
b. Perform a PT/INR test on a patient using a CLIA-waived PT/INR analyzer, and document the results in the chart provided. Circle any values that fall outside the normal range.

CHART	
Date	

767

CHART	
Date	

QUALITY CONTROL HEMOGLOBIN LOG SHEET

Name of Analyzer: _____   **Control Lot Number:** _____

Low-Level Range: _____   **Control Exp. Date:** _____

High-Level Range: _____

Date	Microcuvettes: Lot # and Expiration	Low-Level Value	Accept	Reject	High-Level Value	Accept	Reject	Tech

QUALITY CONTROL PT/INR LOG SHEET

Name of Analyzer: _____

Low-Level Range: _____

High-Level Range: _____

Control Lot Number: _____

Control Exp. Date: _____

Date	Test Strips: Lot # and Expiration	Low-Level Value	Accept	Reject	High-Level Value	Accept	Reject	Tech

770

Procedure 18-A: CLIA-Waived Hemoglobin Test

Name: _____   Date: _____

Evaluated by: _____   Score: _____

Performance Objective

Outcome:	Perform a CLIA-waived hemoglobin test.
Conditions:	Using a Hemoglobin Hb 201 hemoglobin analyzer and operating manual and given the following: disposable gloves, antiseptic wipe, lancet, gauze pad, microcuvette, control solutions, quality control log, and a biohazard sharps container.
Standards:	Time: 10 minutes. Student completed procedure in _____ minutes.
	Accuracy: Satisfactory score on the Performance Evaluation Checklist.

Performance Evaluation Checklist

Trial 1	Trial 2	Point Value	Performance Standards
		•	Sanitized hands.
		•	Assembled equipment.
		•	Checked the expiration date of the microcuvette.
		•	Checked the expiration date of the control solutions.
		•	Applied gloves and ran a low and high control.
		▷	Stated the purpose of running controls.
		•	Removed gloves and sanitized hands.
		•	Documented the control results in the quality control log.
		•	Greeted the patient and introduced yourself.
		•	Identified the patient and explained the procedure.
		•	Pulled out the cuvette tray from the front of the hemoglobin analyzer.
		•	Opened gauze packet.
		•	Cleansed the puncture site and allowed it to air-dry.
		▷	Stated what happens to the blood drop if the site is not dry.
		•	Applied gloves and performed a finger puncture.
		•	Wiped away the first 2 or 3 drops of blood.
		•	Touched the open end of the microcuvette to the drop of blood and filled the microcuvette in one continuous process.
		•	Placed a gauze pad over the puncture site and applied pressure.
		•	Wiped off excess blood from the outside of the microcuvette and placed it in the cuvette holder on the analyzer.

Trial 1	Trial 2	Point Value	Performance Standards
		•	Pushed the tray back into the analyzer when three dashes appear on the LCD screen of the analyzer.
		•	Waited while the hemoglobin analyzer analyzed the blood specimen.
		•	Read the results on the display screen of the analyzer.
		▷	Stated the reference range for a hemoglobin determination for a female (12 to 16 g/dL) and a male (14 to 18 g/dL).
		•	Removed the microcuvette from the analyzer.
		•	Properly disposed of the microcuvette in a biohazard waste container.
		•	Checked the puncture site and applied an adhesive bandage, if needed.
		•	Removed gloves and sanitized hands.
		•	Documented the test results correctly.
		★	The hemoglobin documentation was identical to the reading on the display screen.
		■	Demonstrated critical thinking skills.
		■	Reassured patients.
		★	Completed the procedure within 10 minutes.
			Totals

CHART	
Date	

Evaluation of Student Performance

EVALUATION CRITERIA			COMMENTS
Symbol	**Category**	**Point Value**	
★	Critical Step	16 points	
•	Essential Step	6 points	
■	Affective Competency	6 points	
▷	Theory Question	2 points	

Score calculation: 100 points

−_____ points missed

_____Score

Satisfactory score: 85 or above

CAAHEP Competencies Achieved

Psychomotor (Skills)
- ☑ I. 10. Perform a quality control measure.
- ☑ I. 11. a. Collect specimens and perform CLIA-waived hematology test.
- ☑ II. 2. Record laboratory test results into the patient's record.

Affective (Behavior)
- ☑ A. 1. Demonstrate critical thinking skills.
- ☑ A. 2. Reassure patients.

ABHES Competencies Achieved

- ☑ 9. a. Practice quality control.
- ☑ 9. b. (2). Perform selected CLIA-waived tests that assist with diagnosis and treatment: hematology testing.

Notes

Procedure 18-1: CLIA-Waived Hematocrit Test

Name: _____   Date: _____

Evaluated by: _____   Score: _____

Performance Objective

Outcome:	Perform a CLIA-waived hematocrit test.
Conditions:	Given the following: microhematocrit centrifuge, disposable gloves, lancet, antiseptic wipe, gauze pad, capillary tubes, sealing compound, and a biohazard sharps container.
Standards:	Time: 10 minutes. Student completed procedure in _____ minutes.
	Accuracy: Satisfactory score on the Performance Evaluation Checklist.

Performance Evaluation Checklist

Trial 1	Trial 2	Point Value	Performance Standards
		•	Sanitized hands.
		•	Greeted the patient and introduced yourself.
		•	Identified the patient and explained the procedure.
		•	Assembled equipment.
		•	Opened the gauze packet.
		•	Cleansed the site with an antiseptic wipe and allowed it to air-dry.
		•	Applied gloves.
		•	Performed a finger puncture and discarded the lancet in a biohazard sharps container.
		•	Wiped away the first drop of blood.
		•	Massaged the finger until a large blood drop formed.
		•	Held one end of the capillary tube horizontally but slightly downward next to the free-flowing puncture.
		•	Kept the tip of the pipet in the blood but did not allow it to press against the skin of the patient's finger.
		▷	Explained why the capillary tube should be kept in the blood specimen.
		•	Filled the capillary tube (calibrated tubes filled to the calibration line; uncalibrated tubes filled approximately three-fourths full).
		▷	Explained why a tube with air bubbles is unacceptable.
		•	Filled a second capillary tube.
		▷	Stated why 2 capillary tubes must be filled.
		•	Placed a gauze pad over the puncture site and applied pressure.
		•	Sealed the dry end of each capillary tube.
		•	Checked the puncture site and applied an adhesive bandage, if needed.

775

Trial 1	Trial 2	Point Value	Performance Standards
		•	Placed the capillary tubes in the microhematocrit centrifuge with the sealed end facing toward the outside.
		▷	Explained why the sealed end must face toward the outside.
		•	Balanced one tube with the other tube placed opposite it.
		•	Placed the cover over the capillary tubes and locked it securely.
		•	Centrifuged the blood specimen for 3 to 5 minutes.
		▷	Explained the reason for centrifuging the blood specimen.
		•	Allowed the centrifuge to come to a complete stop.
		•	Removed the protective cover from the capillary tubes.
		•	Read the results using the appropriate reading device.
		•	Determined whether the results agreed within 4 percentage points.
		▷	Explained what to do if the results are not within 4 percentage points.
		•	Averaged the values of the two tubes together to derive the test results.
		★	The results were within 2% of the evaluator's results.
		▷	Stated the normal hematocrit range for a female (37% to 47%) and a male (40% to 54%).
		•	Properly disposed of the capillary tubes in a biohazard sharps container.
		•	Removed gloves and sanitized hands.
		•	Documented the test results correctly.
		•	Returned equipment.
		■	Demonstrated critical thinking skills.
		■	Reassured patients.
		★	Completed the procedure within 10 minutes.
			Totals

CHART

Date	

Evaluation of Student Performance

EVALUATION CRITERIA			COMMENTS
Symbol	**Category**	**Point Value**	
★	Critical Step	16 points	
•	Essential Step	6 points	
■	Affective Competency	6 points	
▷	Theory Question	2 points	

Score calculation: 100 points

− _____ points missed

_____ Score

Satisfactory score: 85 or above

CAAHEP Competencies Achieved

Psychomotor (Skills)
- ☑ I. 10. Perform a quality control measure.
- ☑ I. 11. a. Collect specimens and perform CLIA-waived hematology test.
- ☑ II. 2. Record laboratory test results into the patient's record.

Affective (Behavior)
- ☑ A. 1. Demonstrate critical thinking skills.
- ☑ A. 2. Reassure patients.

ABHES Competencies Achieved

- ☑ 9. a. Practice quality control.
- ☑ 9. b. (2) Perform selected CLIA-waived tests that assist with diagnosis and treatment: hematology testing.

EVALUATION OF COMPETENCY

Procedure 18-2: Preparation of a Blood Smear for a Differential Cell Count

Name: _____   Date: _____

Evaluated by: _____   Score: _____

Performance Objective

Outcome:	Prepare a blood smear for a differential white blood cell count.
Conditions:	Given the following: disposable gloves, supplies to perform a finger puncture or venipuncture, slides with a frosted edge, slide container, biohazard specimen bag, laboratory request form, and a biohazard sharps container.
Standards:	Time: 10 minutes. Student completed procedure in _____ minutes.
	Accuracy: Satisfactory score on the Performance Evaluation Checklist.

Performance Evaluation Checklist

Trial 1	Trial 2	Point Value	Performance Standards
		•	Sanitized hands.
		•	Greeted the patient and introduced yourself.
		•	Identified the patient and explained the procedure.
		•	Assembled equipment.
		•	Labeled the slides.
		•	Opened the gauze packet.
		•	Cleansed the puncture site.
		•	Applied gloves.
		•	Performed a venipuncture (using a lavender-stoppered tube) or a finger puncture.
		•	Placed a drop of blood in the middle of each slide approximately ¼ inch from the frosted edge of the slide.
		•	Held a spreader slide at a 30-degree angle to the first slide in front of the drop of blood.
		▷	Stated what occurs if the angle is more than 30 degrees or less than 30 degrees.
		•	Moved the spreader slide until it touched the drop of blood.
		•	Spread the blood thinly and evenly across slide using the spreader slide.
		•	Prepared the second blood smear.
		•	Disposed of the spreader slide in a biohazard sharps container.
		•	Laid the blood smears on a flat surface and allowed them to dry.
		▷	Explained why the blood smears should be dried immediately.
		•	The length of the smear was approximately 1½ inches.
		•	The smear was smooth and even, with no ridges, holes, lines, streaks, or clumps.
		•	The smear was not too thick or too thin.

Trial 1	Trial 2	Point Value	Performance Standards
		•	There was a feathered edge at the thin end of the smear.
		•	There was a margin on all sides of the smear.
		•	Placed the slides in a protective slide container.
		•	Placed lavender-stoppered tube and slide container in a biohazard specimen bag.
		•	Removed gloves and sanitized hands.
		•	Completed a laboratory request form.
		•	Placed the lab request in the outside pocket of the specimen bag.
		•	Documented the procedure correctly.
		•	Filed a copy of the lab request in the patient's medical record.
		•	Placed the specimen bag in the appropriate location for pickup by a lab courier.
		•	Documented the procedure correctly.
		■	Demonstrated critical thinking skills.
		★	Completed the procedure within 10 minutes.
			Totals

CHART	
Date	

Evaluation of Student Performance

EVALUATION CRITERIA			COMMENTS
Symbol	**Category**	**Point Value**	
★	Critical Step	16 points	
•	Essential Step	6 points	
■	Affective Competency	6 points	
▷	Theory Question	2 points	

Score calculation: 100 points

    −   points missed

        Score

Satisfactory score: 85 or above

CAAHEP Competencies Achieved

Psychomotor (Skills)
☑ I. 10. Perform a quality control measure.

Affective (Behavior)
☑ A. 1. Demonstrate critical thinking skills.

ABHES Competencies Achieved

☑ 9. a. Practice quality control
☑ 9. d. Collect, label, and process specimens

Notes

Procedure 18-B: CLIA-Waived PT/INR Test

Name: _____   Date: _____

Evaluated by: _____   Score: _____

Performance Objective

Outcome:	Perform a PT/INR test.
Conditions:	Using a CLIA-waived CoaguChek XS analyzer and operating manual and given the following: disposable gloves, antiseptic wipe, lancet, gauze pad, test strips, control solutions, quality control log, and a biohazard sharps container.
Standards:	Time: 10 minutes. Student completed procedure in _____ minutes.
	Accuracy: Satisfactory score on the Performance Evaluation Checklist.

Performance Evaluation Checklist

Trial 1	Trial 2	Point Value	Performance Standards
		•	Sanitized hands.
		•	Assembled equipment.
		•	Checked the expiration date of the test strips.
		•	Checked the expiration date of the control solutions.
		•	Applied gloves and ran a low and high control.
		▷	Stated the purpose of running controls.
		•	Removed gloves and sanitized hands.
		•	Documented the control results in the quality control log.
		•	Greeted the patient and introduced yourself.
		•	Identified the patient and explained the procedure.
		•	Placed the test strip in the analyzer.
		•	Opened gauze packet.
		•	Cleansed the puncture site and allowed it to air-dry.
		•	Applied gloves and performed a finger puncture.
		•	Applied the first drop of blood to the test strip.
		•	Placed a gauze pad over the puncture site and applied pressure.
		•	Waited while the analyzer determined the PT test result and calculates the INR.
		•	Read the results on the display screen of the analyzer.
		▷	Stated the reference range for INR results for an adult not on warfarin therapy. (0.9 to 1.2)
		•	Removed the test strip from the analyzer.
		•	Properly disposed of the test strip in a biohazard waste container.

783

Trial 1	Trial 2	Point Value	Performance Standards
		•	Checked the puncture site and applied an adhesive bandage, if needed.
		•	Removed gloves and sanitized hands.
		•	Documented the test results correctly.
		★	The INR result was identical to the reading on the display screen.
		■	Demonstrated critical thinking skills.
		■	Reassured patients.
		★	Completed the procedure within 10 minutes
			Totals

CHART	
Date	

Evaluation of Student Performance

EVALUATION CRITERIA			COMMENTS
Symbol	**Category**	**Point Value**	
★	Critical Step	16 points	
•	Essential Step	6 points	
■	Affective Competency	6 points	
▷	Theory Question	2 points	

Score calculation: 100 points

− _____ points missed

_____ Score

Satisfactory score: 85 or above

CAAHEP Competencies Achieved

Psychomotor (Skills)
☑ I. 10. Perform a quality control measure.
☑ I. 11. a. Obtain specimens and perform CLIA-waived hematology test.
☑ II. 2. Differentiate between normal and abnormal test results.

Affective (Behavior)
☑ A. 1. Demonstrate critical thinking skills.
☑ A. 2. Reassure patients.

ABHES Competencies Achieved

☑ 9. a. Practice quality control.
☑ 9. b. (2). Perform selected CLIA-waived tests that assist with diagnosis and treatment: hematology testing.

19 Blood Chemistry and Immunology

√ After Completing	Date Due	Study Guide Pages	STUDY GUIDE ASSIGNMENTS (CTA = Critical Thinking Activity)	Possible Points	Points You Earned
		789	[?] Pretest	10	
		790	Key Term Assessment	20	
		790-797	Evaluation of Learning questions	47	
		797-798	CTA A: Comprehensive Metabolic Panel Requirements	7	
		798	CTA B: Type 2 Diabetes Information Sheet	40	
		798-799	CTA C: Oral Glucose Tolerance Test Instructions (2 points each)	10	
		799	CTA D: Lipid Panel Reference Ranges	12	
		800	CTA E: Cardiovascular Disease	20	
		800-801	CTA F: Saturated Fat and Cholesterol (5 points each)	15	
			Evolve: The Right Chemistry (Record points earned)		
		801	CTA G: Rh Incompatibility (5 points each)	20	
		802-803	CTA H: Crossword Puzzle	32	
			Evolve: Immunologic Tests (Record points earned)		
			Evolve: Apply Your Knowledge questions	20	
			Evolve: Video Evaluation	16	
		789	[?] Posttest	10	
			ADDITIONAL ASSIGNMENTS		
			Total points		

√ When Assigned By Your Instructor	Study Guide Pages	Practices Required	LABORATORY ASSIGNMENTS (Procedure Number and Name)	Score*
	805-806	3	**Practice for Competency** 19-A: CLIA-Waived Blood Chemistry Test	
	811-812		✎ **Evaluation of Competency** 19-A: CLIA-Waived Chemistry Test	*
	805-807	3	**Practice for Competency** 19-1: CLIA-Waived Fasting Blood Glucose Test	
	813-815		✎ **Evaluation of Competency** 19-1: CLIA-Waived Fasting Blood Glucose Test	*
	805, 809	3	**Practice for Competency** 19-B: CLIA-Waived Rapid Mononucleosis Test	
	817-819		✎ **Evaluation of Competency** 19-B: CLIA-Waived Rapid Mononucleosis Test	*
			ADDITIONAL ASSIGNMENTS	

Notes

Name: _____   Date: _____

True or False

_____ 1. The function of glucose in the body is to build and repair tissue.

_____ 2. Insulin is required for normal utilization of glucose in the body.

_____ 3. An abnormally low level of glucose in the body is known as hypoglycemia.

_____ 4. The hemoglobin A_{1C} test measures the average amount of blood glucose over a 3-month period.

_____ 5. Most of the cholesterol found in the blood comes from the intake of dietary cholesterol.

_____ 6. The primary use of the cholesterol test is to screen for the presence of coronary artery disease.

_____ 7. HDL cholesterol removes excess cholesterol from the walls of arteries and carries it to the liver for removal by the body.

_____ 8. An antibody is a substance that is capable of combining with an antigen.

_____ 9. Mononucleosis is transmitted through coughing and sneezing.

_____10. Blood antigens (A, B, Rh) are located on the surface of red blood cells.

📄 POSTTEST

True or False

_____ 1. Serum is required for most blood chemistry tests.

_____ 2. The normal reference range for a fasting blood glucose test is 120 to 160 mg/dL.

_____ 3. The OGTT is used to assist in the diagnosis of diabetes mellitus.

_____ 4. Before meals, it is recommended that the blood glucose level for a diabetic patient be between 60 and 80 mg/dL.

_____ 5. The ADA recommended hemoglobin A_{1C} level for a diabetic patient is less than 7%.

_____ 6. The buildup of plaque on the walls of arteries is known as thrombophlebitis.

_____ 7. An HDL cholesterol level greater than 50 mg/dL is a risk factor for coronary artery disease.

_____ 8. Most providers prefer that the patient fast for a lipid panel.

_____ 9. The RPR test is a screening test for syphilis.

_____10. The varicella virus causes infectious mononucleosis.

Directions: Match each key term with its definition.

_____ 1. Agglutination

_____ 2. Antibody

_____ 3. Antigen

_____ 4. Antiserum

_____ 5. Cholesterol

6. Donor

_____ 7. Glucose

_____ 8. Glycogen

_____ 9. Glycosylation

_____10. HDL cholesterol

_____11. Hemoglobin A_{1c}

_____12. Hyperglycemia

_____13. Hypoglycemia

_____14. In vitro

_____15. In vivo

_____16. Insulin

_____17. LDL cholesterol

_____18. Lipoprotein

_____19. Prediabetes

_____20. Recipient

A. An abnormally high level of glucose in the blood
B. A complex molecule consisting of protein and a lipid fraction such as cholesterol
C. The form in which glucose is stored in the body
D. A lipoprotein that removes excess cholesterol from the walls of arteries and carries it to the liver for removal by the body.
E. An abnormally low level of glucose in the blood
F. A lipoprotein, that picks up cholesterol from ingested fats and the liver and forms plaques on the walls of arteries.
G. A substance that is capable of combining with an antigen, resulting in an antigen-antibody reaction
H. A substance capable of stimulating the formation of antibodies in an individual.
I. One who receives something, such as a blood transfusion, from a donor
J. Clumping of red blood cells
K. A white, waxy, fatlike substance that is essential for normal functioning of the body.
L. Occurring in the living body or organism
M. The end product of carbohydrate metabolism and is the chief source of energy for the body.
N. A serum that contains antibodies
O. One who furnishes something, such as blood, tissue, or organs, to be used in another individual
P. Occurring in glass; refers to tests performed under artificial conditions, as in the laboratory
Q. The process of glucose attaching to hemoglobin.
R. A compound formed when glucose attaches to the protein in hemoglobin.
S. A hormone secreted by the beta cells of the pancreas and is required for normal utilization of glucose in the body.
T. A condition in which glucose levels are higher than normal, but not high enough to be classified as diabetes.

EVALUATION OF LEARNING

Directions: Fill in each blank with the correct answer.

1. What does blood chemistry testing involve?

2. What information is provided by a comprehensive metabolic panel (CMP)?

3. What type of specimen is usually required for blood chemistry tests?

4. What type of blood specimen is used with a CLIA-waived blood chemistry analyzer?

_____

5. What is the purpose of quality control?

_____

6. What is the purpose of calibrating a blood chemistry analyzer?

_____

_____

7. What is the name of the device used to perform a calibration procedure?

_____

8. What is meant by a blood glucose meter with no-code technology?

_____

9. List and describe the two levels of controls that are performed on a blood chemistry analyzer.

_____

_____

10. What may cause a control to fail to produce expected results?

_____

_____

_____

11. When running controls on a blood chemistry analyzer, what should be done if the controls do not perform as expected?

_____

12. When should the control procedure be performed on a blood chemistry analyzer?

_____

_____

_____

13. What is the function of glucose in the body?

_____

14. What is the function of insulin in the body?

_____

_____

15. What is the purpose of a random blood glucose test?

_____

_____

16. List the abbreviation for each of the following tests:

    a. Fasting blood glucose: _____

    b. Two-hour postprandial blood glucose: _____

    c. Oral glucose tolerance test: _____

17. What type of patient preparation is required for a fasting blood glucose (FBG) test?

_____

_____

18. List two reasons for performing a FBG test.

_____

_____

19. What are the FBG test results for the following?

Hyperglycemia: _____

Hypoglycemia: _____

20. What is prediabetes?

_____

_____

21. What are the ADA recommended values for interpretation of the following FBG classifications?

    a. Normal: _____

    b. Prediabetes: _____

    c. Diabetes: _____

22. What is the purpose of a two-hour postprandial blood glucose (2-hour PPBG) test?

_____

_____

23. What patient preparation is required for a 2-hour PPBG test?

_____

_____

_____

24. Describe the procedure for performing a 2-hour PPBG test.

_____

_____

25. What is the purpose of an oral glucose tolerance test (OGTT)?

_____

_____

26. What patient preparation is required for an OGTT?

_____

_____

_____

27. Describe the procedure for an OGTT.

_____

_____

_____

28. What normal side effects may occur during an OGTT?

_____

29. What are the serious side effects that may occur during an OGTT that should be reported?

_____

_____

30. What are the ADA recommended values for interpretation of the following OGTT classifications?

    a. Normal: _____

    b. Prediabetes: _____

    c. Diabetes: _____

31. What can cause hypoglycemia?

_____

_____

_____

32. What is the purpose of a hemoglobin A_{1c} test?

_____

_____

33. What information is provided by a hemoglobin A_{1c} test?

_____

34. What are the ADA recommended values for the following hemoglobin A_{1c} classifications?

    a. Normal: _____

    b. Prediabetes: _____

    c. Diabetes: _____

35. What are the advantages of diabetic patients maintaining good blood glucose control?

_____

_____

36. What is the ideal testing schedule for an insulin-dependent diabetic patient?

_____

_____

37. What is a continuous monitoring glucose device?

_____

_____

38. What are the ADA recommended target blood glucose levels for a patient with diabetes?

    a. Before meals and snacks: _____

    b. 1 to 2 hours after meals: _____

39. What complications can occur from prolonged high blood glucose levels?

_____

_____

40. What can cause too much insulin in a diabetic patient?

_____

_____

41. What serious life-threatening symptoms occur from untreated hypoglycemia?

_____

_____

42. What is cholesterol and what is its function in the body?

_____

_____

43. List the two main sources of cholesterol in the blood.

_____

_____

44. What determines an individual's blood cholesterol level?

_____

_____

45. What is atherosclerosis, and why is it a health risk?

_____

_____

46. Why is LDL cholesterol referred to as bad cholesterol and HDL referred to as good cholesterol?

    LDL cholesterol: _____

_____

    HDL cholesterol: _____

_____

47. What does a total cholesterol test measure?

_____

48. What tests are included in a lipid panel?

_____

_____

49. What is the primary use of cholesterol test results?

_____

50. What are the recommended values for interpretation the following total cholesterol classifications?

    a. Desirable level: _____

    b. Borderline high level: _____

    c. High level: _____

51. What are the recommended values for interpretation the following LDL cholesterol classifications?

    a. Optimal level: _____

    b. Near optimal level: _____

    c. Borderline high level: _____

    d. High level: _____

    e. Very high level: _____

52. At what level is HDL cholesterol considered an increased risk factor for cardiovascular disease?

Men: _____

Women: _____

53. What are triglycerides?

_____

54. What are the sources of triglycerides in the body?

_____

55. What are the recommended values for interpretation the following triglycerides classifications?

    a. Normal: _____

    b. Borderline high: _____

    c. High: _____

    d. Very high: _____

56. What conditions result in elevated blood triglycerides?

_____

_____

57. What is the purpose of performing a BUN?

_____

58. What is the definition of immunology?

_____

59. List three examples of antigens.

_____

60. What is the purpose of performing each of the following serologic tests?

    a. Hepatitis test: _____

    b. HIV test: _____

    c. Rheumatoid factor test: _____

    d. Antistreptolysin O test: _____

    e. C-reactive protein test: _____

61. How long does it take for HIV antibodies to form in the blood of an adult following infection?

_____

62. What are the two most common screening tests for syphilis?

_____

63. What type of digestive disorders can be caused by *H. pylori*?

_____

_____

64. What is infectious mononucleosis?

_____

65. How is infectious mononucleosis transmitted?

_____

66. What are the symptoms of infectious mononucleosis?

_____

_____

67. What is the most frequent use of an Rh antibody titer test?

_____

68. What is the purpose of performing ABO and Rh blood typing?

_____

_____

69. What happens when a blood antigen and blood antibody combine?

_____

70. Where are the A, B, and Rh blood antigens located?

_____

71. Why is agglutination of red blood cells in vivo a threat to life?

_____

_____

72. If a person has type A blood, what blood antigens and blood antibodies are present?

_____

73. If a person has type AB blood, what blood antigens and blood antibodies are present?

_____

74. If a person has type O blood, what blood antigens and blood antibodies are present?

_____

75. What is the difference between Rh-positive and Rh-negative blood?

_____

_____

CRITICAL THINKING ACTIVITIES

A. Comprehensive Metabolic Panel Requirements

Your provider has ordered a CMP on a patient that will be analyzed at an outside laboratory. You are required to collect the specimen and prepare it for transport to the outside laboratory. Using Figure 19.1 in your textbook as a reference, respond to the following questions in the spaces provided.

1. What is the amount and type of specimen required for this test?

_____

2. What type and capacity of collection container should be used to collect the specimen? *(Note: The tube selected must have a capacity of 2 ½ times the amount of serum required).*

_____

3. What patient preparation is required for this test?

_____

4. What are the collection and processing requirements for this specimen?

_____

_____

_____

797

5. How should your store the specimen while awaiting pickup by the laboratory courier?

_____

6. What would cause the laboratory to reject the specimen?

_____

_____

_____

7. What are the uses of a CMP?

_____

_____

_____

B. Type 2 Diabetes Information Sheet

1. You are working for a provider specializing in internal medicine. The provider is concerned about the increased numbers of patients developing type 2 diabetes. She asks you to design an educational, colorful, and creative information sheet on type 2 diabetes. This information sheet will be published and placed in the waiting room to provide patients with education on type 2 diabetes.

2. Diabetes Internet sites can be used to complete this activity.

3. Include the following topics on your information sheet:

   • Description and cause

   • Symptoms

   • Means of diagnosis

   • Treatment

   • Prevention

C. Oral Glucose Tolerance Test Instructions

Francesa DeLuca has been scheduled for an OGTT to be performed at an outside laboratory. What should you tell Francesa regarding the following topics? Explain the reason for each response.

1. Consumption of food and fluid (other than water)

_____

_____

2. Water consumption

_____

_____

3. Smoking

_____

_____

4. Leaving the test site

_____

_____

5. Activity

_____

_____

6. Normal side effects of the test

_____

_____

7. Serious symptoms that should be reported

_____

_____

D. Lipid Panel Reference Ranges

Refer to the lipid panel laboratory report in your textbook (Figure 19.13). Using the reference ranges listed in this report, determine whether the following test results fall within their normal reference ranges or whether they are high or low. Mark each test result according to the following: N = normal, H = high, L = low.

Female Patient:

_____ 1. Total cholesterol: 180 mg/dL

_____ 2. HDL cholesterol: 65 mg/dL

_____ 3. Triglycerides: 160 mg/dL

_____ 4. LDL cholesterol: 90 mg/dL

_____ 5. VLDL: 28 mg/dL

_____ 6. Cholesterol/HDL Ratio: 2.8

Female Patient:

_____ 1. Total cholesterol: 220 mg/dL

_____ 2. HDL cholesterol: 30 mg/dL

_____ 3. Triglycerides: 140 mg/dL

_____ 4. LDL cholesterol: 110 mg/dL

_____ 5. VLDL: 34 mg/dL

_____ 6. Cholesterol/HDL Ratio: 7.3

E. Cardiovascular Disease

Create a profile of an individual who is at risk for developing cardiovascular disease (CVD) following these guidelines:

1. Using a blank piece of paper, colored pencils, crayons, or markers, draw a figure of an individual exhibiting risk factors for CVD. Be as creative as possible.

2. Do not use any text on your drawing other than to label items you have drawn in your picture. (A picture is worth a thousand words!)

3. Try to include at least ten risk factors for CVD in your drawing. The Highlight on Cardiovascular Disease box in your textbook can be used as a reference source.

4. In the classroom, find a partner and trade drawings. Identify the risk factors for CVD in your partner's drawing and discuss what this individual could do to lower his or her risk of developing CVD.

F. Saturated Fat and Cholesterol

Using a reference source (e.g., Internet) complete the following activities:

1. Create a dinner meal that is as high as possible in saturated fat and cholesterol. Indicate the grams of saturated fat and milligrams of cholesterol in each food item.

Food Item:	Amount of saturated fat and cholesterol:

2. Create a dinner meal that is as low as possible in saturated fat and cholesterol. Indicate the grams of saturated fat and milligrams of cholesterol in each food item.

Food Item:	Amount of saturated fat and cholesterol:

800

3. Choose a fast-food restaurant and plan a meal from its menu that is as low as possible in saturated fat and cholesterol. If possible, indicate the grams of saturated fat and milligrams of cholesterol in each food item. (This can be accomplished through an Internet search. Example: Wendy's Nutrition Facts.)

Food Item: Amount of saturated fat and cholesterol:

_____

_____

_____

_____

G. Rh Incompatibility

Erythroblastosis fetalis (hemolytic disease of the newborn) is a blood disorder of the newborn. It usually is caused by an Rh incompatibility between the infant's blood and the mother's blood. Using reference sources, such as the Internet, answer the following questions regarding erythroblastosis fetalis in the space provided.

1. Explain how Rh incompatibility between the mother and her infant can cause this condition to occur.

_____

_____

_____

_____

_____

2. Indicate the complications experienced by a newborn with erythroblastosis fetalis.

_____

_____

_____

3. Explain the treatment used for this erythroblastosis fetalis.

_____

_____

_____

4. How can this erythroblastosis fetalis be prevented?

_____

_____

_____

801

H. Crossword Puzzle: Blood Chemistry and Immunology

Directions: Complete the crossword puzzle using the clues provided.

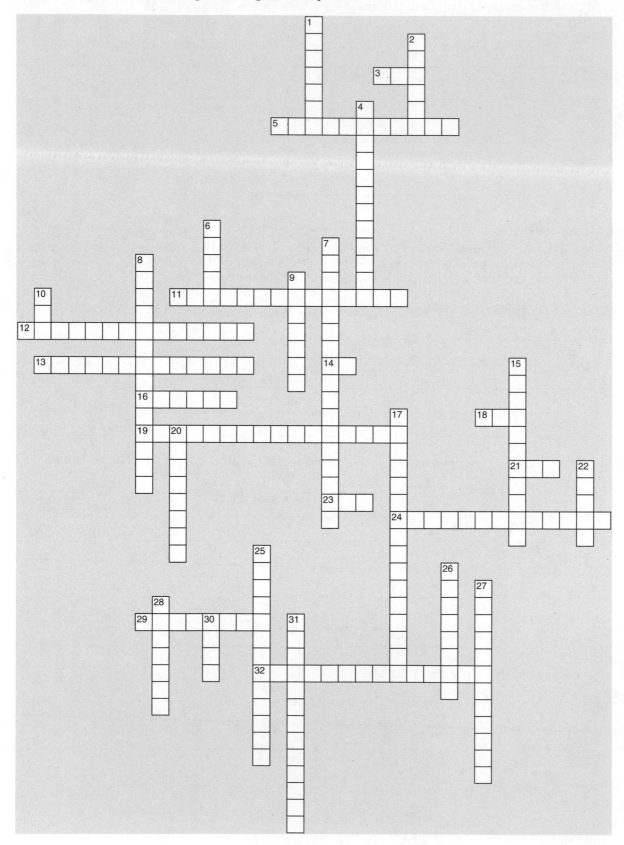

Across

3 Syphilis test
5 Detects ulcers
11 Bulging of aorta
12 Good cholesterol
13 Abnormally high BG
14 Rheumatoid arthritis test
16 Hemoglobin A_{1c}: Less than 5.7%
18 #1 killer in the U.S.
19 Helps prevent CVD
21 Kidney function test
23 Continuously measures BG level
24 Desirable: <150 mg/dL
29 Stored glucose
32 Bad cholesterol

Down

1 Risk factor for CVD
2 Result of no blood to brain
4 Symptom of hypoglycemia
6 Manufacturers cholesterol
7 Body can't use its insulin
8 Total cholesterol: 200-239
9 Produced by beta cells of pancreas
10 Plaque in arteries of heart
15 FBG: 100-125 mg/dL
17 Clot in a vein
20 Combines with an antigen
22 Keep diabetic A_{1c} % below this
25 Kissing disease
26 Calibration device
27 Abnormally low BG
28 Provides energy for body
30 Series of blood glucose tests
31 Clumping of RBCs

Notes

Procedure 19-A: CLIA-Waived Blood Chemistry Test. Perform a CLIA-waived blood chemistry test following the manufacturer's instructions, and document results in the chart provided. Examples of blood chemistry tests: hemoglobin A_{1C}, cholesterol, triglycerides, and BUN.

Procedure 19-1: CLIA-Waived Blood Glucose Test.
a. Run controls on a CLIA-waived glucose meter, and document results on the Blood Glucoses Quality Control Log.
b. Perform a CLIA-waived FBG test, and document the results in the chart provided.

Procedure 19-B: CLIA-Waived Rapid Mononucleosis Test.
a. Run controls on a CLIA-waived rapid mononucleosis test following the manufacturer's instructions, and document results on the Mononucleosis Quality Control Log.
b. Perform a CLIA-waived rapid mononucleosis test following the manufacturer's instructions (presented in your textbook), and document the results in the chart provided.

CHART	
Date	

CHART	
Date	

Chapter **19 Blood Chemistry and Immunology**

Quality Control Log

Blood Glucose Test

NAME OF METER	CONTROLS

Test Strips:

Lot Number:_____

Exp Date:_____

Code Number:_____

Low-Level Control:

Lot Number:_____

Exp Date:_____

Expected Range:_____

High-Level Control:

Lot Number:_____

Exp Date:_____

Expected Range:_____

Date	Level 1 Control	Accept	Reject	Level 2 Control	Accept	Reject	Technician

807

Chapter **19 Blood Chemistry and Immunology**

Quality Control Log

Mononucleosis Test

Date	Name of Test	Control Lot #	Control Expiration Date	External Positive Control	External Negative Control	Technician

Notes

Procedure 19-A: CLIA-Waived Blood Chemistry Test

Name: _____   Date: _____

Evaluated by: _____   Score: _____

Performance Objective

Outcome:	Perform a CLIA-waived blood chemistry test following the manufacturer's instructions.
Conditions:	Given the following: disposable gloves, an antiseptic wipe, lancet, gauze pad, -quality control log, and a biohazard sharps container. Using a CLIA-waived automated blood chemistry analyzer and manufacturer's instructions.
Standards:	Time: 10 minutes. Student completed procedure in _____ minutes.
	Accuracy: Satisfactory score on the Performance Evaluation Checklist.

Performance Evaluation Checklist

Trial 1	Trial 2	Point Value	Performance Standards
		•	Sanitized hands.
		•	Assembled equipment.
		•	Calibrated the blood chemistry analyzer.
		•	Applied gloves and ran controls.
		•	Documented control results in the quality control log.
		•	Sanitized hands.
		•	Greeted the patient and introduced yourself.
		•	Identified patient and explained the procedure.
		•	Applied gloves.
		•	Performed a finger puncture to obtain the blood specimen.
		•	Had the patient hold a gauze pad over the puncture site and apply pressure.
		•	Applied the blood specimen to the testing device (e.g.; test strip, test cassette, or test cartridge) associated with the blood chemistry analyzer according to manufacturer's instructions.
		•	Operated the blood chemistry analyzer according to manufacturer's instructions.
		•	Read the results on digital display screen.
		•	Properly disposed of used materials.
		•	Checked the puncture site and applied adhesive bandage, if needed.
		•	Removed gloves.
		•	Sanitized hands.
		•	Documented the test results correctly.
		★	The documentation was identical to the reading on the digital display screen.

Trial 1	Trial 2	Point Value	Performance Standards
		■	Demonstrated critical thinking skills.
		■	Reassured patients.
		★	Completed the procedure within 10 minutes.
			Totals

CHART	
Date	

Evaluation of Student Performance

EVALUATION CRITERIA			COMMENTS
Symbol	**Category**	**Point Value**	
★	Critical Step	16 points	
•	Essential Step	6 points	
■	Affective Competency	6 points	
▷	Theory Question	2 points	

Score calculation: 100 points

−   points missed
_____

____Score

Satisfactory score: 85 or above

CAAHEP Competencies Achieved

Psychomotor (Skills)

☑   I. 10. Perform a quality control measure.
☑   I. 11. b. Collect specimens and perform CLIA-waived chemistry test.
☑   II. 2. Record laboratory test results into the patient's record.

Affective (Behavior)

☑   A. 1. Record laboratory test results into the patient's record.
☑   A. 2. Reassure patients.

ABHES Competencies Achieved

☑   9. a. Practice quality control.
☑   9. b. (3) Perform selected CLIA-waived tests that assist with diagnosis and treatment: chemistry testing.

EVALUATION OF COMPETENCY

Procedure 19-1: CLIA-Waived Fasting Blood Glucose Test

Name: _____   Date: _____

Evaluated by: _____   Score: _____

Performance Objective

Outcome:	Perform a CLIA-waived FBG test.
Conditions:	Given the following: disposable gloves, Accu-Chek Aviva glucose meter and test strips, control solutions, lancet, antiseptic wipe, gauze pad, and a biohazard sharps container.
Standards:	Time: 10 minutes. Student completed procedure in _____ minutes.
	Accuracy: Satisfactory score on the Performance Evaluation Checklist.

Performance Evaluation Checklist

Trial 1	Trial 2	Point Value	Performance Standards
		•	Sanitized hands.
		•	Assembled equipment.
		•	Checked the expiration date on container of test strips and control solutions.
		▷	Explained what to do when a new bottle of control solution is opened.
		•	Made sure the environmental temperature falls between 57° F (14° C) and 100° F (38° C).
		▷	Stated what occurs if the environmental temperature is outside of the required range.
			Performed the control procedure.
		•	Inserted a test strip into the glucose meter and placed the meter on a flat surface.
		▷	Explained what may occur if the meter is tiled.

		•	Performed level 1 and level 2 control procedures making sure to:
			a. Remove the cap and wipe the tip of the control solution bottle with a tissue.
			b. Squeeze the bottle until a tiny drop forms at the tip of the bottle.
			c. Touch and hold the drop of solution to the front edge of the yellow window until the meter beeps and an hourglass symbol flashes.
			d. Wipe the tip of the bottle with a tissue and recap it tightly.
			e. Mark the control result:
			  • Level 1 control; Press and release the right arrow key once.
			  • Level 2 control: Press the right arrow key twice.
			f. Press the Power/Set button to set the control level in the meter.
			g. Remove and discard the used test strip.

		▷	Stated what occurs if the control result is not within the expected range.
		▷	Stated the purpose for performing the control procedures.
		•	Documented results in the quality control log.
			Performed the FBG test.
		•	Sanitized hands.

Chapter **19 Blood Chemistry and Immunology**

Trial 1	Trial 2	Point Value	Performance Standards
		•	Greeted the patient and introduced yourself.
		•	Identified the patient and explained the procedure.
		•	Asked the patient if he or she prepared properly.
		▷	Stated the preparation required for a fasting blood glucose test.
		•	Removed a test strip from the container and immediately recapped the container.
		▷	Explained why the container should be recapped immediately.
		•	Inserted the test strip into meter in the direction of the arrow with the yellow window facing up.
		•	Placed the meter on a flat surface.
		•	Cleansed the puncture site with an antiseptic wipe and allowed it to dry.
		•	Applied gloves.
		•	Performed a finger puncture and disposed of the lancet in a biohazard sharps container.
		•	Wiped away the first drop of blood with a gauze pad.
		▷	Explained why the first drop of blood should be wiped away.
		•	Placed the patient's hand in a dependent position and gently massaged finger until a large drop of blood formed.
		•	Touched and help the drop of blood to the front edge of the yellow window of the test strip.
		•	Had the patient hold a gauze pad over puncture site and apply pressure.
		•	Observed the digital display of the test results.
		▷	Stated the normal range for a FBG test (70 to 99 mg/dL).
		•	Removed the test strip from the meter and discarded it in a biohazard waste container.
		•	Checked puncture site and applied adhesive bandage, if needed.
		•	Removed gloves and sanitized hands.
		•	Documented the results correctly.
		★	The documentation was identical to the reading on the digital display screen.
		•	Cleaned and disinfected the glucose meter.
		■	Demonstrated critical thinking skills.
		■	Reassured patients.
		★	Completed the procedure within 10 minutes.
			Totals

Evaluation of Student Performance

EVALUATION CRITERIA			COMMENTS
Symbol	**Category**	**Point Value**	
★	Critical Step	16 points	
•	Essential Step	6 points	
■	Affective Competency	6 points	
▷	Theory Question	2 points	

Score calculation: 100 points

−_____ points missed

_____Score

Satisfactory score: 85 or above

CAAHEP Competencies Achieved

Psychomotor (Skills)

☑ I. 10. Perform a quality control measure.
☑ I. 11. b. Collect specimens and perform CLIA-waived chemistry test.
☑ II. 2. Record laboratory test results into the patient's record.

Affective (Behavior)

☑ A. 1. Demonstrate critical thinking skills
☑ A-2 Reassure patients.

ABHES Competencies Achieved

☑ 9. a. Practice quality control.
☑ 9. b. (3) Perform selected CLIA-waived tests that assist with diagnosis and treatment: chemistry testing.

Notes

EVALUATION OF COMPETENCY

Procedure 19-B: CLIA-Waived Rapid Mononucleosis Test

Name: _____   Date: _____

Evaluated by: _____   Score: _____

Performance Objective

Outcome:	Perform a CLIA-waived rapid mononucleosis test.
Conditions:	Given the following: disposable gloves, QuickVue + Mono Test and manufacturer's instructions, controls, lancet, antiseptic wipe, gauze pad, and a biohazard sharps container.
Standards:	Time: 10 minutes. Student completed procedure in _____ minutes.
	Accuracy: Satisfactory score on the Performance Evaluation Checklist.

Performance Evaluation Checklist

Trial 1	Trial 2	Point Value	Performance Standards
		•	Sanitized hands.
		•	Assembled equipment.
		•	Checked the expiration date on the mononucleosis test kit.
		•	Applied gloves and ran a positive and a negative control, if necessary.
		•	Removed gloves and documented results in the quality control log.
		•	Greeted the patient and introduced yourself.
		•	Identified the patient and explained the procedure.
		•	Removed the test cassette from its foil pouch and placed it on a flat surface.
		•	Cleansed the puncture site and allowed it to air dry.
		•	Applied gloves.
		•	Performed a finger puncture.
		•	Disposed of the lancet in a biohazard sharps container.
		•	Wiped away the first drop of blood.
		•	Had the patient hold a gauze pad over puncture site and apply pressure.
		•	Collect the blood specimen: a. *Hanging Drop Procedure*: Add 2 hanging drops of fingertip blood directly to the center of the add well. OR b. *Capillary Tube Procedure*: Filled the capillary tube to the fill line and dispensed all the blood into the add well.
		•	Held the developer bottle vertically and added 5 drops of developing solution to the add well.
		•	Waited 5 minutes and interpreted the test results.
		▷	Described the appearance of a positive, negative, and invalid test result.

Chapter **19 Blood Chemistry and Immunology**

Trial 1	Trial 2	Point Value	Performance Standards
		▷	Stated what can cause an invalid test result.
		•	Did not read the test results after 10 minutes.
		•	Disposed of the test cassette in a biohazard waste container.
		•	Checked puncture site and applied adhesive bandage, if needed.
		•	Removed gloves.
		•	Sanitized hands.
		•	Documented the results correctly.
		•	The results were identical to the evaluator's results.
		■	Demonstrated critical thinking skills.
		■	Reassured patients
		★	Completed the procedure within 10 minutes.
			Totals

CHART

Date	

Evaluation of Student Performance

EVALUATION CRITERIA			COMMENTS
Symbol	**Category**	**Point Value**	
★	Critical Step	16 points	
•	Essential Step	6 points	
■	Affective Competency	6 points	
▷	Theory Question	2 points	

Score calculation: 100 points

       – _____ points missed

       _____ Score

Satisfactory score: 85 or above

CAAHEP Competencies Achieved

Psychomotor (Skills)

- ☑ I. 10. Perform a quality control measure.
- ☑ I. 11. d. Collect specimens and perform CLIA-waived immunology test.
- ☑ II. 2. Record laboratory test results into the patient's record.

Affective (Behavior)

- ☑ A. 1. Demonstrate critical thinking skills.
- ☑ A. 2. Reassure patients.

ABHES Competencies Achieved

- ☑ 9. a. Practice quality control.
- ☑ 9. b. (4) Perform selected CLIA-waived tests that assist with diagnosis and treatment: immunology testing.

20 Medical Microbiology

CHAPTER ASSIGNMENTS

√ After Completing	Date Due	Study Guide Pages	STUDY GUIDE ASSIGNMENTS (CTA = Critical Thinking Activity)	Possible Points	Points You Earned
		825	Pretest	10	
		826	Key Term Assessment	16	
		826-832	Evaluation of Learning questions	62	
		832-833	CTA A: Stages of an Infectious Disease	20	
			Evolve: Microscope Identification (Record points earned)		
		834-835	CTA B: Infectious Disease Information Sheet	20	
		835	CTA C: Patient Education: Influenza	8	
		836	CTA D: Sensitivity Testing	12	
		837	CTA E: Crossword Puzzle	30	
			Evolve: Apply Your Knowledge questions	10	
			Evolve: Video Evaluation	15	
		825	Posttest	10	
			ADDITIONAL ASSIGNMENTS		
			Total points		

√ When Assigned by Your Instructor	Study Guide Pages	Practices Required	LABORATORY ASSIGNMENTS (Procedure Number and Name)	Score*
	839	3	**Practice for Competency** 20-1: Operate a Compound Microscope	
	841-843		**📝 Evaluation of Competency** 20-1: Operate a Compound Microscope	
	839	3	**Practice for Competency** 20-2: Collecting a Throat Specimen	
	845-847		**📝 Evaluation of Competency** 20-2: Collecting a Throat Specimen	
	839	3	**Practice for Competency** 20-3: CLIA-Waived Rapid Strep Testing	
	849-851		**📝 Evaluation of Competency** 20-3: CLIA-Waived Rapid Strep Testing	*
	839-840	3	**Practice for Competency** 20-4: CLIA-Waived Rapid Influenza Testing	
	853-856		**📝 Evaluation of Competency** 20-4: CLIA-Waived Rapid Influenza Testing	
			ADDITIONAL ASSIGNMENTS	

Notes

Name: _____ Date: _____

True or False

_____ 1. Microbiology is the scientific study of microorganisms and their activities.

_____ 2. A disease that can be spread from one person to another is known as an infectious disease.

_____ 3. Droplet infection is the transfer of pathogens from a fine spray emitted from a person already infected with the disease.

_____ 4. Streptococci are round bacteria that grow in pairs.

_____ 5. Chickenpox is caused by a virus.

_____ 6. The coarse adjustment on a microscope is used to obtain precise focusing of an object.

_____ 7. The purpose of transport media is to provide nutrients for the multiplication of the specimen.

_____ 8. A throat specimen should be collected from the tonsillar area and posterior pharynx.

_____ 9. Strep throat is primarily transmitted through droplet infection and by sharing personal items with an infected person.

_____ 10. Antiviral medications can be used to prevent influenza.

? POSTTEST

True or False

_____ 1. Microorganisms that reside in the body but do not cause disease are known as transient flora.

_____ 2. The invasion of the body by a pathogenic microorganism is known as infection.

_____ 3. The interval of time between the invasion by a pathogen and the first symptoms of disease is known as the *prodromal period*.

_____ 4. Staphylococcal infections usually result in pus formation.

_____ 5. *Escherichia coli* normally reside in the urinary tract.

_____ 6. The high-power objective has a magnification of 40x.

_____ 7. Examination of urine sediment requires the use of the oil immersion objective.

_____ 8. A throat specimen is the preferred specimen for a rapid influenza diagnostic test.

_____ 9. A mixed culture contains two or more types of microorganisms.

_____ 10. The purpose of sensitivity testing is to identify the type of microorganism present.

Term KEY TERM ASSESSMENT

Directions: Match each key term with its definition.

_____ 1. Bacilli

_____ 2. Cocci

_____ 3. Contagious

_____ 4. Culture

_____ 5. Culture medium

_____ 6. False-negative result

_____ 7. Incubate

_____ 8. Incubation period

_____ 9. Infection

_____ 10. Infectious disease

_____ 11. Inoculate

_____ 12. Microbiology

_____ 13. Mucous membrane

_____ 14. Normal flora

_____ 15. Specimen

_____ 16. Spirilla

A. A disease caused by a pathogen that produces harmful effects on its host
B. Capable of being transmitted directly or indirectly from one person to another
C. To introduce microorganisms into a culture medium for growth and multiplication
D. Bacteria that have a round shape
E. The scientific study of microorganisms and their activities
F. A mixture of nutrients in which microorganisms are grown in the laboratory
G. The interval of time between invasion by a pathogenic microorganism and the appearance of the first symptoms of the disease
H. Bacteria that have a spiral or curved shape
I. Harmless, nonpathogenic microorganisms that normally reside in many parts of the body but do not cause disease
J. Bacteria that have a rod shape
K. The propagation of a mass of microorganisms in a laboratory culture medium
L. In microbiology, the act of placing a culture in a chamber that provides optimal growth requirements for the multiplication of the organisms.
M. A small sample or part taken from the body to show the nature of the whole
N. A membrane lining body passages or cavities that open to the outside
O. The condition in which the body, or part of it, is invaded by a pathogen.
P. A test result denoting that a condition is absent when it is actually present

EVALUATION OF LEARNING

Directions: Fill in each blank with the correct answer.

1. What are microorganisms?_____

_____

2. What life processes are performed within a unicellular microbe?_____

_____

3. What is meant by the following phrase: "Microorganisms are ubiquitous"?

_____

_____

4. Describe two examples of microorganisms making up the normal flora that are beneficial to the body.

_____

_____

5. What occurs when pathogens invade the body, and what is the response of the body to the invasion?

_____

_____

6. What defense mechanisms are used by the body to stop the invasion of a pathogen once it has entered the body?

_____

_____

7. What is droplet infection?

_____

_____

8. How might the spread of a droplet infection be prevented?

_____

_____

9. What occurs during the incubation period?

_____

_____

10. What is the prodromal period of an infectious disease?

_____

_____

11. What is the acute period of an infectious disease?

_____

_____

12. List three infectious diseases caused by *Staphylococcus aureus.*

_____

_____

13. List three infectious diseases caused by streptococci.

_____

_____

14. List three infectious diseases caused by bacilli.

_____

_____

15. In what part of the body do *E. coli* bacteria normally reside? What can occur if *E. coli* enters the urinary tract?

_____

_____

16. List four infectious diseases caused by a virus.

_____

_____

17. Explain the purpose of each of the following parts of a microscope:

Stage

_____

_____

Condenser

_____

_____

Diaphragm

_____

_____

Coarse adjustment

_____

_____

Fine adjustment

_____

_____

Eyepiece

_____

_____

18. Describe the function of each of the following objective lenses:

Low power

_____

_____

High power

_____

_____

Oil immersion

_____

_____

19. What is the purpose of using oil with the oil-immersion objective?

_____

_____

20. List five guidelines that should be followed for proper care of the microscope.

_____

_____

_____

_____

21. List five common areas of the body from which a microbiologic specimen may be obtained.

_____

_____

22. What are extraneous microorganisms? What may occur if extraneous microorganisms enter a microbiologic specimen?

_____

_____

23. List two ways to prevent contamination of a specimen with extraneous microorganisms.

_____

_____

24. List two precautions a medical assistant should take to prevent infection with a microbiologic specimen.

_____

_____

25. Why should a specimen for microbial culture be processed as soon as possible after it is collected?

_____

26. When collecting a microbiologic specimen, why is it important to indicate on the laboratory request if the patient is receiving antibiotic therapy?

_____

_____

27. Describe the procedure for collecting a wound specimen.

_____

_____

28. What is the purpose of a transport medium?

_____

_____

29. How should a collection and transport system be stored?

_____

_____

829

30. What is strep throat?

_____

_____

31. What is the age range that strep throat is most likely to affect?

_____

32. What are the symptoms of strep throat?

_____

_____

33. How is strep throat transmitted from one person to another?

_____

34. What is a poststreptococcal complication?

_____

_____

35. List two poststreptococcal complications that may occur in a patient with strep throat. How can these complications be prevented?

_____

_____

36. What is the advantage of using a RADT to diagnose strep throat in the medical office?

_____

37. Describe the three different types of influenza viruses:

    a. Influenza Type A:

    _____

    b. Influenza Type B:

    _____

    _____

    c. Influenza Type C:

    _____

38. List two ways in which influenza can be transmitted from one person to another.

_____

_____

39. What is the incubation period for influenza?_____

40. How long is an individual contagious following infection with influenza?

_____

41. How do the symptoms of influenza differ from the symptoms of a cold?

_____

42. What are the symptoms of influenza?

_____

_____

43. What factors can increase an individual's risk of developing serious complications from influenza?

_____

_____

44. What complications may occur from contracting influenza?

_____

_____

45. What is the best means for preventing an influenza infection?

_____

46. Who should receive an influenza vaccine?

_____

47. Why must a new influenza vaccine be produced each year?

_____

_____

48. What are three benefits that are derived from the influenza vaccine?

_____

_____

49. What infection control measures can be taken to prevent the transmission of influenza?

_____

_____

50. What home care measures can be taken to treat the symptoms of influenza?

_____

_____

51. How do antiviral medications work to treat influenza?

_____

_____

52. What is the recommendation for prescribing an antiviral medication against influenza? When is this medication most effective?

_____

_____

53. How is influenza typically diagnosed? Explain your answer.

_____

_____

54. When might a rapid influenza test be performed to diagnose influenza?

_____

55. Why is a nasopharyngeal specimen preferred for a rapid influenza test?

_____

56. What is the advantage of using a flocked swab to collect a nasopharyngeal specimen?

_____

57. How can the depth to insert a nasopharyngeal swab be determined?

_____

58. What is the purpose of culturing a microbiologic specimen?

_____

_____

59. What is the purpose of adding sheep's blood to an agar culture medium?

_____

_____

60. What is the name given to the type of culture that contains two or more types of microorganisms?

_____

61. What is the purpose of performing a sensitivity test on a bacterial culture?

_____

62. How are the test results interpreted when performing a disc diffusion sensitivity test?

_____

_____

_____

CRITICAL THINKING ACTIVITIES

A. Stages of an Infectious Disease

Your provider wants you to design a poster to hang in the office that outlines the stages of an infectious disease. Complete this project using the following diagram in your study guide.

832

STAGES OF INFECTIOUS DISEASE

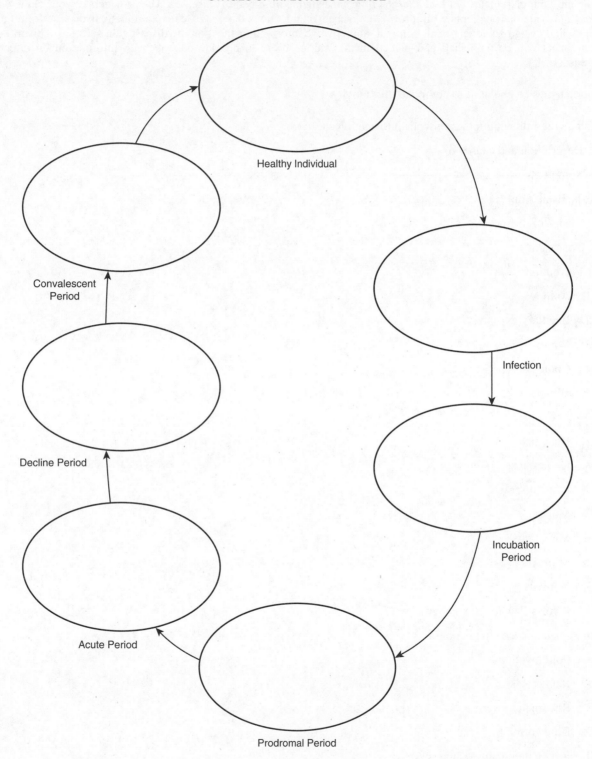

Healthy Individual

Infection

Incubation Period

Prodromal Period

Acute Period

Decline Period

Convalescent Period

B. Infectious Disease Information Sheet

1. You and your classmates work at a large clinic specializing in infectious diseases. The providers at your clinic would like to provide their patients with information sheets on infectious diseases. Select an infectious disease from the list below and design an educational, colorful, and creative information sheet on the disease you selected. This information sheets will be published and placed in the waiting room to provide patients with information on infectious diseases.

2. Internet sites can be used to complete this activity.

3. Include the following topics on your information sheet:

    • Description and cause

    • Symptoms

    • Transmission

    • Means of diagnosis

    • Treatment

    • Prevention

    1. Anthrax

    2. Bacillary dysentery

    3. Botulism

    4. Cholera

    5. Diphtheria

    6. Ebola

    7. Head lice

    8. Herpes zoster (shingles)

    9. Lyme disease

    10. Malaria

    11. Meningitis

    12. Mumps

    13. Norovirus

    14. Pertussis (whooping cough)

    15. Pneumococcal pneumonia

    16. Poliomyelitis

    17. Rabies

    18. Rheumatic fever

    19. Ringworm

    20. Rocky mountain spotted fever

    21. Rotavirus

    22. Rubella

    23. Rubeola

24.   Salmonella food poisoning

25.   Scarlet fever

26.   Smallpox

27.   Tapeworm infection

28.   Tetanus

29.   Typhoid fever

30.   Varicella (chickenpox)

C. Patient Education: Influenza

Answer the following questions that patients may have regarding influenza:

1. How do people catch the flu?

_____

_____

_____

2. When can a person with influenza spread it to other people?

_____

_____

3. How can I tell if I have a cold or the flu?

_____

_____

4. Why can't I take an antibiotic to get rid of the flu?

_____

5. How long does it take go get over the flu?

_____

_____

6. How can I try and avoid getting the flu?

_____

_____

7. After getting a flu vaccine, how long does it take to work?

_____

_____

8. If I don't get the vaccine and am exposed to the flu, can I take antiviral medications to prevent the flu?

_____

_____

D. Sensitivity Testing

Refer to Figure 20-9 in the textbook. Place a check mark next to each antibiotic that is effective against the pathogen growing on the culture medium in the Petri plate.

_____ 1. azithromycin

_____ 2. cephalothin

_____ 3. ciprofloxacin

_____ 4. cefprozil

_____ 5. clarithromycin

_____ 6. doxycycline

_____ 7. erythromycin

_____ 8. nitrofurantoin

_____ 9. norfloxacin

_____ 10. penicillin

_____ 11. sulfisoxazole

_____ 12. tetracycline

E. Crossword Puzzle: Medical Microbiology

Directions: Complete the crossword puzzle using the clues provided.

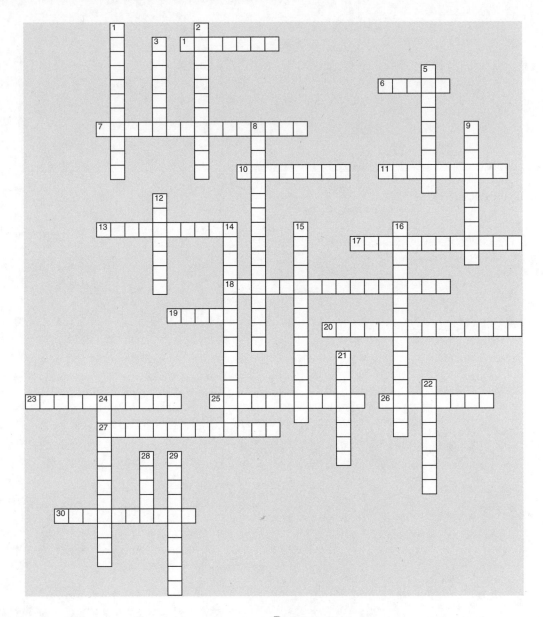

Across

1 Rod-shaped bacteria
6 Disease caused by a virus
7 Prevents drying of specimen
10 Sample of the body
11 Invasion by pathogens
13 It's everywhere!
17 Study of MOs
18 Between invasion and first sym
19 Bacillus that lives in large intestine
20 Poststreptococcal complication
23 Treatment for strep throat
25 Developed microscope
26 Needed for blood clotting
27 Absent when present
30 Can catch it!

Down

1 Disease at its peak
2 Flu virus found here
3 Flu incubation period
5 40x objective
8 Way to transmit contagious diseases
9 Lessens severity of flu
12 Intradermal flu vaccine
14 Which antibiotic to use?
15 For precise focusing
16 First symptoms of disease
21 First line of defense
22 Disease-producing MO
24 Second line of natural defense
28 Round shaped bacteria
29 Virus causing most flu outbreaks

Notes

PRACTICE FOR COMPETENCY

Procedure 20-1: Operate a Compound Microscope

Practice using a microscope.

Procedure 20-2: Collecting a Throat Specimen

Obtain a throat specimen using a sterile cotton swab or a collection and transport system. Document the procedure in the chart provided.

Procedure 20-3: CLIA-Waived Rapid Strep Testing

a. Run controls on a CLIA-waived rapid strep test kit and document results on the quality control log on page 839.

b. Perform a strep test using a CLIA-waived rapid strep test kit, and document results in the chart provided.

Procedure 20-4: CLIA-Waived Rapid Influenza Testing

a. Run controls on a CLIA-waived rapid influenza test and document results on the quality control log on page 840.

b. Perform an influenza test using a CLIA-waived rapid influenza test kit, and document results in the chart provided.

CHART	
Date	

QUALITY CONTROL LOG—STREP TEST

Date	Name of Test	Control Lot #	Control Expiration Date	External Positive Control Results	External Negative Control Results	Technician

QUALITY CONTROL LOG—INFLUENZA TEST

Date	Name of Test	Control Lot #	Control Expiration Date	External Positive Control Results	External Negative Control Results	Technician

Procedure 20-1: Operate a Compound Microscope

Name: _____ Date: _____

Evaluated by: _____ Score: _____

Performance Objective

Outcome:	Operate a compound microscope.
Conditions:	Given a compound microscope with mechanical stage, lens paper, specimen slide, tissue or gauze, immersion oil, xylene, and a soft cloth.
Standards:	Time: 15 minutes. Student completed procedure in _____ minutes.
	Accuracy: Satisfactory score on the Performance Evaluation Checklist.

Performance Evaluation Checklist

Trial 1	Trial 2	Point Value	Performance Standards
		•	Cleaned the ocular and objective lenses with lens paper using a circular motion.
		•	Turned on the light source.
		•	Rotated the nosepiece to the low-power objective and clicked it into place.
		•	Lowered the stage all the way down using the coarse adjustment knob.
		•	Placed the slide on the stage, specimen side up, and secured it.
		•	Using the coarse adjustment knob, raised the stage as far as it would go without letting the slide touch the low-power objective.
		•	Observed this step to prevent the objective from striking the slide.
		▷	Explained why this step should be observed.
		•	Looked through the eyepieces.
		•	Slowly lowered the stage using the coarse adjustment knob.
		•	Observed the specimen until it came into focus.
		•	Used the fine-adjustment knob to bring the specimen into a sharp, clear focus.
		•	Centered the specimen for optimal viewing and adjusted the light as needed using the intensity dial of the illuminator and the diaphragm lever.
		•	Rotated the nosepiece to the high-power objective and clicked it into place.
		•	Used the fine-adjustment knob to bring the specimen into a precise focus.
		•	Did not use the coarse-adjustment knob to focus the high-power objective.
		▷	Explained why the coarse-adjustment knob should not be used for focusing at this point.
		•	Examined the specimen as required by the test or procedure being performed.
		•	Turned off the light after use.

Trial 1	Trial 2	Point Value	Performance Standards
		•	Removed the slide from the stage.
		•	Cleaned the stage with a tissue or gauze and properly cared for and stored the microscope.
			Using the oil-immersion objective:
		•	Brought the specimen into focus with first the low-power objective and then the high-power objective.
		•	Rotated the nosepiece to the oil-immersion objective but did not click it into place.
		•	Placed the objective to one side.
		•	Placed a drop of immersion oil on the slide directly over the center opening in the stage.
		•	Moved the oil-immersion objective into place.
		•	Carefully observed the next steps of the procedure.
		•	Using the fine adjustment knob, slowly positioned the objective until the tip of the lens just touched the oil but did not come into contact with the slide.
		•	Observed the "pop" of light that occurs when the objective lens comes in contact with the oil.
		•	Looked through the eyepieces.
		•	Focused slowly using the fine adjustment knob.
		•	Brought the specimen into a sharp clear focus.
		•	Adjusted the light as needed using the diaphragm lever.
		•	Examined the specimen as required by the test or procedure being performed.
		•	Turned off the light after use.
		•	Removed the slide from the stage making sure not to get oil on the high-power objective lens.
		•	Gently cleaned the oil-immersion objective with lens paper.
		▷	Explained why the lens must be cleaned immediately.
		•	Cleaned the oil from the slide by immersing it in xylene and wiping it with a soft cloth.
		★	Completed the procedure within 15 minutes.
			Totals

Evaluation of Student Performance

EVALUATION CRITERIA			COMMENTS
Symbol	**Category**	**Point Value**	
★	Critical Step	16 points	
•	Essential Step	6 points	
■	Affective Competency	6 points	
▷	Theory Question	2 points	

Score calculation: 100 points

    − _____ points missed

    ____Score

Satisfactory score: 85 or above

CAAHEP Competencies Achieved

Psychomotor (Skills)
☑   I. 9. Assist provider with a patient exam.

ABHES Competencies Achieved

☑   8. c. Assist provider with general/physical examination.

Notes

Procedure 20-2: Collecting a Throat Specimen

Name: _____ Date: _____

Evaluated by: _____ Score: _____

Performance Objective

Outcome:	Collect a throat specimen for transport to an outside laboratory.
Conditions:	Given the following: disposable gloves, tongue depressor, sterile swab, sterile transport container, laboratory request form, biohazard specimen bag and a waste container.
Standards:	Time: 5 minutes. Student completed procedure in _____ minutes.
	Accuracy: Satisfactory score on the Performance Evaluation Checklist.

Performance Evaluation Checklist

Trial 1	Trial 2	Point Value	Performance Standards
		•	Sanitized hands.
		•	Assembled equipment.
		•	Checked the expiration date on the swab envelope.
		•	Labeled the transport container.
		•	Completed the laboratory request form.
		•	Greeted the patient and introduced yourself.
		•	Identified the patient and explained the procedure.
		•	Positioned the patient and adjusted the light.
		•	Applied gloves.
		•	Removed the sterile swab from its peel-apart package, being careful not to contaminate it.
		•	Depressed the patient's tongue with a tongue depressor.
		▷	Stated the function of the tongue depressor.
		•	Placed the swab at the back of the patient's throat and firmly rubbed it over lesions or white or inflamed areas of the tonsillar area and posterior pharynx.
		▷	Explained why the swab should be rubbed over suspicious-looking areas.
		•	Constantly rotated the swab as the specimen was being obtained.
		▷	Described why a rotating motion should be used.
		•	Did not allow the swab to touch any area other than the throat.
		▷	Explained why the swab should not be allowed to touch any areas other than the throat.
		•	Kept the patient's tongue depressed and withdrew the swab and removed the tongue depressor.

845

Trial 1	Trial 2	Point Value	Performance Standards
		•	Disposed of the tongue depressor.
		•	Properly handled and prepared the specimen for transport to an outside laboratory.
		•	Removed gloves and sanitized hands.
		•	Documented the information.
		■	Demonstrated critical thinking skills.
		■	Reassured patient.
		★	Completed the procedure within 5 minutes.
			Totals

CHART

Date	

Evaluation of Student Performance

EVALUATION CRITERIA			COMMENTS
Symbol	**Category**	**Point Value**	
★	Critical Step	16 points	
•	Essential Step	6 points	
■	Affective Competency	6 points	
▷	Theory Question	2 points	

Score calculation: 100 points

− _____ points missed

_____ Score

Satisfactory score: 85 or above

CAAHEP Competencies Achieved	
Psychomotor (Skills)	
☑	I. 11. e. Collect specimens and perform CLIA-waived microbiology test.
Affective (Behavior)	
☑	A. 1 Demonstrate critical thinking skills.
☑	A. 2. Reassure patient.

ABHES Competencies Achieved	
☑	9. d. (4) Collect, label, and process specimens: Obtain throat specimen.

Chapter **20** **Medical Microbiology**

Procedure 20-3: CLIA-Waived Rapid Strep Testing

Name: _____   Date: _____

Evaluated by: _____   Score: _____

Performance Objective

Outcome:	Perform a CLIA-waived rapid strep test.
Conditions:	Given the following: QuickVue rapid strep test kit, sterile throat swab, disposable gloves, tongue depressor, external controls, manufacturer's instructions, quality control log, and a biohazard waste container.
Standards:	Time: 10 minutes. Student completed procedure in _____ minutes.
	Accuracy: Satisfactory score on the Performance Evaluation Checklist.

Performance Evaluation Checklist

Trial 1	Trial 2	Point Value	Performance Standards
		•	Sanitized hands.
		•	Assembled equipment.
		•	Checked the expiration date on the test kit.
		•	Applied gloves and ran a positive and negative control, if needed.
		▷	Stated when controls should be run.
		•	Disposed of test cassettes and control swabs in a biohazard waste container.
		•	Removed gloves and sanitized hands.
		•	Documented results in the quality control log.
		•	Greeted the patient and introduced yourself.
		•	Identified the patient and explained the procedure.
		•	Positioned the patient and adjusted the light.
		•	Sanitized hands and applied gloves.
		•	Removed the test cassette from its foil pouch, and placed it on a clean, dry, level surface.
		•	Checked the expiration date of the sterile swab and removed the swab from its peel-apart package.
		•	Depressed the patient's tongue with the tongue depressor.
		•	Placed the swab at the back of the patient's throat and firmly rubbed it over lesions or white or inflamed areas of the tonsillar area and posterior pharynx.
		•	Constantly rotated the swab as the specimen was being obtained.
		•	Did not allow the swab to touch any area other than the throat.

Chapter **20 Medical Microbiology**

Trial 1	Trial 2	Point Value	Performance Standards
		•	Kept the patient's tongue depressed and withdrew the swab.
		•	Removed the tongue depressor and discarded it.
		•	Inserted the swab completely into the swab chamber.
		•	Squeezed the extraction bottle once to break the glass ampule.
		•	Vigorously shook the extraction bottle five times.
		▷	Stated what color the solution should turn after the ampule is broken.
		•	Removed the cap of the extraction bottle and quickly filled the swab chamber to the rim.
		▷	Stated the purpose of the extraction solution.
		•	Started the timer for 5 minutes.
		•	Did not move the test cassette.
		▷	Stated what should be done if the liquid has not moved across the result window within 1 minute.
		•	Waited 5 minutes and read the results.
		▷	Described the appearance of a positive and negative result.
		▷	Described the appearance of an invalid result.
		▷	Explained what to do if an invalid result occurs.
		•	The results were identical to the evaluator's results.
		•	Disposed of the test cassette and swab in a biohazard waste container.
		•	Removed gloves and sanitized hands.
		•	Documented results in the patient's medical record.
		■	Demonstrated critical thinking skills.
		■	Reassured patients.
		■	Demonstrated empathy for patients' concerns.
		★	Completed the procedure within 10 minutes.
			Totals

CHART

Date	

Evaluation of Student Performance

EVALUATION CRITERIA			COMMENTS
Symbol	**Category**	**Point Value**	
★	Critical Step	16 points	
•	Essential Step	6 points	
■	Affective Competency	6 points	
▷	Theory Question	2 points	

Score calculation: 100 points

−_____ points missed

_____Score

Satisfactory score: 85 or above

CAAHEP Competencies Achieved

Psychomotor (Skills)
☑ I. 10. Perform a quality control measure.
☑ I. 11. d. Collect specimens and perform CLIA-waived immunology test.
☑ II. 2. Record laboratory test results into the patient's record.

Affective (Behavior)
☑ A. 1. Demonstrate critical thinking skills.
☑ A. 2. Reassure patients.
☑ A. 3. Demonstrated empathy for patients' concerns.

ABHES Competencies Achieved

☑ 9. a. Practice quality control.
☑ 9. b. Perform selected CLIA-waived tests that assist with diagnosis and treatment: (5) Microbiology testing.

Notes

Procedure 20-4: CLIA-Waived Rapid Influenza Testing

Name: _____   Date: _____

Evaluated by: _____   Score: _____

Performance Objective

Outcome:	Collect a nasopharyngeal swab specimen and perform a CLIA-waived rapid influenza diagnostic test.
Conditions:	
Standards:	Given the following: CLIA-waived Binax Now Influenza A and B test kit, sterile nasopharyngeal flocked swab, disposable gloves, face mask, protective eyewear, external controls, manufacturer's instructions, quality control log, tissues, biohazard waste container.
	Time: 20 minutes. Student completed procedure in _____ minutes.
	Accuracy: Satisfactory score on the Performance Evaluation Checklist

Performance Evaluation Checklist

Trial 1	Trial 2	Point Value	Performance Standards
		•	Sanitized hands.
		•	Assembled equipment.
		•	Checked the expiration date on the test kit.
		▷	Stated the reason for checking the expiration date.
		•	Applied gloves and ran a positive and negative control, if necessary.
		▷	Stated when controls should be run.
		•	Disposed of test devices and control swabs in a biohazard waste container.
		•	Removed gloves and sanitized hands.
		•	Documented the control results in a quality control log.
			Collected the nasopharyngeal swab specimen:
		•	Greeted the patient and introduced yourself.
		•	Identified the patient and explained the collection procedure.
		•	Explained to the patient that the collection procedure may cause coughing, sneezing, or tearing of the eyes.
		•	Positioned the patient in a sitting position.
		•	Asked the patient to blow his or her nose to remove nasal secretions.
		•	Sanitized hands and applied personal protective equipment.
		▷	Stated why personal protective equipment must be applied.
		•	Tilted the patient's head back slightly.

Trial 1	Trial 2	Point Value	Performance Standards
		▷	Stated the reason for tilting the patient's head back.
		•	Removed the cap from the extraction vial using a twisting motion.
		•	Checked the expiration date of the nasopharyngeal swab.
		•	Removed the sterile swab from its peel-apart package, being careful not to contaminate it.
		•	Estimated the depth for insertion of the swab.
		▷	Stated the reason for estimating the depth for insertion of the swab.
		•	Gently inserted the swab straight back into one nostril along the floor of the nasal passage.
		•	Slowly pushed the swab forward into the nasal passage until resistance is encountered.
		•	The depth of insertion was equal to approximately one-half of the distance from the corner of the nose to the ear lobe.
		•	Did not force the swab.
		▷	Stated what should be done if an obstruction or resistance is encountered.
		•	Rotated the swab against the mucosa of the nasopharynx between 3 and 5 times.
		▷	Stated the reason for rotating the swab.
		•	Left the swab in place for a few seconds.
		▷	Stated what can occur if an insufficient number of cells is collected.
		•	Gently removed the swab from the patient's nose with a rotating motion.
		•	Provided the patient with tissues, as required.
			Performed the Binax Now Influenza A and B Test:
		•	Inserted the swab into the extraction vial.
		•	Rinsed the swab in the extraction solution by vigorously rotating it three times without creating a lot of bubbles.
		▷	Stated the reason for vigorously rotating the swab in the solution.
		•	Removed the swab from the vial by rolling it with pressure against the inside of the vial.
		•	Properly disposed of the swab in a biohazard waste container.
		•	Removed the test device from its foil pouch and set it on a clean, dry, level surface.
		•	Filled the pipet.
		•	Checked to make sure the pipet was full and that there were no air spaces in the lower part of the pipet.
		▷	Stated what may occur if too little sample is added to the test.
		•	Slowly added the contents of the pipet to the middle of the white pad on the test strip
		•	Did not allow the pipet to touch the pad.

854

Trial 1	Trial 2	Point Value	Performance Standards
		•	Immediately peeled off the brown adhesive liner from the test device.
		•	Closed and securely sealed the test device.
		•	Waited 15 minutes and read the results.
		▷	Stated why the results should not be read before or after 15 minutes have elapsed.
		•	Interpreted the test results.
		▷	Described the appearance of negative and positive test results.
		▷	Explained what to do if an invalid result occurs.
		★	The results were identical to the evaluator's results.
		•	Disposed of the test device in a biohazard waste container.
		•	Removed personal protective equipment and sanitized hands.
		•	Documented results in the patient's medical record.
		■	Demonstrated critical thinking skills.
		■	Reassured patients.
		■	Demonstrated empathy for patients' concerns.
		★	Completed the procedure within 20 minutes.
			Totals

CHART

Date	

Evaluation of Student Performance

EVALUATION CRITERIA			COMMENTS
Symbol	**Category**	**Point Value**	
★	Critical Step	16 points	
•	Essential Step	6 points	
■	Affective Competency	6 points	
▷	Theory Question	2 points	

Score calculation: 100 points

— _____ points missed

_____ Score

Satisfactory score: 85 or above

855

CAAHEP Competencies Achieved

Psychomotor (Skills)

☑ I.10. Perform a quality control measure.

☑ I. 11.d. Collect specimens and perform CLIA-waived immunology test.

☑ II. 2. Record laboratory test results into the patient's record.

Affective (Behavior)

☑ A. 1. Demonstrate critical thinking skills.

☑ A. 2. Reassure patients.

☑ A. 3. Demonstrate empathy for patients' concerns.

ABHES Competencies Achieved

☑ 9. a. Practice quality control.

☑ 9.b. Perform selected CLIA-waived tests that assist with diagnosis and treatment: 4. Immunology testing.

21 Nutrition

CHAPTER ASSIGNMENTS

√ After Completing	Date Due	Study Guide Pages	STUDY GUIDE ASSIGNMENTS (CTA = Critical Thinking Activity)	Possible Points	Points You Earned
		861	Pretest	10	
		862-863	Key Term Assessment A. Definitions B. Word Parts (Add 1 point for each key term)	28 20	
		864-876	Evaluation of Learning questions	105	
		876	CTA A: Nutrition Density	8	
		877	CTA B: Sodium	10	
		877-879	CTA C: MyPlate	10	
		879	CTA D: Nutrition Facts Panel Analysis	13	
		880	CTA E: Nutrition and Disease	13	
		880	CTA F: Ingredients List	15	
		881	CTA G: Crossword Puzzle	34	
			Evolve: Apply Your Knowledge Questions	10	
		861	Posttest	10	
			ADDITIONAL ASSIGNMENTS		
			Total points		

√ When Assigned By Your Instructor	Study Guide Pages	Practices Required	LABORATORY ASSIGNMENTS (Procedure Number and Name)	Score*
		3	**Practice for Competency** 21-A: Instruct a Patient According to Patient's Special Dietary Needs	
	883-886		**Evaluation of Competency** 21-A: Instruct a Patient According to Patient's Special Dietary Needs	*

Chapter **21** **Nutrition**

Name _____ Date _____

True or False

_____ 1. A food with a high nutrient density is high in calories and low in nutrients.

_____ 2. Carbohydrates provide 4 kilocalories of energy per gram.

_____ 3. Ingested glucose that is not needed for energy is stored for later use in the form of glycogen.

_____ 4. Fat transports water soluble vitamins in the body.

_____ 5. Saturated fat is liquid at room temperature and comes primarily from plant sources.

_____ 6. The fat soluble vitamins include A, D, E, and K.

_____ 7. Food labeling is required for most packaged foods.

_____ 8. One pound of body fat is equal to 2000 calories.

_____ 9. An individual with lactose intolerance is allergic to milk.

_____10. Common food allergens include milk, eggs, wheat, and peanuts.

?≡ **POSTTEST**

True or False

_____ 1. An enriched food has vitamins and minerals added to it to replace those lost during the processing of that food.

_____ 2. Micronutrients include vitamins and minerals.

_____ 3. Lactose is a monosaccharide.

_____ 4. Soluble fiber helps to lower the blood cholesterol level.

_____ 5. The function of protein is to build, maintain, and repair body tissue.

_____ 6. Minor minerals are found in the body in levels of 5 grams or higher.

_____ 7. Approximately 60 to 65% of an adult's total body weight is made up of water.

_____ 8. The treatment of obesity involves a combination of nutrition therapy, a physical exercise program, and a behavior modification plan.

_____ 9. The TLC eating plan provides recommendations for a heart healthy diet.

_____10. Celiac disease results in damage to the intestinal villi of the small intestine.

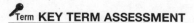
A. Definitions

Directions: Match each key term with its definition.

_____ 1. Antioxidant

_____ 2. Atherosclerosis

_____ 3. Bariatrics

_____ 4. Cholesterol

_____ 5. Complete protein

_____ 6. Disaccharide

_____ 7. Empty calorie food

_____ 8. Essential amino acid

_____ 9. Gluten

_____ 10. Glycogen

_____ 11. Incomplete protein

_____ 12. Kilocalorie

_____ 13. Lactose

_____ 14. Macronutrient

_____ 15. Micronutrient

_____ 16. Mineral

_____ 17. Monosaccharide

_____ 18. Nonessential amino acid

_____ 19. Nutrient

_____ 20. Nutrition

_____ 21. Nutrition therapy

_____ 22. Obesity

_____ 23. Percent daily value

_____ 24. Polysaccharide

_____ 25. Saturated fat

_____ 26. Triglycerides

_____ 27. Unsaturated fat

_____ 28. Vitamin

A. A food that provides calories but little or no nutrients. Also known as a low nutrient density food.

B. The amount of heat needed to raise the temperature of 1 kilogram of water 1 degree Celsius. (Often referred to as a calorie).

C. A chemical substance found in food that is needed by the body for survival and well-being.

D. The percentage of a nutrient provided by a single serving of a food item compared to how much is required for the entire day.

E. Buildup of fibrous plaques of fatty deposits and cholesterol on the inner walls of an artery that causes narrowing, obstruction, and hardening of the artery.

F. An organic compound that is required in small amounts by the body for normal growth and development.

G. A white waxy, fatlike substance that is essential for normal functioning of the body.

H. A type of protein found in certain grains such as wheat, rye, and barley.

I. The application of the science of nutrition to promote optimal health and treat illness.

J. The chemical form in which most fat exists in food, as well as in the body.

K. A molecule that inhibits the oxidation of other molecules.

L. A medical condition in which there is an excessive accumulation of body fat to the extent where it may have an adverse effect on the health and well-being of an individual.

M. A simple carbohydrate consisting of two sugar units.

N. A nutrient required in relatively large amounts by the body. Includes carbohydrates, fat, and protein.

O. A naturally occurring inorganic substance this is essential to the proper functioning of the body.

P. The branch of medicine that deals with the treatment and control of obesity and diseases associated with obesity.

Q. An amino acid that is required by the body but cannot be manufactured by the body and must be obtained from food.

R. A protein that contains all of the essential amino acids needed by the body.

S. The study of nutrients in food including how the body uses them and their relationship to health.

T. A simple carbohydrate consisting of one sugar unit.

U. The form in which carbohydrate is stored in the body.

V. An amino acid that is required by the body that can be synthesized by the body in sufficient quantities to meet its needs.

W. A protein that lacks one or more of the essential amino acids needed by the body.

X. A type of fat that is liquid at room temperature and comes primarily from plant sources.

Y. A disaccharide which consists of two sugar units and is found in milk and milk products.

Z. A type of fat that is solid at room temperature and comes primarily from animal sources.

AA. A nutrient required in very small amounts by the body. Includes vitamins and minerals.

BB. A complex carbohydrate made up of many sugar units strung together in a long chain.

B. Word Parts

Directions: Indicate the meaning of each word part in the space provided. List as many medical terms as possible that incorporate the word part in the space provided.

Word Part	Meaning of Word Part	Medical Terms That Incorporate Word Part
1. anti-		
2. ox/I		
3. ather/o		
4. -sclerosis		
5. bar/o		
6. -iatrics		
7. di-		
8. -saccharide		
9. glyc/o		
10. -gen		
11. kilo-		
12. lact/o		
13. -ose		
14. macr/o		
15. micr/o		
16. mono-		
17. non-		
18. satur-		
19. tri-		
20. vit/a		

Directions: Fill in each blank with the correct answer.

NUTRIENTS AND TOOLS FOR HEALTHY NUTRITION

1. What benefits can be derived from good nutrition?

_____

_____

2. List examples of tasks performed by the medical assistant that required a knowledge of basic nutrition principles.

_____

_____

_____

3. Define the term diet.

_____

4. What are the responsibilities of a dietitian?

_____

5. What is the difference between an enriched food and a fortified food?

a. Enriched food: _____

_____

b. Fortified food: _____

_____

6. What is malnutrition?

_____

_____

7. What is nutrient density? What is the difference between a food with a high nutrient density and one with a low nutrient density?

Nutrient density: _____

High nutrient density: _____

Low nutrient density: _____

8. How many kilocalories per gram are provided by each of the following macronutrients?

a. Carbohydrate: _____

b. Fat: _____

c. Protein: _____

9. Why does the body prefer to use carbohydrate as an energy source rather than protein?

_____

_____

10. List specific examples of body functions that require an energy source.

_____

_____

_____

11. What are two functions of insulin in the body?

_____

_____

12. What is the difference between a simple carbohydrate and a complex carbohydrate?

    a. Simple carbohydrate: _____

    b. Complex carbohydrate: _____

13. What sugar units are included in the following simple carbohydrates?

    a. Monosaccharides: _____

    b. Disaccharides: _____

14. What are some examples of empty calorie foods?

_____

_____

15. Why do complex carbohydrates lead to a less dramatic rise in the blood sugar?

_____

16. What are some examples of foods that are classified as complex carbohydrates?

_____

_____

17. Why can't fiber be used as an energy source by the body?

_____

_____

18. What are the advantages of soluble fiber in the diet? What are some examples of food sources containing soluble fiber?

    Advantages:_____

    Food sources:_____

19. What are the advantages of insoluble fiber in the diet? What are some examples of food sources containing insoluble fiber?

    Advantages:_____

    Food sources: _____

20. What functions are performed by fat in the body?

_____

_____

21. What is the difference between saturated and unsaturated fat?

_____

_____

22. What are some examples of foods that are high in saturated fat?

_____

_____

23. List examples of food sources that include the following type of fat.

   a. Monounsaturated fat: _____

   b. Polyunsaturated fat: _____

24. What is the disadvantage of trans fat?

_____

_____

25. What is the function of cholesterol in the body? What are some examples of foods that contain cholesterol?

   a. Function: _____

            _____

   b. Foods: _____

            _____

26. What may occur in an individual with a high blood cholesterol level?

_____

_____

27. Indicate the total blood cholesterol levels for each of the following categories:

   a. Desirable: _____

   b. Borderline high: _____

   c. High: _____

28. What occurs if there is an excess of blood triglycerides in the body?

_____

29. What conditions may result in elevated triglycerides levels?

_____

_____

30. What are the functions of protein in the body? What are some rich food sources of protein?

Functions: _____

_____

Food sources: _____

_____

31. What does protein break down into through the process of digestion?

_____

32. What is the difference between an essential amino acid and a nonessential amino acid?

a. Essential amino acid: _____

b. Nonessential amino acid: _____

33. What is the difference between a complete protein and an incomplete protein? List food sources of each.

a. Complete protein: _____

b. Food sources: _____

c. Incomplete protein: _____

d. Food sources: _____

34. What is the difference between a water soluble vitamin and a fat soluble vitamin?

a. Water soluble vitamin: _____

b. Fat soluble vitamin: _____

35. What is the overall function of the B vitamins?

_____

_____

36. What are rich food sources of many of the B vitamins?

_____

_____

37. What is the function of vitamin C?

_____

_____

38. Identify diseases and conditions that may result from a deficiency of the following vitamins.

a. B_1 (Thiamine): _____

b. B_2 (Riboflavin): _____

c. B_3 (Niacin): _____

d. B_5 (Pantothenic acid): _____

e. B_6 (Pyridoxine): _____

f. B_7 (Biotin): _____

867

g. B$_9$ (Folic acid): _____

h. B$_{12}$ (Cobalamin): _____

i. C (Ascorbic acid): _____

39. What may result from an excessive consumption of the fat soluble vitamins?

_____

_____

40. Identify the function, food sources, and deficiency diseases and conditions of each of the following fat soluble vitamins.

a. Vitamin A

Function: _____

Food sources: _____

Deficiency diseases/conditions: _____

_____

b. Vitamin D

Function: _____

Food sources: _____

Deficiency diseases/conditions: _____

_____

c. Vitamin E

Function: _____

Food sources: _____

Deficiency diseases/conditions: _____

_____

d. Vitamin K

Function: _____

Food sources: _____

Deficiency diseases/conditions: _____

_____

41. What effect do free radicals have on body cells? What may occur as a result of this?

_____

_____

42. What is the difference between a major mineral and a trace mineral?

a. Major mineral: _____

b. Trace mineral: _____

43. Identify the function, food sources, and deficiency diseases and conditions of each of the following major minerals.

    a. Calcium

        Function: _____

        Food sources: _____

        Deficiency diseases/conditions: _____

        _____

    b. Magnesium

        Function: _____

        Food sources: _____

        Deficiency diseases/conditions: _____

        _____

    c. Phosphorus

        Function: _____

        Food sources: _____

        Deficiency diseases/conditions: _____

        _____

    d. Potassium

        Function: _____

        Food sources: _____

        Deficiency diseases/conditions: _____

        _____

    e. Chloride

        Function: _____

        Food sources: _____

        Deficiency diseases/conditions: _____

        _____

    f. Sodium

        Function: _____

        Food sources: _____

        Deficiency diseases/conditions: _____

        _____

44. Identify the function, food sources, and deficiency diseases and conditions of each of the following minor minerals.

    a. Iron

        Function: _____

        Food sources: _____

        Deficiency diseases/conditions: _____

        _____

869

b. Copper

Function: _____

Food sources: _____

Deficiency diseases/conditions: _____

_____

c. Zinc

Function: _____

Food sources: _____

Deficiency diseases/conditions: _____

_____

d. Manganese

Function: _____

Food sources: _____

Deficiency diseases/conditions: _____

_____

e. Fluoride

Function: _____

Food sources: _____

Deficiency diseases/conditions: _____

_____

f. Selenium

Function: _____

Food sources: _____

Deficiency diseases/conditions: _____

_____

g. Iodine

Function: _____

Food sources: _____

Deficiency diseases/conditions: _____

_____

h. Chromium

Function: _____

Food sources: _____

Deficiency diseases/conditions: _____

_____

45. What percentage of an adult's total body weight is made up of water?

_____

46. What are the functions of water in the body?

_____

_____

_____

47. How is water lost from the body?

_____

_____

48. What are the symptoms of dehydration in the adult?

_____

_____

49. What conditions or diseases may warrant the use of a vitamin and mineral supplement?

_____

_____

_____

50. What is the major objective of the MyPlate and the Dietary Guidelines for Americans?

_____

_____

_____

51. What are the recommended MyPlate proportions for the following food groups?

    a. Fruits and vegetables: _____

    b. Protein: _____

    c. Grains: _____

    e. Dairy: _____

52. What is the focus of the Dietary Guidelines for Americans?

_____

_____

53. What type of food requires a food label and what type does not require a food label?

    a. Food requiring a food label: _____

    b. Food not requiring a food label: _____

54. What are the sections of the Nutrition Facts panel?

_____

_____

_____

_____

55. How does the serving size section of a food label assist consumers?

_____

_____

56. What kcal/day is the %DV based upon? _____

57. What are the interpretation guidelines for the percent daily value of the following?

    a. Low nutrient level: _____

    b. Good nutrient level: _____

    c. High or rich nutrient level: _____

58. What nutrients should be limited in the diet?

_____

59. What nutrients should be obtained in adequate amounts (100% DV) in the diet?

_____

60. Why must the grams of trans fat be included on the Nutrition Facts panel?

_____

_____

_____

61. Why is the %DV for protein not required on the Nutrition Facts panel?

_____

62. In what order are the ingredients listed on a food label (in the ingredients list)?

_____

63. What benefits are provided by the ingredients list?

_____

_____

_____

64. List some terms that are used to describe added sugars in the ingredients list.

_____

_____

65. What type of foods typically have a short ingredients list? What type of foods typically have a lengthy ingredients list?

    a. Short ingredients list: _____

    b. Lengthy ingredients list: _____

NUTRITION THERAPY

1. What is the importance of nutrition therapy?

   _____

2. What is weight management?

   _____

   _____

3. What is the primary cause of obesity?

   _____

4. What diseases are associated with overweight and obesity?

   _____

   _____

5. What three components should be included in the treatment of obesity?

   _____

6. What is a calorie deficit and how does it contribute to weight loss?

   _____

   _____

7. How many calories make up one pound of body fat? _____

   _____

8. What are the disadvantages of a fad diet?

   _____

   _____

9. What are the characteristics of a fad diet?

   _____

   _____

10. How does physical exercise contribute to weight loss?

    _____

    _____

11. What is the American Heart Association's (AHA) recommendations for exercise?

    _____

    _____

12. How does a behavior modification plan assist in weight loss?

    _____

    _____

873

13. What is the leading cause of death in the United States? _____

14. What may eventually occur as atherosclerosis progresses?

_____

_____

15. According to the TLC eating plan, what is the daily recommended intake for each of the following?

   a. Total fat: _____

   b. Saturated fat: _____

   c. Dietary fiber: _____

   d. Dietary cholesterol: _____

   e. Sodium: _____

16. What are some examples of foods that are high in cholesterol?

_____

17. What is the most important dietary factor leading to high blood cholesterol?

_____

18. How does soluble fiber lower the cholesterol level?

_____

19. What can occur if hypertension is not brought under control?

_____

_____

20. The DASH eating plan recommends a balanced eating plan that is low in which nutrients?

_____

_____

21. How does a low sodium diet help to lower blood pressure?

_____

_____

22. What causes type 1 diabetes?

_____

_____

23. What are the six food groups included in the diabetic exchange list system?

_____

_____

24. What is the biggest risk factor for the development of type 2 diabetes?

_____

874

25. What is insulin resistance?

_____

_____

26. What are the two key factors involved in the dietary management of type 2 diabetes?

_____

27. What is lactose intolerance?

_____

28. What is the cause of lactose intolerance?

_____

29. What are the symptoms of lactose intolerance?

_____

_____

30. What is the treatment for lactose intolerance?

_____

31. What is gluten intolerance?

_____

32. What is celiac disease?

_____

33. What are the symptoms of gluten intolerance?

_____

_____

34. What are some examples of foods that:

    a. Contain gluten: _____

    b. Are gluten-free: _____

35. What are the most common food allergens?

_____

_____

36. What are the symptoms of a food allergy? When do they usually occur?

_____

_____

37. What is an elimination diet? When is it usually recommended?

_____

_____

875

38. What is a rotation diet? When is it usually recommended?

_____

_____

39. How does denaturation assist in treating food allergies?

_____

_____

40. How do supplemental digestive enzymes assist in treating food allergies?

_____

_____

CRITICAL THINKING ACTIVITIES

A. Nutrient Density

1. List 3 examples of snacks you consume that have a high nutrient density.

    a. _____

    b. _____

    c. _____

2. List 3 examples of snacks you consume that have a low nutrient density (empty calorie foods).

    a. _____

    b. _____

    c. _____

3. List advantages and disadvantages of high nutrient density snacks.

_____

_____

_____

4. List advantages and disadvantages of empty calorie foods.

_____

_____

_____

B. Sodium

Review the Nutrition Facts Panel on five packaged foods. In the space provided, list the name of the food item and the amount of sodium included in one serving. Place a checkmark next to each food item that is high in sodium.

Name of Food   Amount of Sodium

a. _____

b. _____

c. _____

d. _____

e. _____

C. MyPlate

Create a breakfast, lunch, and dinner meal for yourself according to the MyPlate guidelines. Indicate your food group choices in the spaces provided in the appropriate (breakfast, lunch, or dinner) MyPlate illustration.

1. Breakfast

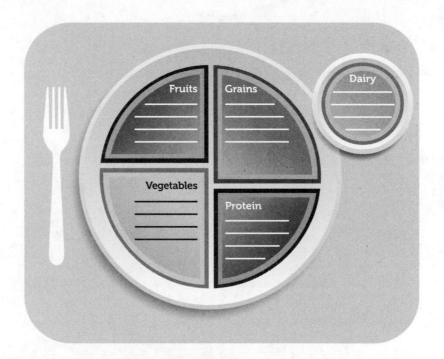

(Modified from U.S. Department of Agriculture: ChooseMyPlate, 2011, www.choosemyplate.gov.)

877

2. Lunch

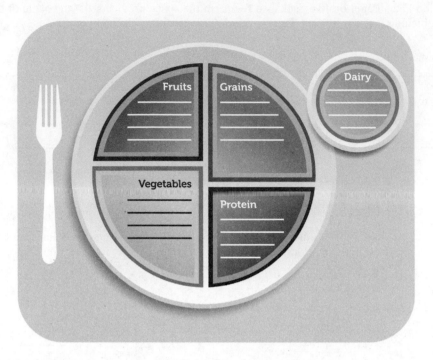

(Modified from U.S. Department of Agriculture: ChooseMyPlate, 2011, www.choosemyplate.gov.)

3. Dinner

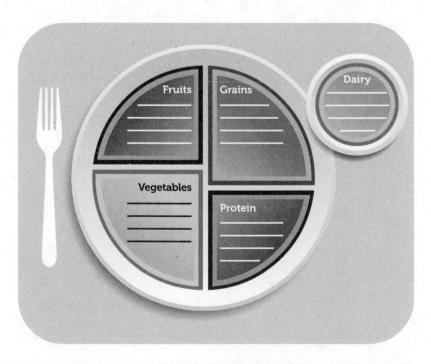

(Modified from U.S. Department of Agriculture: ChooseMyPlate, 2011, www.choosemyplate.gov.)

Compare each of the breakfast, lunch, and dinner MyPlate meals with the meals you typically consume. In the space provided below, discuss the similarities and differences between the meals.

_____

_____

_____

_____

_____

D. Nutrition Facts Panel Analysis

Refer to the Nutrition Facts Panel in your textbook (Figure 21.10) and answer the following questions:

1. How many calories are in one serving of this food item? _____

2. How many servings are included in the entire container? _____

3. What makes up one serving of this food item? _____

4. How many calories are in the entire container? How many calories are in 1/2 serving of this food item?

   _____

5. How many grams of saturated fat are in one serving of this food item? _____

6. What is the %DV of saturated fat in this food item? _____

7. What is the %DV of sodium in this food item? _____

8. Is this food item a low (<5%DV), good (10-19%DV), or rich (>20%DV) source of dietary fiber?

   _____

9. Is this food item a low, good, or rich source of vitamin D? _____

10. Is this food item a low, good, or rich source of calcium? _____

11. Is this food source a low, good, or rich source of iron? _____

12. Should an individual on a low sodium diet avoid this food item? _____

13. Do you consider this food item a healthy food choice? Explain the rationale for your answer.

    _____

    _____

    _____

    _____

E. Nutrition and Disease

The chart below lists the nutrients included on a nutrition facts panel. For each nutrient, indicate a disease or condition that may require a modification in consumption of that nutrient. Indicate if the nutrient should be increased or decreased by placing a checkmark in the appropriate box.

Nutrient	Disease or Condition	Increase	Decrease
1. Total fat			
2. Saturated fat			
3. Natural trans fat			
4. Cholesterol			
5. Sodium			
6. Total carbohydrate			
7. Dietary fiber			
8. Added sugars			
9. Protein			
10. Vitamin D			
11. Calcium			
12. Iron			
13. Potassium			

F. Ingredients List

1. Obtain an ingredients list from an unprocessed healthy food (usually has a short ingredients list) and list the ingredients of the food item below:

_____

_____

_____

2. Obtain an ingredients list from a highly processed food (usually has a long ingredients list) and list the ingredients of the food item below:

_____

_____

_____

3. Compare the ingredients in these two lists (unprocessed food and processed food) and discuss your findings below:

_____

_____

_____

G. Crossword Puzzle: Nutrition

Directions: Complete the crossword puzzle using the clues provided.

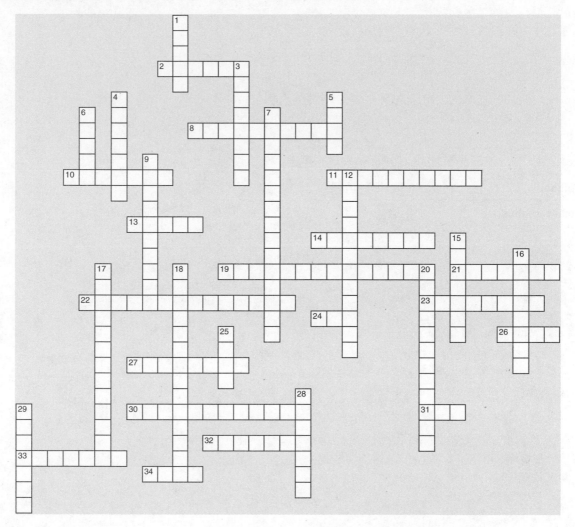

Across

2 Wheat protein
8 Treatment of obesity
10 Builds, maintains, and repairs tissue
11 Makes up protein
13 Makes up 60% to 65% of an adult
14 Makes teeth strong
19 Vitamins and minerals
21 Mineral for healthy bones
22 Vitamin A deficiency
23 FDA banned fat
24 Correlates with total body fat
26 Calcium food source
27 Storage form for glucose
30 Two sugar units
31 Provides 9 kcal/gram
32 Enables glucose to enter a cell
33 Milk sugar
34 Daily food and drink

Down

1 Celiac disease damages this
3 Chemical substance in food needed by body
4 Vitamin D deficiency
5 Eating plan to prevent and control hypertension
6 Iron food source
7 Condition of artery plaque
9 Fat found in food
12 Poor nutrition
15 Breaks down lactose
16 Antioxidant vitamin
17 Chemical form of fat
18 Contains many sugar units
20 Solid fat
25 Fat soluble vitamins
28 Common food allergen
29 Provides portion control

Notes

Procedure 21-A: Instruct a Patient According to Patient's Special Dietary Needs

Name: _____ Date: _____

Evaluated by: _____ Score: _____

Performance Objective

Outcome:	Instruct a patient regarding a dietary change related to a patient's special dietary needs.
Conditions:	Given the following: Nutrition scenario, a Nutrition Facts Panel (Figure 21.10 in textbook), and Ingredients List (Figure 21.11 in textbook).
	Nutrition scenario: Based upon a thorough health history, physical examination, and laboratory test results, Dr. Jada Jordan has determined that her patient, Josefina Perez, is malnourished because of unhealthy food choices. Josephina consumes a lot of salty, sugary, and fried foods. Her test results indicate that she has prediabetes, stage 1 hypertension, and a borderline high cholesterol level. Josephina consumes approximately 2,000 kcal per day and has a BMI of 24 which is normal. Dr. Jordan wants you to instruct Josephina in reading a food label to assist her in making healthier food choices by decreasing the intake of added sugars, sodium, saturated fat, and cholesterol in her diet. Dr. Jordan also wants Josephina to increase the amount of dietary fiber and calcium in her diet.
Standards:	Time: 10 minutes. Student completed procedure in _____ minutes.
	Accuracy: Satisfactory score on the performance evaluation checklist.

Performance Evaluation Checklist

Trial 1	Trial 2	Point Value	Performance Standards
		•	Greeted the patient and introduced yourself.
		•	Identified the patient.
		•	Informed the patient that you will be providing instructions on reading a food label to assist the patient in making healthier food choices.
		•	Explained that the food label is required for most packaged food.
			Using Figure 21.10 in your textbook, instructed the patient on each section of the nutrition facts panel
		•	1. **Servings:** Explained the serving size and servings per package section including the following:
		•	a. The serving size represents the size of a single serving.
		•	b. The total number of servings in the package are included in this section.
		•	c. A packaged food frequently contains more than one serving.
		•	d. The serving size is presented in common household measures such as cup, tablespoon, pieces or slice. The serving size reflects the amount people typically eat or drink. It is not a recommendations on how much a person should eat or drink.
		•	e. The amount of calories and nutrients listed on the remainder of the label are based on one serving.
		•	f. This section allows a comparison of similar foods with the same serving size to determine which is a healthier choice.

Trial 1	Trial 2	Point Value	Performance Standards
		•	2. **Amount of Calories:** Explained the amount of calories section including the following:
		•	a. The amount of calories represents the total number of calories in one serving in large, bold letters.
		•	b. It is important to pay attention to the number of calories consumed. If two servings are consumed, this doubles the amount of calories and nutrients consumed.
		•	3. **Percent Daily Value:** Explained the percent daily value section including the following:
		•	a. Indicates the percentage of a nutrient provided by a single serving of a food item compared with how much is required for the entire day.
		•	b. Provides information on whether a nutrient in one serving contributes a little or a lot of that nutrient to the total daily diet which helps to make informed food choices.
		•	c. The %DV is based on a 2,000 kcal/day diet and each nutrient is based on 100% of the recommended daily amount for that nutrient.
		•	d. Interpretation guidelines for %DV include the following: • Low nutrient level: 5% DV or less • Good nutrient level: 10% to 19% DV • High or rich nutrient level: 20% DV or more
		•	4. **Nutrients That Should be Limited:** Explained which nutrients are important to health but should be limited in the diet. Included the following:
		•	a. Nutrients to limit include saturated fat, trans fat, cholesterol, sodium, and added sugars.
		•	These nutrients should be limited because they contribute to health problems such as heart disease, some cancers, obesity, and hypertension.
		•	b. Foods should be selected with a low %DV of these nutrients (5% DV or less).
		•	5. **Nutrients That Should be Obtained in Adequate Amounts:** Explained which nutrients should be obtained in adequate amounts. Included the following:
		•	a. Nutrients to obtain in adequate amounts include dietary fiber, vitamin D, calcium, iron, and potassium.
		•	Consuming adequate amounts of these nutrients improves health and helps reduce the risk of certain diseases and conditions.
		•	b. The patient should strive to achieve a 100% DV of these nutrients each day.
		•	c. Foods should be selected with a high %DV of these nutrients (20% DV or more).
		•	6. **Footnote:** Explained the the footnote section explains the meaning of the %DV and identifies the number of calories used (2,000 kcal/day) for general nutrition advice.
		•	7. **Additional Nutrients:** Explained the additional nutrients section including the following:

884

Trial 1	Trial 2	Point Value	Performance Standards
		•	a. Total carbohydrates consist of both simple and complex carbohydrates.
		•	b. Sugars include the simple carbohydrates.
		•	c. Dietary fiber is a complex carbohydrate.
		•	d. The remaining carbohydrate comes from starches.
		•	e. A %DV for protein is not required on a food label since most Americans consume more protein than they need.
			Using Figure 21.11 in your textbook, instructed the patient on the ingredients list. Include the following:
		•	The ingredients are listed in descending order of weight from highest to lowest.
		•	The first ingredient makes up the largest proportion of the food by weight than any other ingredient
		•	The ingredients list can assist in making healthy food choices.
		•	Added sugars appear in the ingredients list under a number of different names.
		•	Provide the patient with examples of names used to describe added sugars.
		•	The ingredients list allows the consumer to scan for ingredients that may cause food allergies.
		•	Unprocessed foods typically have a short and simple ingredients list.
		•	Processed foods typically have a lengthy list of ingredients that include chemical terms.
		•	Answered any questions the patient had regarding food labels.
		■	Reassured patients.
		■	Demonstrated empathy for patients' concerns.
		•	Documented the procedure correctly.
		★	Completed the procedure within 10 minutes.
			Totals
CHART			
Date			

Evaluation of Student Performance

EVALUATION CRITERIA			COMMENTS
Symbol	Category	Point Value	
★	Critical Step	16 points	
•	Essential Step	6 points	
■	Affective Competency	6 points	
▷	Theory Question	2 points	

Score calculation: 100 points

− _____ points missed

_____ Score

Satisfactory score: 85 or above

2015 CAAHEP Competencies Achieved

Psychomotor (Skills)

☑ IV. 1. Instruct a patient regarding a dietary change related to a patient's special dietary needs.

Affective (Behavior)

☑ A. 2. Reassure patients.
☑ A. 3. Demonstrate empathy for patients' concerns.

ABHES Competencies Achieved

☑ 2. d. Provide patient education by identifying diet and nutrition requirements.

22 Emergency Preparedness and Protective Practices

CHAPTER ASSIGNMENTS

√ After Completing	Date Due	Study Guide Pages	STUDY GUIDE ASSIGNMENTS (CTA = Critical Thinking Activity)	Possible Points	Points You Earned
		891	Pretest	10	
		892	Term Key Term Assessment	14	
		892-898	Evaluation of Learning questions	60	
		898	CTA A: Disasters	20	
		899	CTA B: Personal Safety Plan	30	
		899-900	CTA C: Disaster Planning in the Medical Office	30	
		900	CTA D: Fire Hazards	20	
		900	CTA E: Methods of Fire Protection and Prevention	20	
		901	CTA F: Use of Fire Extinguisher	20	
		901-903	CTA G: Table-Top Fire Drill	60	
		904	CTA H: Table-top Mock Emergency Events	60	
		904	CTA I: Community Resources	9	
		905	CTA J: Crossword Puzzle	20	
			Evolve: Apply Your Knowledge Questions	10	
		891	Posttest	10	
			ADDITIONAL ASSIGNMENTS		
			Total points		

√ When Assigned By Your Instructor	Study Guide Pages	Practices Required	LABORATORY ASSIGNMENTS (Procedure Number and Name)	Score*
	907	5	**Practice for Competency** 22-1: Demonstrating Proper Use of a Fire Extinguisher	
	909-910		**Evaluation of Competency** 22-1: Demonstrating Proper Use of a Fire Extinguisher	*
	907	4	**Practice for Competency** 22-2: Participating in a Mock Exposure Event: Fire Drill	
	911-914		**Evaluation of Competency** 22-2: Participating in a Mock Exposure Event: Fire Drill)	*
			ADDITIONAL ASSIGNMENTS	

Notes

Name: _____   Date: _____

True or False

_____ 1. A flood is an example of a man-made disaster.

_____ 2. A positive reaction to a disaster involves the triggering of resources to meet the challenge.

_____ 3. During the alarm phase of the general adaptation syndrome (GAS), the body prepares for fight or flight.

_____ 4. During the recovery phase of the GAS, epinephrine is released into the bloodstream.

_____ 5. Hyperventilation may occur during severe anxiety.

_____ 6. Emergency exit routes must be at least 60 inches wide.

_____ 7. An oxygen tank is an example of an ignition source.

_____ 8. A fire door prevents the spread of fire from one area of a building to another.

_____ 9. The number, size, location, and type of fire extinguishers in a medical office are determined by the owner of the building.

_____ 10. The sequence of events that should be included in responding to a fire includes: rescue, activate, confine, and extinguish/evacuate.

?☰ **POSTTEST**

True or False

_____ 1. A man-made disaster is caused by the natural processes of the earth.

_____ 2. Stress is the body's response to threat or change.

_____ 3. Epinephrine causes a decrease in the blood pressure.

_____ 4. Anxiety is a feeling of worry or uneasiness.

_____ 5. The responsibility of an emergency evacuation coordinator is to take charge of and manage evacuation procedures.

_____ 6. A secondary exit route is the quickest and easiest way to exit a building in an emergency.

_____ 7. The elements that must exist in order for a fire to occur include a fuel source, ignition source, and carbon dioxide.

_____ 8. A flammable material catches fire easily.

_____ 9. A portable fire extinguisher can be used to fight a large fire that is out of control.

_____ 10. The batteries in a smoke detector should be changed every 6 months.

Directions: Match each key term with its definition.

_____ 1. Anxiety

_____ 2. Disaster

_____ 3. Emergency action plan

_____ 4. Emergency preparedness

_____ 5. Evacuation

_____ 6. Evacuation procedures

_____ 7. Exit route

_____ 8. Fire extinguisher

_____ 9. Fire prevention plan

_____ 10. Fire protection

_____ 11. HAZMAT

_____ 12. Man-made disaster

_____ 13. Natural disaster

_____ 14. Stress

A. The process of making plans to prevent, respond, and recover from an emergency situation

B. A feeling of worry or uneasiness, often triggered by an event that is perceived as having an uncertain outcome

C. The implementation of safety measures to reduce the unwanted effects of fire

D. A sudden event that causes damage or loss of life

E. A catastrophic event that is caused by nature or the natural process of the earth

F. A written document that describes the actions that employees should take to ensure their safety if a fire or other emergency situation occurs

G. A continuous and unobstructed path of travel from any point within a workplace to a place of safety

H. A planned systemic retreat of people to safety in an emergency situation

I. An event that causes serious damage through intentional or negligent human actions or the failure of a man-made system

J. The body's response to threat or change

K. A written document that identifies flammable and combustible materials stored in the workplace and ways to control workplace fire hazards

L. A portable device that discharges an agent designed to extinguish a fire

M. An acronym that refers to materials that pose a danger to health or the environment and that must be handled with protective equipment

N. Clear step-by-step procedures for the rapid, efficient, and safe removal of individuals from a building during an emergency

---

EVALUATION OF LEARNING

Directions: Fill in each blank with the correct answer.

1. Why is it important for a medical office to plan ahead for a disaster or serious emergency?

_____

_____

2. What causes a natural disaster?

_____

_____

3. What are some examples of natural disasters?

_____

_____

4. What is a man-made disaster?

_____

5. What are some examples of man-made disasters?

_____

_____

6. What does a positive reaction to a disaster involve?

_____

_____

7. When do individuals react negatively to a disaster?

_____

8. What characteristics of a disaster tend to cause the most serious psychological effects?

_____

_____

_____

9. What occurs during the alarm phase of the GAS?

_____

10. What changes occur in the body when epinephrine stimulates the sympathetic nervous system?

_____

_____

11. What occurs during the resistance phase of the GAS?

_____

_____

12. How long does the resistance phase last? _____

13. What are some examples of stress-related symptoms that may occur during the resistance phase?

_____

_____

14. What occurs during the recovery phase of the GAS?

_____

_____

15. What occurs during the exhaustion phase of GAS?

_____

_____

16. What is anxiety?

_____

_____

893

17. Why is it important to learn and practice emergency procedures?

_____

_____

18. How might severe anxiety be a problem in an emergency situation?

_____

_____

19. What are the symptoms of severe anxiety?

_____

_____

20. How should the medical assistant respond to a patient exhibiting severe anxiety?

_____

_____

21. What should the medical assistant do if an emergency occurs at his or her workplace?

_____

_____

22. What is the purpose of an emergency action plan?

_____

_____

23. What methods are typically used in the medical office to report emergency situations and/or to alert employees to the presence of an emergency situation?

_____

_____

_____

24. According to OSHA, when is it acceptable to use direct voice communication to alert employees of an emergency situation?

_____

_____

25. What is the responsibility of an emergency evacuation coordinator?

_____

_____

26. According to OSHA, what three components must be included in an emergency evacuation plan?

_____

_____

_____

27. What type of evacuation is typically required for the following?

   a. Large fire: _____

   b. Small wastebasket fire: _____

   c. Tornado: _____

28. List five guidelines (as stipulated by OSHA) that must be followed with respect to exit routes.

   _____

   _____

29. What is the difference between a primary and secondary exit route?

   a. Primary exit route: _____

   b. Secondary exit route: _____

30. What information should be included on an evacuation floor plan?

   _____

   _____

   _____

31. Why is it important to account for all building occupants following an emergency evacuation?

   _____

   _____

32. What is an evacuation warden?

   _____

33. List examples of how a fire may start in the medical office.

   _____

   _____

34. What three elements must exist in order for a fire to occur?

   _____

35. Explain the difference between a flammable and a combustible material, and list examples of each.

   a. Flammable material: _____

      Examples: _____

   b. Combustible material: _____

      Examples: _____

36. List five examples of fuel sources that may be found in the medical office.

   _____

   _____

895

37. List examples of common ignition sources.

_____

38. What effect will oxygen released from an oxygen tank have on a fire?

_____

39. What is the purpose of a fire prevention plan?

_____

_____

40. List methods of fire prevention in the medical office for each of the following categories.

   a. Flammable and combustible materials:

   _____

   _____

   b. Electrical equipment and appliances:

   _____

   _____

   c. Inspection and maintenance:

   _____

   _____

41. What is the purpose of fire protection?

_____

_____

42. Explain how sprinklers are activated.

_____

43. What is the purpose of a fire door?

_____

44. What occurs when a fire alarm is activated?

_____

45. What type of testing and maintenance should be performed on battery-operated smoke detectors?

_____

46. What are some examples of fire extinguishing agents?

_____

47. What are the two primary functions of a fire extinguisher?

_____

_____

48. List the fuel sources included in the following fire classifications:

Class A: _____

Class B: _____

Class C: _____

Class D: _____

Class K: _____

49. Where are fire extinguishers usually located?

_____

50. Why is it important to properly maintain a fire extinguisher?

_____

51. What is the purpose of the tag attached to a fire extinguisher?

_____

52. Identify the steps that should be taken in operating a fire extinguisher following the PASS format.

P: _____

A: _____

S: _____

S: _____

53. Describe the steps that should be taken in responding to a fire following the RACE format.

R: _____

A: _____

C: _____

E: _____

54. What information should be included in the training of employees on the emergency action plan as required by OSHA?

_____

_____

_____

_____

55. When must the emergency action plan be reviewed with each employee?

_____

_____

_____

56. What is the purpose of an emergency practice drill?

_____

_____

57. Why is it important to conduct fire drills?

_____

_____

58. Who determines whether or not fire drills must be held at a facility?

_____

59. What is the difference between a fire drill and a disaster drill?

_____

_____

60. What role does the medical assistant serve in developing and implementing an emergency action plan?

_____

_____

CRITICAL THINKING ACTIVITIES

A. Disasters

1. Indicate a major natural disaster and a man-made disaster that have occurred in your community and/or state.

2. Provide a brief description of each disaster and the damage that resulted. (*Note:* An Internet search using the terms "Disasters in (name of your state)" will assist you in completing this activity.)

3. Natural disaster:

_____

_____

_____

_____

4. Man-made disaster:

_____

_____

_____

_____

B. Personal Safety Plan

1. Choose a natural disaster (e.g., tornado, hurricane, flood, blizzard) or man-made disaster (e.g., fire, power outage, burglary) that might occur in your locale.

2. Develop and outline a personal safety plan for responding to the disaster in your home environment. Include information on what you would do before, during, and after the disaster occurred. The following websites can assist you in locating information to complete this activity: www.redcross.org; www.fema.gov

   a. Name of disaster: _____

   b. Personal Safety Plan Response:

      Before:

      _____
      _____
      _____
      _____
      _____
      _____

      During:

      _____
      _____
      _____
      _____
      _____
      _____

      After:

      _____
      _____
      _____
      _____
      _____
      _____

C. Disaster Planning in the Medical Office

1. Choose a natural disaster or man-made disaster that might occur in your locale.

2. Outline step-by-step emergency procedures for responding to the disaster in a medical office setting using the form presented below. The following websites can assist you in locating information to complete this activity: www.redcross.org; www.fema.gov; www.osha.gov/Publications/osha3088.pdf; www.osha.gov/SLTC/emergencypreparedness

DISASTER PLANNING IN THE MEDICAL OFFICE

Name of Disaster: _____

Step-by-Step Emergency Procedure Response:

1.	
2.	
3.	
4.	
5.	
6.	
7.	
8.	
9.	
10.	
11.	
12.	

D. Fire Hazards

Perform a survey of your home to determine if there are any fire hazards. If so, list these hazards and what steps should be taken to correct them. Table 22.1 in your textbook and the following websites will assist you in completing this activity: www.fire-extinguisher101.com/hazards.html; https://www.usfa.fema.gov/prevention/

Fire Hazard: Steps Needed to Correct:

_____

_____

_____

_____

_____

_____

E. Methods of Fire Protection and Prevention

Survey the interior of a health care facility (or other type of commercial building) in your community, and observe the fire protection and prevention methods in place at this facility. List these below:

_____

_____

_____

_____

F. Use of Fire Extinguisher

Perform an Internet search for a video of the operation of a fire extinguisher. Write a short paragraph below describing the video.

_____

_____

_____

_____

G. Table-Top Fire Drill

Participate in a table-top fire drill by completing the following:

1. Each student should create a small "paper doll" figure out of paper, cardboard, felt, and other materials (e.g., a tongue blade or a wood craft stick). The figure should be free-standing (be able to stand by itself).

2. Form a group of students and assemble around a table or other flat surface.

3. Place the evacuation floor plan (provided on page 903 of this study guide) in the center of the table.

4. Locate and review the purpose of the following using the evacuation floor plan:

   a. Primary exit route

   b. Secondary exit route

   c. Fire alarm pull stations

   d. Portable fire extinguishers

   e. Emergency exit doors

   f. Wheelchair-accessible exits

   g. Assembly areas

   h. Shelter-in-place areas

5. Choose a student (paper doll) to play the role of the emergency evacuation coordinator, which includes the following responsibilities:

   a. Calling emergency responders

   b. Identifying safe evacuation routes

   c. Ensuring that evacuation wardens are performing their duties

   d. Coordinating with emergency responders

6. Select students (paper dolls) to play the roles of patients with various types of conditions.

7. Select students (paper dolls) to play the roles of evacuation wardens. Assign various duties to these students as outlined in Table 22.1 of your textbook.

8. Place the various paper doll figures in various rooms on the evacuation floor plan.

9. Designate a fire that has erupted in one of the rooms on the floor plan.

10. Locate _Procedure 22-2: Participating in a Mock Exposure Event_ in your textbook, and go to the following subheading: Conduct the Fire Drill.

Chapter **22 Emergency Preparedness and Protective Practices**

11. Conduct a table-top fire drill following the step-by-step procedures listed under *Conduct the Fire Drill*. Explain the principle for performing each step in the drill after performing it.

12. Evaluate the fire drill by completing the *Fire Drill Evaluation Form* below.

FIRE DRILL EVALUATION FORM

Date: _____   Completed By: _____

S	U	Evaluation Criteria:
		The fire drill was completed in an orderly, efficient, and timely manner.
		Building occupants and emergency responders were immediately alerted to the emergency situation.
		Evacuation wardens effectively completed their duties.
		Patients and visitors were escorted to the nearest exits and assembly area.
		Each building occupant was accounted for following the evacuation.
		Emergency responders were provided with appropriate information.

STRENGTHS:

CONCERNS:	MEANS OF IMPROVEMENT:

EVACUATION FLOOR PLAN

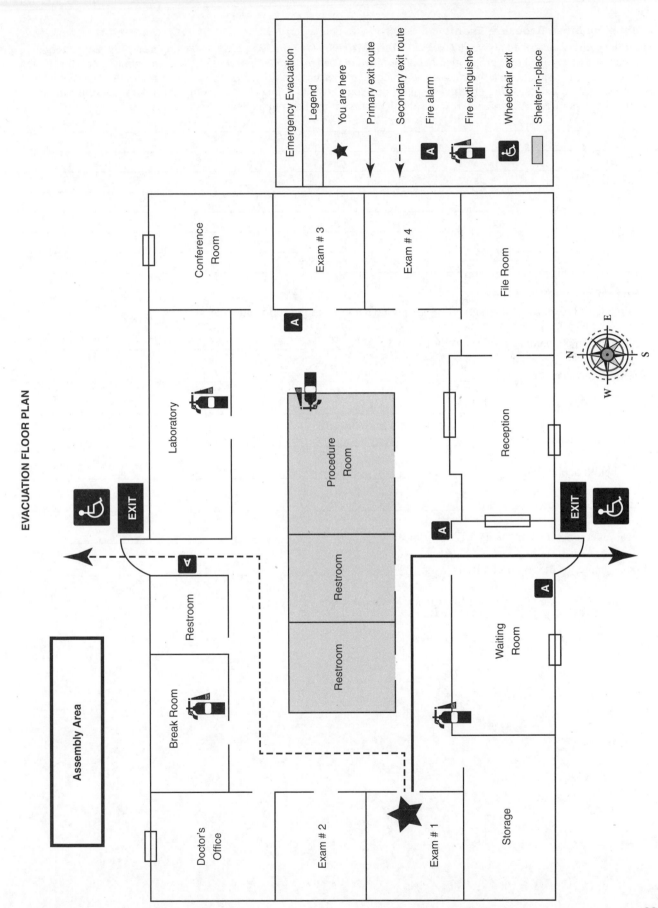

H. Table-Top Mock Exposure Events

Repeat the activity described above in *Critical Thinking Activity G: Table-Top Fire Drill* using a step-by-step emergency procedure plan developed by a group member as outlined in *Critical Thinking Activity C*. The group member who created the emergency plan should take the role of the evacuation coordinator. If time permits, participate in as many mock exposure events as possible, using emergency plans developed by other members of your group. Evaluate the timeliness and effectiveness of each emergency response, and document the key points below:

_____

_____

_____

_____

_____

_____

_____

_____

I. Community Resources

Look up and indicate below the names and telephone numbers of the following:

1. Emergency management services (will usually be 911): _____

2. Poison control center: _____

3. Local hospital(s): _____

4. Local health department: _____

5. State health department: _____

6. State HAZMAT response team: _____

7. Local emergency management (LEMA) office: _____

8. Local chapter of the American Red Cross: _____

9. Citizen Corps Council or Citizen Emergency Response Team (if any): _____

J. Crossword Puzzle: Emergency Preparedness and Protective Practices

Directions: Complete the crossword puzzle using the clues provided.

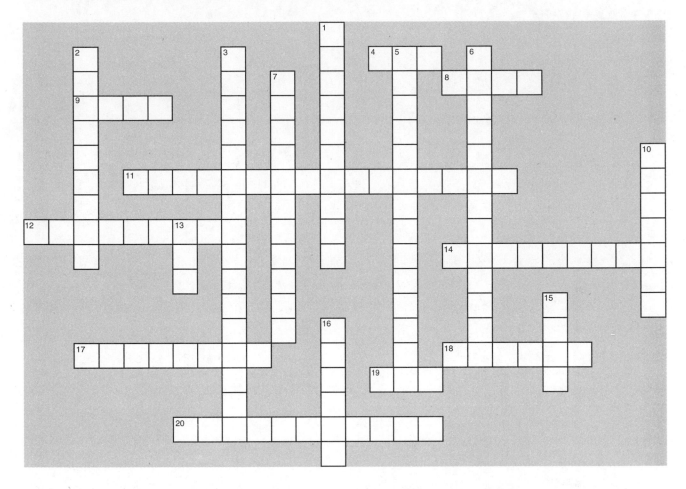

Across

4 Actions to take in an emergency
8 Man-made disaster
9 Response to a fire
11 Severe anxiety symptom
12 Natural disaster
14 Catches on fire easily
17 Increases blood glucose
18 Caused by threat or change
19 Reaction to stress
20 Helps to control anxiety

Down

1 Planned emergency retreat
2 Fire alerter
3 Quickest way to exit
5 Releases epinephrine
6 Alarm reaction response
7 Stimulates sympathetic NS
10 Worry or uneasiness
13 Multipurpose fire extinguisher
15 Fire extinguisher procedure
16 Fire element

Chapter **22** **Emergency Preparedness and Protective Practices**

Notes

PRACTICE FOR COMPETENCY

Procedure 22-1: Demonstrating Proper Use of a Fire Extinguisher

Demonstrate the proper use of a fire extinguisher in a role-playing situation using a discharged fire extinguisher.

Using the information printed on the label of the fire extinguisher (or owner's manual), complete the information requested below:

1. What is the brand name of the extinguisher?

   _____

2. What type of extinguishing agent is contained in the extinguisher (e.g., dry chemical, foam, carbon dioxide)?

   _____

3. What types of fire classification(s) is this extinguisher capable of extinguishing?

   _____

4. What type of precautions should be observed with this extinguisher?

   _____

   _____

5. What are the storage requirements for the fire extinguisher?

   _____

   _____

6. What should be done with the fire extinguisher after it has been discharged?

   _____

   _____

7. What type of care and maintenance is required for this extinguisher?

   _____

   _____

   _____

Procedure 22-2: Participating in a Mock Exposure Event: Fire Drill

a. Prepare for participating in a mock exposure (fire drill) event by first completing *Critical Thinking Activity G: Table-Top Fire Drill.*

b. Participate in a mock exposure (fire drill) event at a facility designated by your instructor.

907

Copyright © 2023 by Elsevier Inc. All rights reserved.

Chapter 22 Emergency Preparedness and Protective Practices

Notes

EVALUATION OF COMPETENCY

Procedure 22-1: Demonstrating Proper Use of a Fire Extinguisher

Name: _____   Date: _____

Evaluated by: _____   Score: _____

Performance Objective

Outcome:	Demonstrate use of a fire extinguisher in a role-playing situation.
Conditions:	Given the following: portable multipurpose (ABC) fire extinguisher that has been discharged and a poster, flashing light, or other indicator to indicate the location of the fire.
Standards:	Time: 5 minutes. Student completed procedure in _____ minutes.
	Accuracy: Satisfactory score on the Performance Evaluation Checklist.

Performance Evaluation Checklist

Trial 1	Trial 2	Point Value	Performance Standards
		•	Identified a safe evacuation route before approaching the fire.
		▷	Stated the reason for identifying a safe evacuation route.
		•	Removed the fire extinguisher from its mounting device.
		•	Held the fire extinguisher upright with the nozzle pointing away from you.
		•	Stood 6 to 8 feet from the fire, keeping the back to the exit.
		▷	Explained the reason for standing at 6 to 8 feet from the fire and keeping the back to the exit.
		•	Performed a quick assessment of the fire to determine whether an attempt should be made to extinguish it with a fire extinguisher.
		▷	Stated when an attempt to extinguish a fire with a fire extinguisher should not be made.
		•	Pulled the safety pin straight out from the handle of the fire extinguisher.
		▷	Stated the purpose of the tamper-proof seal and the safety pin.
		•	Aimed the nozzle at the base of the fire (not the flames).
		▷	Stated why the nozzle should be directed at the base of the fire.
		•	Squeezed the handle slowly and continuously to release the extinguishing agent.
		▷	Stated what occurs if the pressure is released from the handle.
		•	Swept the extinguisher evenly from side to side at the base of the fire.
		▷	Stated why a sweeping motion should be used.
		•	Moved closer to the fire gradually as it began to smolder.
		•	Continued to discharge the extinguishing agent until the fire was completely out.
		▷	Stated what should be done if the fire grows larger.
		•	Backed away from the extinguished fire and continued to watch the area.

Chapter **22** **Emergency Preparedness and Protective Practices**

Trial 1	Trial 2	Point Value	Performance Standards
☐		▷	Stated the reason for continuing to watch the area.
☐		■	Demonstrated critical thinking skills.
☐		★	Completed the procedure within 5 minutes.
☐			**Totals**

Evaluation of Student Performance

EVALUATION CRITERIA			COMMENTS
Symbol	**Category**	**Point Value**	
★	Critical Step	16 points	
•	Essential Step	6 points	
■	Affective Competency	6 points	
▷	Theory Question	2 points	

Score calculation: 100 points

−   points missed

___ Score

Satisfactory score: 85 or above

CAAHEP Competencies Achieved

Psychomotor (Skills)
☑ XII. 1. Comply with safety practices.
☑ XII. 2. b. Demonstrate proper use of fire extinguishers.

Affective (Behavior)
☑ A. 1. Demonstrate critical thinking skills.

ABHES Competency Achieved

☑ 8. g. Recognize and respond to medical office emergencies.

Procedure 22-2: Participating in a Mock Exposure Event: Fire Drill

Name: _____ Date: _____

Evaluated by: _____ Score: _____

Performance Objective

Outcome: Participate in a fire drill.

Conditions: Given the following: a scenario; a poster, flashing light, or other indicator to indicate the location of the fire; evacuation floor plan; employee roster; patient log-in sheet; pen; and paper.

Standards: Time: 20 minutes.   Student completed procedure in _____ minutes.

  Accuracy: Satisfactory score on the Performance Evaluation Checklist.

Performance Evaluation Checklist

Trial 1	Trial 2	Point Value	Performance Standards
			Predrill activities:
		•	Made a list of the names and phone numbers that may be needed in the event of a fire.
		•	Located and reviewed the purpose of the following using the evacuation floor plan: a. Primary exit route b. Secondary exit route c. Fire alarm pull stations d. Portable fire extinguishers e. Emergency exit doors f. Wheelchair-accessible exits g. Shelter-in-place areas h. Assembly areas
		•	Located and reviewed the purpose of the following: a. Sprinklers b. Smoke detectors c. Fire doors d. Exit signs
		•	Evaluated primary and secondary exit routes for the following: a. Clearly marked and well-lit b. Unobstructed and free of clutter c. Exit doors are free of decorations or signs that obscure the visibility of the exit d. Exit doors are unlocked from the inside e. Exit doors open outward f. Fire extinguishers are in place and clearly identified g. Evacuation floor plans are posted in multiple locations
		•	Assigned an emergency evacuation coordinator to perform the following: a. Calling emergency responders b. Identifying safe evacuation routes c. Ensuring that evacuation wardens are performing their duties d. Coordinating with emergency responders
		•	Compiled an employee roster.
		•	Assigned evacuation wardens.
		•	Assigned individuals to play the roles of patients.

911

Trial 1	Trial 2	Point Value	Performance Standards
		•	Compiled a patient log-in sheet.
			Conducted the fire drill:
		•	Rescued anyone in immediate danger of the fire.
		•	Performed the following if an individual's clothes are on fire: a. Instructed the person to stop, drop, and roll. b. Covered the person with a blanket or clothing to extinguish the flames.
		•	Activated the fire alarm.
		•	Immediately notified emergency responders.
		▷	Stated the information that should be relayed to the medical dispatcher.
		•	Closed doors and windows in the immediate area of the fire.
		▷	Stated the purpose of closing doors and windows.
		•	Extinguished the fire with a fire extinguisher if it is small and confined.
		▷	Explained what to do if the fire is too large to extinguish.
		•	Performed evacuation duties and evacuated the area immediately.
		▷	Stated why it is important to evacuate immediately.
		•	Shut down all electrical equipment and appliances in the immediate area.
		•	Before exiting a door, felt the door with the back of the hand. Performed the following if an exit door is warm: a. Did not open the door. b. Called 911 to report your location. c. Placed clothing or towels along the bottom of the door. d. Stayed calm and waited to be rescued. e. Did not break the window.
		•	Exited by the primary exit route.
		▷	Explained what to do if the primary route is blocked.
		•	Exited by stairways only.
		▷	Explained why an elevator should not be used during a fire.
		•	Closed doors after a room is evacuated and placed an "X" on the door.
		•	Escorted patients to the designated assembly area.
		•	Accounted for all building occupants.
		▷	Stated the reason for accounting for all building occupants.
		•	Kept building occupants together in the assembly area and did not allow them to block access to the building.
		•	Did not allow building occupants to reenter the building nor to leave until dismissed.
		•	Provided emergency responders with necessary information.
			Postdrill activities:
		•	Evaluated the effectiveness of the fire drill.

912

Trial 1	Trial 2	Point Value	Performance Standards
		•	Identified the strengths, concerns, and means of improvement of the fire drill.
		•	Documented the results of the fire drill.
		▷	Stated the purpose of evaluating and documenting the results of the fire drill.
		■	Demonstrated critical thinking skills.
		■	Reassured patients.
		★	Completed the procedure within 20 minutes.
			Totals

FIRE DRILL EVALUATION FORM

Date: _____   Completed By: _____

S	U	Evaluation Criteria:
		The evacuation was completed in an orderly, efficient, and timely manner.
		Building occupants and emergency responders were immediately alerted to the situation.
		Evacuation wardens effectively completed their duties.
		Patients and visitors were escorted to the nearest exits and assembly area.
		Each building occupant was accounted for following the evacuation.
		Emergency responders were provided with appropriate information.

STRENGTHS:	
CONCERNS:	**MEANS OF IMPROVEMENT:**

Evaluation of Student Performance

EVALUATION CRITERIA			COMMENTS
Symbol	**Category**	**Point Value**	
★	Critical Step	16 points	
•	Essential Step	6 points	
■	Affective Competency	6 points	
▷	Theory Question	2 points	

Score calculation: 100 points
— _____ points missed
_____ Score
Satisfactory score: 85 or above

Chapter **22** Emergency Preparedness and Protective Practices

CAAHEP Competencies Achieved

Psychomotor (Skills)

☑ I. 13. Provide first aid procedures for a. bleeding e. environmental emergencies.
☑ V. 3. b. Coach patients regarding medical encounters.
☑ V. 7. Use a list of community resources to facilitate referrals.
☑ XII. 1. Comply with safety practices.
☑ XII. 2. b. Demonstrate proper use of fire extinguishers.
☑ XII. 4. Evaluate an environment to identify unsafe conditions.

Affective (Behavior)

☑ A. 1. Demonstrate critical thinking skills.
☑ A. 2. Reassure patients.

ABHES Competencies Achieved

☑ 4. e. Perform risk management procedures.
☑ 8. g. Recognize and respond to medical office emergencies.
☑ 8. i. Identify community resources and Complementary and Alternative medicine (CAM) practice.
☑ 8. j. Accommodate patients with special needs (psychological or physical limitations).

23 Emergency Medical Procedures and First Aid

√ After Completing	Date Due	Study Guide Pages	STUDY GUIDE ASSIGNMENTS (CTA = Critical Thinking Activity)	Possible Points	Points You Earned
		917	🔲 Pretest	10	
		918	⚷Term Key Term Assessment	16	
		919-923	📄 Evaluation of Learning questions	27	
		924	CTA A: First-Aid Kit	10	
		924	CTA B: EMD Information	5	
		924	CTA C: Emergency Care (2 points each)	6	
		925-926	CTA D: Emergency Situations (3 points each)	33	
		927	CTA E: Crossword Puzzle	37	
			Evolve: Apply Your Knowledge questions	10	
		917	📄 Posttest	10	
			ADDITIONAL ASSIGNMENTS		
			TOTAL POINTS		

Notes

Name _____ Date _____

True or False

_____ 1. A specially equipped cart for holding and transporting medications, equipment, and supplies needed in an emergency is known as a crash cart.

_____ 2. Symptoms of an asthmatic attack include dyspnea and wheezing.

_____ 3. Symptoms of a heart attack include sudden weakness on one side of the body.

_____ 4. Another name for a stroke is a coronary occlusion.

_____ 5. Arterial bleeding is characterized by a slow and steady flow of blood that is dark red.

_____ 6. A laceration is an example of a closed wound.

_____ 7. Symptoms of a fracture include pain, swelling, deformity, and loss of function.

_____ 8. A sprain is a tearing of ligaments at a joint.

_____ 9. Heat stroke is a life-threatening emergency.

_____ 10. Insulin enables glucose to enter the body's cells and be converted to energy.

?≣ POSTTEST

True or False

_____ 1. When providing emergency care, you should obtain information about what happened from bystanders.

_____ 2. Emphysema is a progressive lung disorder in which there is a loss of elasticity of the alveoli of the lungs.

_____ 3. Symptoms that may occur with hyperventilation include rapid and deep respirations and tachycardia.

_____ 4. The first priority for hypovolemic shock is to control bleeding.

_____ 5. Status asthmaticus is the type of shock caused by a reaction of the body to a substance to which an individual is highly allergic.

_____ 6. Another name for a nosebleed is epistaxis.

_____ 7. The type of fracture in which the broken ends of the bone are forcefully jammed together is a greenstick fracture.

_____ 8. The type of seizure in which the abnormal electrical activity is localized into very specific areas of the brain is a tonic-clonic seizure.

_____ 9. Chipmunks have a high incidence of rabies.

_____ 10. Emergency care for insulin shock is to give the patient sugar immediately.

Chapter **23 Emergency Medical Procedures and First Aid**

Directions: Match each key term with its definition.

_____ 1. Burn

_____ 2. Crash cart

_____ 3. Crepitus

_____ 4. Dislocation

_____ 5. Emergency medical services

_____ 6. First aid

_____ 7. Fracture

_____ 8. Hypothermia

_____ 9. Poison

_____ 10. Pressure point

_____ 11. Seizure

_____ 12. Shock

_____ 13. Splint

_____ 14. Sprain

_____ 15. Strain

_____ 16. Wound

A. A network of community resources, equipment, and personnel that provides care to victims of injury or sudden illness

B. Any substance that causes illness, injury, or death if it enters the body

C. An injury to the tissues caused by exposure to thermal, chemical, electrical, or radioactive agents

D. Any device that immobilizes a body part

E. A grating sensation caused by fractured bone fragments rubbing against each other

F. A sudden episode of involuntary muscular contractions and relaxation, often accompanied by changes in sensation, behavior, and level of consciousness

G. A stretching or tearing of muscles or tendons caused by trauma

H. The immediate care that is administered to an individual who is injured or suddenly becomes ill before complete medical care can be obtained

I. A break in the continuity of an external or internal surface caused by physical means

J. A specially equipped cart for holding and transporting medications, equipment, and supplies needed for performing lifesaving procedures in an emergency

K. Any break in a bone

L. The failure of the cardiovascular system to deliver enough blood to all the vital organs of the body

M. An injury in which one end of a bone making up a joint is separated or displaced from its normal anatomic position

N. A life-threatening condition in which the temperature of the entire body falls to a dangerously low level

O. A site on the body where an artery lies close to the surface of the skin and can be compressed against an underlying bone to control bleeding

P. Trauma to a joint that causes tearing of ligaments

EVALUATION OF LEARNING

Directions: Fill in each blank with the correct answer.

1. What is the purpose of first aid?

   _____

   _____

   _____

   _____

2. What is the purpose of the office crash cart?

   _____

   _____

   _____

   _____

3. What is the difference between an EMT-basic and an EMT-paramedic?

   _____

   _____

   _____

4. What are the responsibilities of an emergency medical dispatcher?

   _____

   _____

   _____

5. List five OSHA Standards that should be followed when administering first aid.

   _____

   _____

   _____

   _____

6. What is the reason for performing each of the following during an emergency situation?

   a. Remaining calm and speaking in a normal tone of voice

   _____

   _____

   b. Making sure it is safe before approaching the patient

   _____

   _____

c. Following OSHA Standards when providing emergency care

_____

_____

d. Activating the emergency medical services

_____

_____

e. Not moving the patient unnecessarily

_____

_____

f. Checking the patient for a medical alert tag

_____

_____

7. What are the symptoms of asthma?

_____

_____

8. What is emphysema?

_____

_____

9. What are the symptoms of hyperventilation?

_____

_____

10. What are the symptoms of a heart attack?

_____

_____

11. What are the symptoms of a stroke?

_____

_____

12. What is the cause of the following types of shock?

a. Hypovolemic

_____

_____

b. Cardiogenic

_____

_____

c. Neurogenic

_____

_____

d. Anaphylactic

_____

_____

e. Psychogenic

_____

_____

13. What are the characteristics of each of the following types of external bleeding?

a. Capillary

_____

_____

b. Venous

_____

_____

c. Arterial

_____

_____

14. What is the difference between an open wound and a closed wound?

_____

_____

15. What are the signs and symptoms of a fracture?

_____

_____

16. What are the characteristics of each of the following types of fractures?

a. Impacted

_____

_____

b. Greenstick

_____

_____

c. Transverse

_____

_____

d. Oblique

_____

_____

e. Comminuted

_____

_____

f. Spiral

_____

_____

17. What are the characteristics of each of the following types of burns?

a. Superficial

_____

_____

b. Partial thickness

_____

_____

c. Full thickness

_____

_____

18. What is the difference between a partial seizure and a generalized seizure?

_____

_____

19. List two examples of each of the following types of poisoning:

a. Ingested

_____

_____

b. Inhaled

_____

_____

c. Absorbed

_____

_____

d. Injected

_____

_____

20. What spiders (found in the United States) have bites that can result in serious or life-threatening reactions?

_____

_____

21. What species of snakes (found in the United States) are poisonous?

_____

_____

22. What animals tend to have a high incidence of rabies?

_____

_____

23. What factors place an individual at higher risk for developing heat- and cold-related injuries?

_____

_____

24. What areas of the body are most susceptible to frostbite?

_____

_____

25. What is the difference between type 1 diabetes and type 2 diabetes?

_____

_____

26. What is insulin shock, and what causes it to occur?

_____

_____

27. What is a diabetic coma, and what causes it to occur?

_____

_____

CRITICAL THINKING ACTIVITIES

A. First-Aid Kit

You are assembling a first-aid kit. What supplies should be included in your kit? Identify one use for each of the supplies you list.

_____

_____

_____

_____

_____

_____

_____

_____

_____

B. EMD Information

Jeff Stickler suddenly develops weakness in his left arm and leg, has difficulty speaking, and has a severe headache and dizziness. You immediately call the Emergency Medical Services (EMS). What information should you be prepared to relay to the emergency medical dispatcher (EMD)?

_____

_____

_____

_____

C. Emergency Care

In which of the following emergency situations would you be legally permitted to administer first aid? Explain your answers.

1. A patient is unconscious and bleeding profusely.

   _____

   _____

2. You identify yourself and state your level of training and what you plan to do. You ask the patient if it is alright to administer emergency care. The patient responds by saying, "Yes, please help me."

   _____

   _____

3. You ask the patient if you can administer emergency care, but the patient refuses your help.

   _____

   _____

D. Emergency Situations

Explain what you would do in each of the following situations.

1. Holly Murphy falls while roller skating. She comes down hard on her left arm, which begins to swell and discolor. Holly guards her arm and complains of intense pain.

_____

_____

_____

_____

2. John Phillips is mowing the grass and mows over a yellow jacket nest. He is stung twice and soon starts complaining of intense itching and exhibits erythema and hives on his arms, torso, and face.

_____

_____

_____

_____

3. Steve Williams complains of severe indigestion and squeezing pain in the chest. He is short of breath and perspiring profusely.

_____

_____

_____

_____

4. Clara Miller is playing basketball and is accidentally hit in the face with the ball. Her nose begins bleeding profusely.

_____

_____

_____

_____

5. Debbie Carter, age 4 years, finds some children's chewable vitamins that have been left open on a table. She eats about 10 of them.

_____

_____

_____

_____

6. Rita Preston accidentally cuts her finger with a knife while preparing dinner. Her finger begins bleeding profusely.

_____

_____

_____

_____

Chapter **23** Emergency Medical Procedures and First Aid

7. Jose Perez is jogging on a cinder track. He falls and scrapes his left knee on the cinders.

_____

_____

_____

_____

8. Charlotte Lambert is getting ready to perform a piano recital for her entire church congregation. Suddenly she starts breathing very rapidly and deeply and complains that she feels light-headed and dizzy.

_____

_____

_____

9. Bruce Jones is a diabetic. He is in a hurry and forgets to eat breakfast. He begins exhibiting behavior similar to that of someone who is intoxicated.

_____

_____

_____

_____

10. Debra Murray is delivering newspapers and is bitten by a strange dog. The bite causes several puncture marks and slight bleeding.

_____

_____

_____

_____

11. Tanya Howe is playing tennis on a hot and humid day and begins to feel weak and nauseous. Her skin feels cold and clammy, and she is sweating profusely and complains of dizziness.

_____

_____

_____

_____

E. Crossword Puzzle: Emergency Medical Procedures and First Aid

Directions: Complete the crossword puzzle using the clues provided.

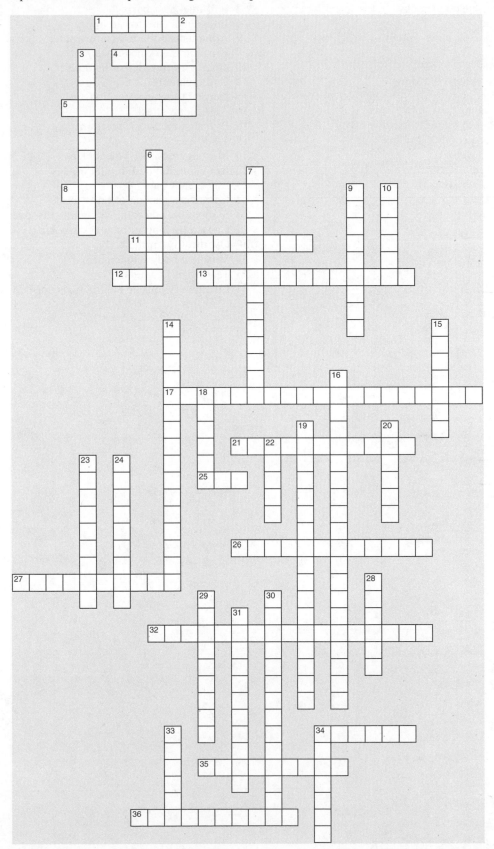

927

Across
1 Transmitted in animal saliva
4 Treatment of insulin shock
5 Broken bone
8 Spider producing toxic venom
11 Poisonous snake
12 Answers emergency calls
13 Site used to control bleeding
17 Trouble breathing
21 Displaced joint
25 Provides care to injured victim
26 Caused by not enough insulin
27 Ragged edge wound
32 Severe allergic reaction
34 Immobilizes a body part
35 AKA nosebleed
36 Number to activate EMS

Down
2 Brain artery is blocked or ruptured
3 Full-thickness burn
6 Immediate care for an injury
7 Administer for a puncture wound
9 Break in the skin surface
10 Tearing of muscles or tendons
14 Overbreathing
15 Needed to administer first aid
16 AKA heart attack
18 Psychogenic shock position
19 1-800-222-1222
20 Most aggressive Hymenoptera
22 Not enough blood to vital organs
23 Emergency cart
24 Localized freezing of body tissue
28 Symptoms: wheezing, coughing, dyspnea
29 Caused by long-term heavy smoking
30 Overheating of the body
31 Very low body temperature
33 Tearing of ligaments
34 Involuntary muscle contractions episode